Renal Cancer

Christopher Anderson • Mehran Afshar
Editors

Renal Cancer

Current Status and Innovations

Springer

Editors
Christopher Anderson
Department Urology
St Georges University Hospital NHS
Foundation Trust
London, UK

Mehran Afshar
Department Uro-Oncology
St Georges University Hospital NHS
Foundation Trust
London, UK

ISBN 978-3-030-84755-5   ISBN 978-3-030-84756-2 (eBook)
https://doi.org/10.1007/978-3-030-84756-2

This Springer imprint is published by the registered company Springer Nature Switzerland AG
The registered company address is: Gewerbestrasse 11, 6330 Cham, Switzerland

This book is dedicated to our Families for their unwavering support and our Patients who we shall always feel privileged to care for and for whom this book was ultimately written.

Contents

Introduction

Christopher Anderson and Mehran Afshar

The management of renal cancer has seen transformative innovations over the last 2 decades, in both the realms of diagnosis and management. The pace of change has been such that much of the literature becomes historical soon after it is made available to the wider clinical community. These advances are not only a sign of the progress of modern medicine, but rather the longstanding human endeavour to cure disease. For example, the management of metastatic renal cancer saw a paradigm shift in the twenty-first century with the discovery of drugs targeting angiogenesis, whereas identifying angiogenesis itself dates back to the British surgeon John Hunter in 1787 [1]. To put that into perspective, it was nearly a century prior to the publication of *On the Origin of Species* by Charles Darwin. The use of robotic surgery is becoming more prevalent in the surgical arena, and often touted as a novel development, whereas Kwoh *et al* [2] used the PUMA 560 robot system to undertake neurosurgical biopsies with greater accuracy as far back as almost half a century ago. In renal cancer surgery, the use of the robot has now become established and surgical technique and technology is advancing rapidly. The treatment of renal cancer, in all stages of disease, is an exciting area of development in the field of oncology.

Although it is clear that progress has been sustained over many years, it is undoubtedly very recent history that has seen the fastest developments. It is with this in mind that the authors have collated a series of chapters which endeavour to deliver both a global education on renal cancer and a review of modern developments. The book will cover all areas needed by any clinician treating renal

C. Anderson (✉)
Department Urology, St Georges University Hospital NHS Foundation Trust, London, UK
e-mail: chris.anderson@stgeorges.nhs.uk

M. Afshar
Department Uro-Oncology, St Georges University Hospital NHS Foundation Trust, London, UK
e-mail: Mehran.Afshar@stgeorges.nhs.uk

C. Anderson, M. Afshar (eds.), *Renal Cancer*,
https://doi.org/10.1007/978-3-030-84756-2_1

cancer or students wanting to learn with an appetite for an understanding of technological advancements and their relationship to current gold standard management. The text will cover a wide range of topics from epidemiology and screening, diagnostics and biomarkers, to complex surgical issues such as renal parenchymal preservation, to psychological approaches to patient care, and the role of big data. The driver for the development of this book was the multidisciplinary management approach in the treatment of renal cancer in the United Kingdom where the authors practice. The holistic, comprehensive overview taken by a multidisciplinary team affords bespoke care for the patient with renal cancer, and the importance given to the wide-ranging topics covered in this book are inspired by this approach. This breadth of topics covered provides an ideal text book to be used as an adjunct to conventional reading in each of the domains of renal oncology.

References

1. Folkman J. History of angiogenesis. In: Figg WD, Folkman J, editors. Angiogenesis: an integrative approach from science to medicine. New York: Springer; 2008. p. 1–14.
2. Kwoh YS, Hou J, Jonckheere EA, et al. A robot with improved absolute positioning accuracy for CT guided stereotactic brain surgery. IEEE Trans Biomed Eng. 1988;35:153–61.

Epidemiology and Screening in RCC

Sabrina H. Rossi and Grant D. Stewart

Epidemiology

Renal cell carcinoma (RCC) is the sixth most common cancer in men and tenth most common cancer in women worldwide [1]. Incidence is 15 times higher in developed countries compared to the developing world [2] and RCC is one of the fastest accelerating cancers. Indeed, RCC incidence rates have increased by 47% in the last 10 years [1]. The rise in incidence has been postulated to be, at least in part, due to rising rates of risk factors such as obesity and the aging population [2–4]. In addition, a major contributor is the increased use of abdominal imaging for the investigation of other abdominal symptoms, which leads to incidental detection [5]. On one hand, survival rates are poor (10 year overall survival: 52%) [6] meaning there is a drive to improve patient outcomes (Fig. 1) [8]. On the other hand, although the overall incidence is increasing, the incidence of metastatic disease and mortality rates have remained static, suggesting that a proportion of detected cancers will not impact patient survival and have led to concerns regarding overdiagnosis [9]. RCC mortality continues to rise in Eastern Europe however [10]. These epidemiological data highlight the need for improved understanding of the pathophysiology of RCC.

Risk Factors

The main risk factors and associated relative risks (RR) for RCC are [1, 6, 11, 12]:

- Increasing age: peak incidence is 60-70 years
- Male sex (RR = 1.5 to 2)

S. H. Rossi (✉) · G. D. Stewart
Department of Surgery, University of Cambridge, Cambridge, UK
e-mail: sr725@cam.ac.uk; gds35@cam.ac.uk

C. Anderson, M. Afshar (eds.), *Renal Cancer*,
https://doi.org/10.1007/978-3-030-84756-2_2

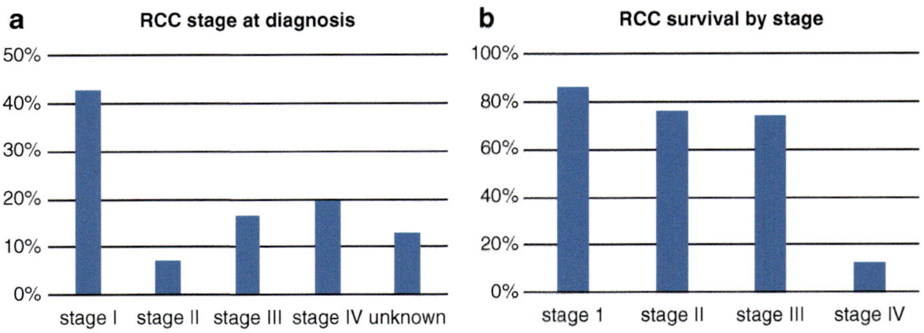

Fig. 1 (**a** and **b**): Stage at diagnosis (**a**) and five-year survival by stage (**b**). (**a**) stage at diagnosis in England for patients diagnosed between 2012 and 2017 [7]. (**b**) Five-year survival by stage in the UK for 2013–2017 [6]

- Race: Higher risk in African Americans compared to Caucasians
- Obesity (RR = 1.7 for BMI >35 kg/m^2 vs <25 kg/m^2)
- Smoking (RR = 1.3 to 1.5 smokers vs never smokers)
- Hypertension (RR = 1.7)
- Renal disease: acquired cystic kidney disease, end stage renal failure and renal transplant (RCC affects the native kidney).
- Family history
  - A number of inherited rare cancer syndromes predispose to RCC. In sporadic RCC, having an affected first degree relative is associated with a RR of 2. A number of single nucleotide polymorphisms (SNPs) have been identified, which can be combined into a polygenic risk score (three fold increased risk of RCC in the highest decile compared to the lowest decile) [13].
- Diabetes type 2 (RR = 1.6)

Moderate alcohol consumption and high physical activity are considered protective [14–17]. A number of potential risk factors have been identified which are less well established and require further research. According to the International Agency for Research on Cancer (IARC) exposure to trichloroethylene, gamma and x radiation are associated with an increased risk of RCC; whilst other occupational exposures have limited evidence [18]. Conflicting results have been observed for: renal stones, parity/hormonal factors, fruit/vegetable intake and analgesic use.

Rationale for Screening

Earlier detection and screening for RCC has been identified as a key research focus by two independent priority setting initiatives, as well as patient advocacy groups [19–22]. This is because the disease is often asymptomatic, resulting in delayed diagnosis, and there is a clear association between stage at detection and survival. In fact, 60% of cases of RCC are asymptomatic at diagnosis, and this rate is even higher (87%) for stage T1a RCC, which have the most favourable prognosis (cancer specific survival >95% in surgically treated T1a RCC) [23, 24]. Approximately 20–25% cases have metastases at diagnosis, and five-year cancer specific survival for these individuals is 12% [6, 7].

It has therefore been postulated that earlier diagnosis, and treatment of the disease at a curable stage, would lead to overall improved survival rates. In addition, the relatively high cost of systemic therapies for advanced disease means that investing resources into screening could potentially be cost-effective.

However, no randomised controlled trials (RCT) have been performed to date, so it is yet unclear what the ideal screening modality and target population would be, and if screening would impact survival [8, 11]. Any screening programme must be considered in the context of the Wilson and Jungner criteria and weigh up potential benefits and harms (Table 1) [28].

Screening Test

A number of modalities have been proposed as potential screening tools (Table 2). These include primary screening with imaging or a staged approach, where a non-invasive blood or urine test (such as urinary dipstick or biomarkers) may be used to identify individuals who warrant further investigation. A number of studies were performed in the 1990s evaluating ultrasound as a screening tool, however none were randomised in nature, nor powered to assess survival (Table 2). Screening using ultrasound or low dose CT remain the most likely candidates. Offering screening for RCC in combination with other existing or possible future screening programs (e.g. ultrasound for aortic aneurysms or CT for lung cancer) may increase cost-effectiveness and is viewed positively by the public [48].

Although a number of blood and urinary biomarkers (such as proteins, micro RNAs, circulating tumour DNA and circulating tumour cells) have been studied, none have been validated and adopted for use in clinical practice. Biomarker studies are heterogeneous, adopt small sample sizes, lack external validation and on occasion generate conflicting results [47]. A main limitation of existing biomarkers has been the lack of sensitivity and specificity for RCC. In addition, studies use techniques such as western blotting (e.g. for proteins) or expensive next generation sequencing approaches (e.g. for circulating tumour DNA) which are not scalable in the context of a population screening program. Further research in this fields remains promising.

The Screening Population

The ideal screening population has yet to be determined. One potential strategy would be to screen individuals based on age and sex. Further work should elucidate the ideal starting age, and if this should be different for men and women. One of the

Table 1 Wilson and Jungner criteria applied to screening for RCC (adapted from [11]), highlighting key research questions

Criteria for screening	
1. The condition sought should be an important health problem	• Screening for RCC is a key research priority • RCC is the seventh most common cancer in Europe [25] and overall 5-year survival is 52%. • 20%–25% of patients have metastases at diagnosis and 5 year-survival in this group is 12%, suggesting early detection could improve survival.
2. There should be an accepted treatment for patients with recognised disease	• Early detection of smaller tumours may preferentially allow minimally invasive techniques, reducing rates of open surgery and therefore associated morbidity and length of hospital stay, and improving quality of life and renal function.
3. Facilities for diagnosis and treatment should be available	• Screening would increase disease incidence. Further research on cost and resource implications of this are key.
4. There should be a recognizable latent or early symptomatic stage	• The natural history of small renal masses is not completely understood. However, since >50% of RCCs are detected incidentally, this suggests there is a latent asymptomatic stage at which to intervene.
5. There should be a suitable test	• Currently, screening with ultrasound or low dose CT seems the most viable option. Ideally screening would adopt a staged approach to increase efficiency and cost-effectiveness. First a risk-stratification tool/prediction model would identify high-risk individuals from the general population. These individuals would be invited to have an initial urine or blood based biomarker test (ideally a point of care test at home or in the community), followed by further imaging in secondary care.
6. The test should be acceptable to the population	• Surveys demonstrate public acceptability and willingness to attend screening.
7. The natural history of the condition, including development from latent to declared disease, should be adequately understood	• This area is the highest research priority.
8. There should be an agreed policy on whom to treat as patients.	• Clear European Association of Urology guidelines on the management of RCC have been published [26], including active surveillance, ablative and surgical options for localised disease.
9. The cost of case finding (including diagnosis and treatment of patients diagnosed) should be economically balanced in relation to possible expenditure on medical care as a whole	• A cost-effectiveness analysis of screening for RCC using ultrasound suggested that screening could potentially be cost-effective in men [27]. The low prevalence was a key determinant of cost-effectiveness, suggesting risk-stratified screening would be an ideal option.
10. Case finding should be a continuing process and not a "once and for all" project	• It is unclear if screening should be performed as a one-off or repeated at regular intervals.

Table 2 Potential screening tools

Tool	Advantages	Disadvantages
Ultrasound	– Non-invasive – Well tolerated – Relatively inexpensive – Widely available (most departments have ultrasound) – Does not involve ionizing radiation – Most well researched screening tool. A number of observational studies have been performed, however these collected only limited data, none were randomised, and all were published more than a decade ago [29–36]. – Potential for combination with the existing ultrasound-based abdominal aortic aneurysm screening program [36]. – Focused renal ultrasound has the advantage of imaging the kidney exclusively, therefore reducing the number of incidental findings in other abdominal organs. Conversely, imaging of the whole abdomen may identify other conditions, thus maximising benefit of screening.	– Operator dependent – Accuracy depends on lesion size: Detection of 85–100% tumours >3 cm in size, but only 67–82% of tumours 2-3 cm in size, therefore there is a potential for false negatives [37, 38]. – Dependent on anatomical factors such as obesity and presence of overlying bowel gas.
Low-dose non-contrast CT	– Most sensitive and specific of the proposed screening tools. – CT chest performed as part of lung cancer screening may be extended to include the kidneys. The Yorkshire kidney cancer screening trial, currently underway, is investigating the feasibility of this approach (ref: https://www.isrctn.com/ISRCTN18055040).	– Ionizing radiation – High cost and significant number of incidental findings suggest whole-body CT for the simultaneous detection of a number of conditions is unlikely to be cost-effective [39–41].
Urinary dipstick	– Non-invasive, quick, cheap – Can be performed in primary care with minimal training or at home by the patient themselves. – Can be used to screen for urological malignancies in combination. – In patients with non-visible haematuria, cancer detection rates are: 0%–16% for bladder cancer, 0%–3.5% for upper tract urothelial cancer and 0%–9.7% for RCC [42].	– Non-visible haematuria is a very common and non-specific finding, meaning screening using dipstick would generate a high volume of participants requiring further investigation, to detect only a very small number of RCCs [11]. – High number of false negatives as only 35% of individuals with RCC have visible or non-visible haematuria, compared to 94% in patients with urothelial carcinoma [43]. – A feasibility study of population screening utilising home urinary dipstick in 1747 men aged 50 to 75 years demonstrated that the prevalence of non-visible haematuria was 23%. However, only one RCC was detected and one RCC was missed [44].

(continued)

Table 2 (continued)

Tool	Advantages	Disadvantages
Plasma and urinary biomarkers	– Non-invasive – Perhaps the most promising biomarkers are: Urinary Aquaporin-1 and perilipin-2 [45] and plasma KIM-1 [46].	– A number of plasma and urinary biomarkers have been investigated including proteins [47], urinary exosomes and circulating tumour DNA (ctDNA), however none have been adopted into clinical practice.

main challenges associated with screening is the relatively low prevalence of RCC [29]; with prevalence being a major determinant of cost-effectiveness [27]. Targeted screening may overcome this, by identifying individuals at high risk, who would therefore benefit the most from screening, thus maximising efficiency [49]. A comprehensive systematic review of risk prediction models for RCC identified 11 models in which performance measures were reported; however only 6 models had been validated and only two had done so using external populations [50]. The majority of risk models incorporated a combination of demographic/lifestyle factors that are easily determined through medical records or self-assessment questionnaires, and/or biomarkers. Only one study considered genetic risk (e.g. single nucleotide polymorphisms). None of the biomarker risk factors were included in more than one study and a high risk of bias was noted, highlighting once again the challenges of biomarker research. Most of the models had acceptable-to-good discrimination (area under the receiver-operating curve >0.7) in development and validation. The risk factors that were included most commonly were: age, smoking status and BMI. One key challenge is that none of the risk factors for RCC are disease specific. Further external validation of risk prediction models is a priority.

Screening Implementation and Public Acceptability

The optimal frequency of screening for RCC is yet to be determined (e.g. one-off screening *vs* repeated screening at regular intervals). No studies have addressed this question thus far and insufficient evidence is known regarding the natural history and growth rates of undiagnosed disease to postulate regarding the value of repeated screening [11]. Once the optimal screening strategy has been identified, it will be crucial to determine whether the health care system has adequate resources to support implementation.

Although the general public have a relatively low awareness of RCC (82% knew nothing about RCC or had only heard of the condition), a high willingness to attend screening has been noted [48]. The vast majority of participants stated that they would be 'very likely' or 'likely' to undergo each of the following screening tests: urine test: 94%; blood test: 90%; ultrasound: 90%; low-dose CT: 79%; low-dose CT offered as part of lung screening: 95% [48]. Whether this translates to high attendance rates is unknown. Risk-stratified screening is viewed positively by the public.

Varying the starting age of RCC screening based on estimated risk from models incorporating phenotypic or genetic risk factors would be acceptable to most (83%) individuals, and is preferable to using sex alone. This may increase uptake, as 85% of participants reported they would be more likely to attend screening if the score suggested they were high-risk [51].

Current Nuances

As with any screening programme, potential harms include costs to the individual (both physical and psycho-social) and society (opportunity costs: monetary, resource allocation).

The ideal screening strategy would consist of a highly sensitive and specific test, which is non-invasive, cost-effective and well accepted by the population. A high test sensitivity is key to avoid missing cancers (false negatives) and falsely reassuring individuals with the disease and maintaining public confidence in the screening process.

A high specificity is crucial because screening large numbers of individuals (such as the whole population) may lead to a high number of people who require further investigations and potentially treatment, with subsequent risk of morbidity, anxiety and reduction in of quality of life. For example, even if the specificity of the test is 99%, screening a hypothetical cohort of 500,000 people/annum would lead to 5000 false positives/annum. There is a drive to reduce over-investigation and over-treatment of healthy individuals and to prevent over-medicalisation of the worried well [9]. This needs to be balanced against the relatively low prevalence of RCC, meaning that any potential harms would occur to detect only a small number of individuals with cancer. Two systematic reviews and meta-analyses have been performed evaluating the prevalence of undiagnosed RCC in asymptomatic individuals undergoing screening with ultrasound and CT respectively. The pooled prevalence was 0.21% (95% CI, 0.14–0.28%) in a North American cohort undergoing CT and 0.17% (95% CI 0.09–0.27%) in a European and North American cohort undergoing ultrasound [29, 52]. This suggests screening 1000 individuals would lead to the detection of between 1 and 3 cancers; thus screening our hypothetical cohort of 500,000 individuals would detect up to 1500 cases of RCC. As already mentioned, risk-stratified screening may help overcome this challenge.

A unique screening consideration is linked to our current understanding of the natural history of RCC and our ability to accurately determine diagnosis and prognosis. Unlike other malignancies that have an existing screening program, RCC does not have an identifiable pre-malignant state (such as carcinoma in situ in the breast, cervical intraepithelial neoplasia and adenomatous polyps of the colon). It is postulated that all RCCs must start off as small renal masses (SRM), and genomic studies suggest copy number aberrations affecting the VHL pathway occur as early as adolescence [53]. However, once a SRM is detected, there are difficulties in differentiating malignant from benign disease (especially fat poor angiomyolipoma and oncocytoma) despite imaging and renal biopsy, meaning 20% of SRM treated surgically are found of be benign post-operatively [54]. More recent studies suggest this may be as high as 30% [55].

In addition to diagnostic challenges relating to SRM, there are also complexities relating to patient risk stratification and prognosis. 30% of SRM display aggressive growth (rapid growth or doubling time < 12 months), whilst the remainder grow slowly or remain stable [56, 57]. 3–12% of SRM will either present with concurrent metastases or will develop metastases at a later date [58], however there is a lack of validated scores for risk stratification. Linear growth rate has been proposed as a marker for aggressiveness, but this has recently been challenged, as it did not correlate with overall outcomes, and similar average growth rates were observed for benign and malignant (low and high grade) SRM [59, 60].

As such, a potential consequence of screening is the over-diagnosis of SRM with indolent potential which would not have otherwise affected patient survival. In screening, lead time bias refers to an artificially inflated survival time noted simply through earlier diagnosis of a cancer rather than truly affecting mortality. Length time bias refers to artificially inflated survival time noted in screening secondary to the detection of indolent and therefore slow growing disease (relative to aggressive disease which is more likely to be detected by the symptomatic patient pathway) [8]. RCCs detected incidentally have a lower grade and stage and better survival than cancers detected due to symptoms [61]. Our understanding of the natural history of the disease has improved in recent years thanks to increasing use of diagnostic biopsies, patient registries and trials of active surveillance. Improvements in imaging (such as contrast enhanced ultrasound and MRI) as well as more nuanced treatment strategies (use of active surveillance, ablation and nephron sparing surgery) aim to reduce over-treatment and offer risk-based management. In addition, it is crucial to determine if screening would lead to an increase in the detection of RCC beyond that already noted due to the increased use of abdominal imaging. 43% of individuals aged 65–85 years on Medicare in the USA undergo either a CT chest or CT abdomen over a 5-year period [5], although the numbers are likely to be lower in non-privatised healthcare systems. Ultimately, a RCT would enable us to tease out if screening would lead to a stage shift and if this would impact survival.

Depending on the screening tool used (focused renal ultrasound vs imaging of the whole abdomen), incidental findings will be identified. Although some of these will have uncertain clinical significance and may lead to increased investigations and worry/anxiety, this could be balanced by the added benefit from the identification of other abdominal malignancies or potentially life-threatening benign disease (e.g. aortic aneurysms). No studies have been performed to investigate the potential impact of screening for RCC itself on participants' quality of life [29], although studies in other conditions suggest that the impact of screening is either negligible or short lived (Aneurysms [62], breast [63] and ovarian cancer [64, 65]).

Key Points

- The incidence of RCC is highest in the developing world and rates are rising – partially due to increases in risk factors, but also secondary to incidental detection during abdominal imaging for other conditions
- The main risk factors for RCC are: advancing age, male sex, obesity, hypertension and smoking
- Screening for RCC has been identified as a top research priority by clinicians, researchers and the public.
- It is postulated that screening for RCC may improve survival outcomes through earlier detection, however the ideal screening modality and screening population have yet to be elucidated. No RCT of screening for RCC have been performed.
- The most likely potential screening tools would be imaging-based, with either ultrasound or low-dose CT (potentially in combination with other screening programs). Although promising, no blood or urine biomarkers have been approved for clinical use.
- The relatively low prevalence of RCC limits cost-effectiveness. Risk-stratified screening may overcome this, however established risk factors for RCC are not disease specific, limiting accuracy.
- Screening for RCC is acceptable to the public and there is public appetite for a screening study.
- Important screening considerations include: risk of overdiagnosis, management of incidental findings, nuances associated with limited understanding of the natural history of small renal masses.

References

1. Capitanio U, Bensalah K, Bex A, Boorjian SA, Bray F, Coleman J, et al. Epidemiology of renal cell carcinoma. Eur Urol. 2019;75(1):74–84.
2. Znaor A, Lortet-Tieulent J, Laversanne M, Jemal A, Bray F. International variations and trends in renal cell carcinoma incidence and mortality. Eur Urol. 2015;67(3):519–30.
3. Hock LM, Lynch J, Balaji KC. Increasing incidence of all stages of kidney cancer in the last 2 decades in the United States: an analysis of surveillance, epidemiology and end results program data. J Urol. 2002;167(1):57–60.
4. Lightfoot N, Conlon M, Kreiger N, Bissett R, Desai M, Warde P, et al. Impact of noninvasive imaging on increased incidental detection of renal cell carcinoma. Eur Urol. 2000;37(5):521–7.
5. Welch HG, Skinner JS, Schroeck FR, Zhou W, Black WC. Regional variation of computed tomographic imaging in the United States and the risk of nephrectomy. JAMA Intern Med. 2018;178(2):221–7.
6. Cancer Research UK Kidney Cancer Statistics. Available from: http://www.cancerresearchuk.org/health-professional/cancer-statistics/statistics-by-cancer-type/kidney-cancer
7. Service Public Health England and the English National Cancer Registration Service. National Cancer Registration and Analysis Service: TNM stage group by CCG by tumour type for 10+3 tumour types, 2012–2017. Available from: http://www.ncin.org.uk/view?rid=3864

8. Usher-Smith J, Simmons RK, Rossi SH, Stewart GD. Current evidence on screening for renal cancer. Nat Rev Urol. 2020;17(11):637–42.
9. Welch HG, Kramer BS, Black WC. Epidemiologic signatures in cancer. N Engl J Med. 2019;381(14):1378–86.
10. Wong MCS, Goggins WB, Yip BHK, Fung FDH, Leung C, Fang Y, et al. Incidence and mortality of kidney cancer: temporal patterns and global trends in 39 countries. Sci Rep. 2017;7(1):15698.
11. Rossi SH, Klatte T, Usher-Smith J, Stewart GD. Epidemiology and screening for renal cancer. World J Urol. 2018;36(9):1341–53.
12. Macleod LC, Hotaling JM, Wright JL, Davenport MT, Gore JL, Harper J, et al. Risk factors for renal cell carcinoma in the VITAL study. J Urol. 2013;190(5):1657–61.
13. Scelo G, Purdue MP, Brown KM, Johansson M, Wang Z, Eckel-Passow JE, et al. Genome-wide association study identifies multiple risk loci for renal cell carcinoma. Nat Commun. 2017;8:15724.
14. Wozniak MB, Brennan P, Brenner DR, Overvad K, Olsen A, Tjonneland A, et al. Alcohol consumption and the risk of renal cancers in the European prospective investigation into cancer and nutrition (EPIC). Int J Cancer. 2015;137(8):1953–66.
15. Bellocco R, Pasquali E, Rota M, Bagnardi V, Tramacere I, Scotti L, et al. Alcohol drinking and risk of renal cell carcinoma: results of a meta-analysis. Ann Oncol. 2012;23(9):2235–44.
16. Song DY, Song S, Song Y, Lee JE. Alcohol intake and renal cell cancer risk: a meta-analysis. Br J Cancer. 2012;106(11):1881–90.
17. Behrens G, Leitzmann MF. The association between physical activity and renal cancer: systematic review and meta-analysis. Br J Cancer. 2013;108(4):798–811.
18. International Agency for Research on Cancer list of classifications by cancer sites with sufficient or limited evidence in humans 2017 [2]. Available from: http://monographs.iarc.fr/ENG/Classification/Table4.pdf
19. Rossi SH, Blick C, Handforth C, Brown JE, Stewart GD. Renal cancer gap analysis C. essential research priorities in renal cancer: a modified Delphi consensus statement. Eur Urol. Focus. 2020;6(5):991–8.
20. Rossi SH, Fielding A, Blick C, Handforth C, Brown JE, Stewart GD. Setting research priorities in partnership with patients to provide patient-centred urological cancer care. Eur Urol. 2019;75(6):891–3.
21. Jones J, Bhatt J, Avery J, Laupacis A, Cowan K, Basappa N, et al. The kidney cancer research priority-setting partnership: identifying the top 10 research priorities as defined by patients, caregivers, and expert clinicians. Can Urol Assoc J. 2017;11(12):379–87.
22. The Kidney Cancer UK patient survey report 2018 2018 Available from: https://www.kcuk.org.uk/wp-content/uploads/2018/01/2018-Kidney-Cancer-UK-Patient-Survey-Report-1.pdf
23. Vasudev NS, Wilson M, Stewart GD, Adeyoju A, Cartledge J, Kimuli M, et al. Challenges of early renal cancer detection: symptom patterns and incidental diagnosis rate in a multi-centre prospective UK cohort of patients presenting with suspected renal cancer. BMJ Open. 2020;10(5):e035938.
24. Pierorazio PM, Johnson MH, Patel HD, Sozio SM, Sharma R, Iyoha E, et al. Management of Renal Masses and Localized Renal Cancer: systematic review and meta-analysis. J Urol 2016.
25. Kidney cancer incidence statistics: Kidney cancer incidence in Europe and worldwide 2014 [19/01/2017]. Available from: http://www.cancerresearchuk.org/health-professional/cancer-statistics/statistics-by-cancer-type/kidney-cancer/incidence#heading-Ten
26. Ljungberg B, Albiges L, Abu-Ghanem Y, Bensalah K, Dabestani S, Fernandez-Pello S, et al. European Association of Urology guidelines on renal cell carcinoma: the 2019 update. Eur Urol. 2019;75(5):799–810.
27. Rossi SH, Klatte T, Usher-Smith JA, Fife K, Welsh SJ, Dabestani S, et al. A decision analysis evaluating screening for kidney cancer using focused renal ultrasound. Eur Urol Focus 2019.
28. Wilson JM, Jungner YG. Principles and practice of mass screening for disease. Bol Oficina Sanit Panam. 1968;65(4):281–393.

29. Rossi SH, Hsu R, Blick C, Goh V, Nathan P, Nicol D, et al. Meta-analysis of the prevalence of renal cancer detected by abdominal ultrasonography. Br J Surg. 2017;104(6):648–59.
30. Spouge AR, Wilson SR, Wooley B. Abdominal sonography in asymptomatic executives: prevalence of pathologic findings, potential benefits, and problems. J Ultrasound Med. 1996;15(11):763–7. quiz 9-70
31. Fujii Y, Ajima J, Oka K, Tosaka A, Takehara Y. Benign renal tumors detected among healthy adults by abdominal ultrasonography. Eur Urol. 1995;27(2):124–7.
32. Mihara S, Kuroda K, Yoshioka R, Koyama W. Early detection of renal cell carcinoma by ultrasonographic screening–based on the results of 13 years screening in Japan. Ultrasound Med Biol. 1999;25(7):1033–9.
33. Tsuboi N, Horiuchi K, Kimura G, Kondoh Y, Yoshida K, Nishimura T, et al. Renal masses detected by general health checkup. Int J Urol. 2000;7(11):404–8.
34. Mizuma Y, Watanabe Y, Ozasa K, Hayashi K, Kawai K. Validity of sonographic screening for the detection of abdominal cancers. J Clin Ultrasound. 2002;30(7):408–15.
35. Filipas D, Spix C, Schulz-Lampel D, Michaelis J, Hohenfellner R, Roth S, et al. Screening for renal cell carcinoma using ultrasonography: a feasibility study. BJU Int. 2003;91(7):595–9.
36. Malaeb BS, Martin DJ, Littooy FN, Lotan Y, Waters WB, Flanigan RC, et al. The utility of screening renal ultrasonography: identifying renal cell carcinoma in an elderly asymptomatic population. BJU Int. 2005;95(7):977–81.
37. Warshauer DM, McCarthy SM, Street L, Bookbinder MJ, Glickman MG, Richter J, et al. Detection of renal masses: sensitivities and specificities of excretory urography/linear tomography, US, and CT. Radiology. 1988;169(2):363–5.
38. Jamis-Dow CA, Choyke PL, Jennings SB, Linehan WM, Thakore KN, Walther MM. Small (< or = 3-cm) renal masses: detection with CT versus US and pathologic correlation. Radiology. 1996;198(3):785–8.
39. Beinfeld MT, Wittenberg E, Gazelle GS. Cost-effectiveness of whole-body CT screening. Radiology. 2005;234(2):415–22.
40. Ishikawa S, Aoki J, Ohwada S, Takahashi T, Morishita Y, Ueda K. Mass screening of multiple abdominal solid organs using mobile helical computed tomography scanner–a preliminary report. Asian J Surg. 2007;30(2):118–21.
41. Wernli KJ, Rutter CM, Dachman AH, Zafar HM. Suspected extracolonic neoplasms detected on CT colonography: literature review and possible outcomes. Acad Radiol. 2013;20(6):667–74.
42. Jubber I, Shariat SF, Conroy S, Tan WS, Gordon PC, Lotan Y, et al. Non-visible haematuria for the detection of bladder, upper tract, and kidney cancer: an updated systematic review and meta-analysis. Eur Urol. 2020;77(5):583–98.
43. Sugimura K, Ikemoto SI, Kawashima H, Nishisaka N, Kishimoto T. Microscopic hematuria as a screening marker for urinary tract malignancies. Int J Urol. 2001;8(1):1–5.
44. Bangma CH, Loeb S, Busstra M, Zhu X, El Bouazzaoui S, Refos J, et al. Outcomes of a bladder cancer screening program using home hematuria testing and molecular markers. Eur Urol. 2013;64(1):41–7.
45. Morrissey JJ, Mellnick VM, Luo J, Siegel MJ, Figenshau RS, Bhayani S, et al. Evaluation of urine Aquaporin-1 and Perilipin-2 concentrations as biomarkers to screen for renal cell carcinoma: a prospective cohort study. JAMA Oncol. 2015;1(2):204–12.
46. Scelo G, Muller DC, Riboli E, Johansson M, Cross AJ, Vineis P, et al. KIM-1 as a blood-based marker for early detection of kidney cancer: a prospective nested case-control study. Clin Cancer Res. 2018;24(22):5594–601.
47. Jordan Flitcroft JV, Tarun Vemulkar, Emma Welbourne, Sabrina H Rossi, Sarah J Welsh, Russell Cowburn, Grant D Stewart Early detection of kidney cancer using urinary proteins: a truly non-invasive strategy. BJU Int 2021.
48. Harvey-Kelly LLW, Harrison H, Rossi SH, Griffin SJ, Stewart GD, Usher-Smith JA. Public attitudes towards screening for kidney cancer: an online survey. BMC Urol. 2020;20(1):170.
49. Shea MW. A proposal for a targeted screening program for renal cancer. Front Oncol. 2013;3:207.

50. Harrison H, Thompson RE, Lin Z, Rossi SH, Stewart GD, Griffin SJ, et al. Risk prediction models for kidney cancer: a systematic review. Eur Urol Focus 2020.
51. Usher-Smith JA, Harvey-Kelly LLW, Rossi SH, Harrison H, Griffin SJ, Stewart GD. Acceptability and potential impact on uptake of using different risk stratification approaches to determine eligibility for screening: a population-based survey. Health Expect 2020.
52. Fenton JJ, Weiss NS. Screening computed tomography: will it result in overdiagnosis of renal carcinoma? Cancer. 2004;100(5):986–90.
53. Mitchell TJ, Turajlic S, Rowan A, Nicol D, Farmery JHR, O'Brien T, et al. Timing the landmark events in the evolution of clear cell renal cell cancer: TRACERx renal. Cell. 2018;173(3):611–23 e17.
54. Johnson DC, Vukina J, Smith AB, Meyer AM, Wheeler SB, Kuo TM, et al. Preoperatively misclassified, surgically removed benign renal masses: a systematic review of surgical series and United States population level burden estimate. J Urol. 2015;193(1):30–5.
55. Kim JH, Li S, Khandwala Y, Chung KJ, Park HK, Chung BI. Association of Prevalence of benign pathologic findings after partial nephrectomy with preoperative imaging patterns in the United States from 2007 to 2014. JAMA Surg. 2019;154(3):225–31.
56. Jewett MA, Mattar K, Basiuk J, Morash CG, Pautler SE, Siemens DR, et al. Active surveillance of small renal masses: progression patterns of early stage kidney cancer. Eur Urol. 2011;60(1):39–44.
57. Volpe A, Panzarella T, Rendon RA, Haider MA, Kondylis FI, Jewett MA. The natural history of incidentally detected small renal masses. Cancer. 2004;100(4):738–45.
58. Pierorazio PM, Hyams ES, Mullins JK, Allaf ME. Active surveillance for small renal masses. Rev Urol. 2012;14(1–2):13–9.
59. Jang A, Patel HD, Riffon M, Gorin MA, Semerjian A, Johnson MH, et al. Multiple growth periods predict unfavourable pathology in patients with small renal masses. BJU Int. 2018;121(5):732–6.
60. Gordetsky J, Eich ML, Garapati M, Del Carmen Rodriguez Pena M, Rais-Bahrami S. Active surveillance of small renal masses. Urology. 2019;123:157–66.
61. Ficarra V, Prayer-Galetti T, Novella G, Bratti E, Maffei N, Dal Bianco M, et al. Incidental detection beyond pathological factors as prognostic predictor of renal cell carcinoma. Eur Urol. 2003;43(6):663–9.
62. Ashton HA, Buxton MJ, Day NE, Kim LG, Marteau TM, Scott RA, et al. The multicentre aneurysm screening study (MASS) into the effect of abdominal aortic aneurysm screening on mortality in men: a randomised controlled trial. Lancet. 2002;360(9345):1531–9.
63. Tosteson AN, Fryback DG, Hammond CS, Hanna LG, Grove MR, Brown M, et al. Consequences of false-positive screening mammograms. JAMA Intern Med. 2014;174(6): 954–61.
64. Barrett J, Jenkins V, Farewell V, Menon U, Jacobs I, Kilkerr J, et al. Psychological morbidity associated with ovarian cancer screening: results from more than 23,000 women in the randomised trial of ovarian cancer screening (UKCTOCS). BJOG. 2014;121(9):1071–9.
65. Reade CJ, Riva JJ, Busse JW, Goldsmith CH, Elit L. Risks and benefits of screening asymptomatic women for ovarian cancer: a systematic review and meta-analysis. Gynecol Oncol. 2013;130(3):674–81.

Hereditary Renal Cancer Predisposition Syndromes

Scott T. C. Shepherd and Samra Turajlic

Renal cell carcinoma (RCC) comprises a heterogenous group of cancers with distinct histopathological appearance and molecular drivers. In addition to smoking, obesity and hypertension, genetic factors are implicated in the pathogenesis of the disease. Pathogenic germline variants in at least 12 genes (Table 1) are associated with an increased lifetime risk of RCC, accounting for 4–6% of all RCC diagnoses [1]. It is likely that other undescribed genes and background germline genetic factors contribute to the development of familial RCC.

Hereditary RCC syndromes are usually inherited in an autosomal dominant manner, although a lack of family history of RCC may occur if there is incomplete penetrance or if the mutation has arisen *de novo*.

Most guidance agree that individuals with bilateral and/or multicentric disease; early age of onset (<= 46 years of age [1]); or a first or second degree relative with any renal tumour should be referred for genetic counselling [2]. In addition, the presence of additional non-RCC clinical features in a patient or histopathological features might suggest the diagnosis of a specific hereditary RCC syndrome and guide molecular genetic investigations (Table 1).

Herein, we discuss the well described clinical syndromes, their molecular pathogenesis and clinical management strategies. The clinical features, suggested renal screening and management recommendations are summarised in Table 2.

S. T. C. Shepherd · S. Turajlic (✉)
The Royal Marsden NHS Foundation Trust, London, UK

The Francis Crick Institute, London, UK
e-mail: Samra.Turajlic@crick.ac.uk

C. Anderson, M. Afshar (eds.), *Renal Cancer*,
https://doi.org/10.1007/978-3-030-84756-2_3

Table 1 Summary of known hereditary RCC syndromes, the associated variant germline gene and RCC histological subtype

Syndrome	*Gene*	Locus	Protein	Type	Renal Cancer Histology	Lifetime risk of RCC
von Hippel-Lindau (vHL) disease	*VHL*	3p25	pVHL	Tumour suppressor	ccRCC Clear cell papillary Cysts	60–70%
Hereditary papillary RCC	*MET*	7q31	Hepatocyte growth factor	Proto-oncogene	Type 1 papillary	100%
Hereditary leiomyomatosis and renal cell carcinoma (HLRCC)	*FH*	1q43	Fumerate hydratase	Tumour suppressor	HLRCC-associated RCC (formally papillary type 2)	15–35%
Hereditary paraganglioma-phaeochromocytoma syndrome	*SDHA* *SDHB* *SDHC* *SDHD*	5p15 1p36 1q23 11q23	Succinate dehydrogenase complex, subunit A Succinate dehydrogenase complex, subunit B Succinate dehydrogenase complex, subunit C Succinate dehydrogenase complex, subunit D	Tumour suppressor	SDH-deficient RCC	–
Birt-Hogg-Dubé	*FLCN*	17p11	Folliculin	Tumour suppressor	Chromophobe oncocytic hybrid Oncocytoma Papillary ccRCC	15–29%
BAP1 tumour predisposition syndrome	*BAP1*	3p21	BRCA1-associated protein 1	Tumour suppressor	Clear cell	–
Tuberous sclerosis	*TSC1* *TSC2*	9q34 16p13	Hamartin Tuberin	Tumour suppressor Tumour suppressor	Angiomyolipoma Oncocytoma Chromophobe ccRCC	2–3%
Cowden syndrome	*PTEN*	10q23	Phosphatase and tensin homolog	Tumour suppressor	Papillary Chromophobe ccRCC	34% [1]

Table 2 Clinical features and summarised renal screening and management reccomendations

Syndrome	*Gene*	Extrarenal manifestations	Suggested RCC surveillance imaging	Management of renal manifestations
von Hippel-Lindau (vHL) syndrome	*VHL*	– Phaeochromocytoma/paraganglioma – Pancreatic neuroendocrine tumours – Retinal/CNS hemangioblastomas – Cystic disease: Pancreatic, broad ligament, epididymal – Endolymphatic sac tumours	– From age 16 years [1] – Annual MRI abdomen alternating with USS [1]	– Active surveillance with delayed intervention when >3 cm – Nephron sparing surgical approach or thermal/cryoablation may be considered [1]
Hereditary papillary RCC syndrome	*MET*	– None	– Abdominal imaging at least every 36 months (MRI preferred) [2]	– Active surveillance with delayed intervention when >3 cm [2] – Nephron sparing approach/ enucleation favoured over ablation [2]
Hereditary leiomyatosis and renal cell carcinoma (HLRCC) syndrome	*FH*	– Uterine leiomyomas – Cutaneous leiomyomas – Uterine leiomyosarcoma	– From age 10 [3] – Annual MRI (preferred) or contrast enhanced CT	– Low threshold for surgical intervention [2] – Wide surgical margins
Hereditary paraganglioma-phaeochromocytoma syndrome	*SDHA* *SDHB* *SDHC* *SDHD*	– Phaeochromocytoma – Paraganglioma – GIST	– Abdominal MRI every 2 years [4]	– Immediate extirpative surgery
Birt-Hogg-Dubé (BHD) syndrome	*FLCN*	– Cutaenous fibrofolliculomas – Cystic disease: Lung and kidney	– Abdominal imaging at least every 36 months (MRI preferred) [2]	– Active surveillance with delayed intervention when >3 cm – Nephron sparing surgical approach or thermal/cryoablation may be considered [1]

(continued)

Table 2 (continued)

Syndrome	*Gene*	Extrarenal manifestations	Suggested RCC surveillance imaging	Management of renal manifestations
BAP1 tumour predisposition syndrome	*BAP1*	– Uveal melanoma – Cutaneous melanoma – Mesothelioma	– Abdominal MRI every 2 years [5]	– No specific published guidance – Immediate extirpative surgery advised [6]
Tuberous sclerosis complex (TSC)	*TSC1* *TSC2*	– Cutaneous lesions: Hypopigmented macules, angiofibromas and others – CNS lesions: Cortical dysplasia, hamartomas, giant cell astrocytoma – Retinal haemartomas – Cardiac rhabdomyomas	– Abdominal MRI every 1–3 years [7]	– Consider biopsy to differentiate RCC vs AML – mTOR inhibitor (e.g. sirolimus) is preferred therapy for AML – Nephron sparing surgery for RCC
Cowden syndrome	*PTEN*	– Cutaneous lesions: Hamartomas, trichilemmomas, oral fibromas, and punctate palmoplantar keratoses – Breast cancer – Thyroid cancer – Endometrial cancer – Colorectal polyps/carcinoma	– Abdominal MRI every 2 years [8]	– No specific published guidance

Von Hippel Lindau (VHL) Disease

Clinicopathological Hallmarks

VHL disease is an autosomal dominant multi-organ tumour predisposition syndrome caused by inactivating germline variants in the von Hippel-Lindau tumour suppressor gene (*VHL*). Incidence is approximately 1:34,000 live births and penetrance approaches 100% by age 60 [3, 4]. Affected individuals can develop a variety of VHL deficient lesions across differing tissue contexts, including many hundreds of renal cysts and clear cell renal cacners (ccRCCs) in addition to benign pancreatic cysts, central nervous system (CNS) and retinal haemangioblastomas (HB), and neuroendocrine tumors (NET) such as pheochromocytoma. Classifications have been proposed based on predilection for phaeochromocytoma (Table 3) although clinical phenotypes vary considerably between and within families [5].

The lifetime risk of developing a renal cancer is 60–70% at a mean age onset of 44 years (two decades earlier than sporadic ccRCC) although cases affecting teenagers have been described [6]. In-situ RCC growth is typically indolent [7] and primary tumour size appears to be an important determinant of outcome with the risk of metastasis virtually nil below 3 cm in size [8].

Genetics and Molecular Pathogenesis

The *VHL* gene is located on the short arm of chromosome 3 (3p25) [9] and encodes a 213 amino acid product, pVHL. pVHL forms the substrate recognition component of a E3 ubiquitin ligase complex with Elongin B and C (collectively, VCB complex) and plays a central role in cellular oxygen sensing and orchestrating the transcriptional response to hypoxia (Fig. 1). The VCB complex targets the hypoxia-inducible

Table 3 VHL disease subgroup categorisation and genotype/phenotype correlations (see further [1, 2]). HB, haemangioblastoma; PCC/PGL, phaeochromocytoma/paraganglioma; ccRCC clear cel renal cell carcinoma; VHL, von Hippel-Lindau

VHL Subtype	*VHL* Variant Type	Clinical phenotype	
		High Risk	Low Risk
Type 1	Deletions, insertions, truncations, missense	CNS/retinal HB, ccRCC	PCC/PGL
Type 1B	Contiguous gene deletions encompassing VHL	CNS/retinal HB	PCC/PGL, ccRCC
Type 2A	Missense	CNS/retinal HB, PCC/PGL	ccRCC
Type 2B	Missense	CNS/retinal HB, PCC/PGL, ccRCC	
Type 2C	Missense	PCC/PGL	CNS/retinal HB, ccRCC absent

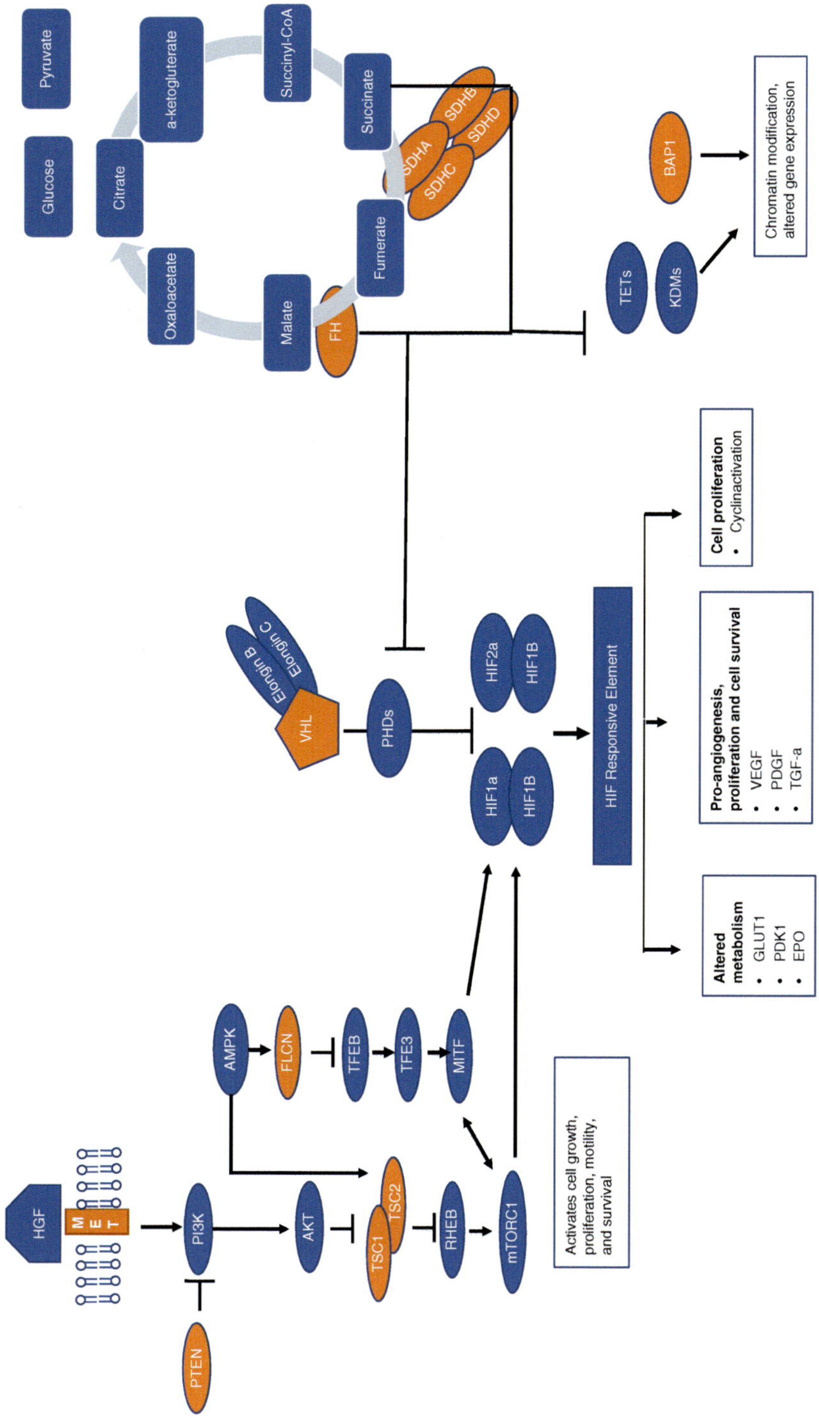
Pyruvate
Glucose
Citrate
a-ketogluterate
Succinyl-CoA
Succinate
SDHA
SDHB
SDHC
SDHD
Fumerate
Malate
FH
Oxaloacetate
TETs
KDMs
BAP1
Chromatin modification, altered gene expression
Elongin B
Elongin C
VHL
PHDs
HIF2a
HIF1B
HIF1a
HIF1B
HIF Responsive Element
Cell proliferation
• Cyclinactivation
Pro-angiogenesis, proliferation and cell survival
• VEGF
• PDGF
• TGF-a
Altered metabolism
• GLUT1
• PDK1
• EPO
HGF
M E T
PI3K
PTEN
AKT
TSC1
TSC2
RHEB
mTORC1
AMPK
FLCN
TFEB
TFE3
MITF
Activates cell growth, proliferation, motility, and survival

Fig. 1 Pathogenic germline variants in a number of genes (coloured red figure) are associated with increased lifetime risk of RCC. pVHL loss in tumors results in the inability of the VHL E3 ubiquitin ligase complex to target the HIF transcription factors for proteosomal degradation, leading to stabilisation of HIF and activation of the hypoxia response. Pseudohypoxia is pro-tumourigenic through expression of growth factors that induce proliferation, survival, and angiogenesis, including VEGF, PDGF, and TGFα, and increases expression of proteins that regulate glucose metabolism and cell proliferation, including GLUT1, LDHA, PDK1, and CCND1. Activating mutations of *MET*, inactivating mutations of *PTEN*, *TSC1*, *TSC2*, and *FLCN* in tumors result in increased activation of the PI3K/AKT/mTOR pathway which regulates cell growth, proliferation, and survival. Dysregulation of the PI3K/AKT/mTOR pathway results in increased production of the HIF transcription factors via MTORC1 and MITF signalling, indirectly influencing the VHL/HIF oxygen-sensing pathway. Loss of fumarate hydratase (FH) or components of succinate dehydrogenase (SDHB, SDHC, SDHD) changes the activity ofthe TCA cycle, leading to altered metabolism, and the accumulation of the oncometabolites fumarate and succinate, respectively. Fumarate or succinate can both inhibit α-ketoglutarate–dependent prolylhydroxylase enzymes that regulate the HIF transcription factors, resulting in inhibition of the VHL/HIF oxygen-sensing pathway. Other α-ketoglutarate–dependent enzymes include the Ten-eleven translocation (TET) and Lysine-specific demethylase (KDM) enzymes that regulate DNA/histone methylation, acetylation and effect chromatin remodeling. Loss of chromatin remodelling protein, BAP1 also alters gene-expression profiles in RCC

factors (HIF1a and HIF2a) for proteasomal degradation in an oxygen dependant fashion. Under hypoxic conditions, there is an accumulation of HIF leading to transcriptional activation of the so-called hypoxia response element (HRE) genes, resulting in metabolic re-programming, increased proliferation, angiogenesis and cellular survival. Inactivation of *VHL* leads to HRE activation in the absence of hypoxia, 'pseudohypoxia', and is characteristic of both sporadic and hereditary ccRCCs.

More than 500 unique germline pathogenic variants have been described in over 900 families with VHL disease [10, 11] from specific missence mutations to exon or whole gene deletions (Table 3). Genotype/phenotype correlations have been described based on predilection for phaeochromocytoma but these are imperfect and manifestations of VHL vary considerably between and within kindred with an identical inactivating mutation [5].

Clinical Management and Therapeutic Approaches

Regular radiological surveillance is the mainstay of management in individuals found to have or be at risk of carrying a pathogenic variant in *VHL*. Surveillance imaging protocols to monitor renal and non-renal manifestations of the disease have been published and recommend imaging modalities that limit exposure to ionising radiation [12].

In the kidney, management involves serial radiological monitoring and surgical intervention when the dominant lesion reaches 3 cm in maximal diameter [8].

The risk of metastasis is minimal in lesions <3 cm in size, with the risk of systemic spread increasing stepwise beyond this cut off [8]. Nephron sparing approaches (partial nephrectomy or enucleation) are undertaken wherever feasible to preserve renal clearance (surgical approach reviewed in [13]). Kidney transplantation in patients with end-stage renal disease appears to be safe and does not appear to be associated with worse graft or overall survival outcomes than non-VHL patients [14].

Receptor tyrosine kinase inhibitors targeting the VEGF-pathway have shown clinical activity in patients with clinically localised disease [15, 16]. Objective response to pazopanib was seen in 42% of VHL patients in one non-randomised phase 2 tral; partial responses were observed in 52% of RCCs, 53% of pancreatic lesions but only 4% of CNS haemangioblastomas. Median shrinkage varied between organ site and was 40·5% (IQR 21–53) in the renal lesions, 30·5% (IQR 18–36) in pancreatic lesions, and 13% (IQR 7–23) in the haemangioblastomas suggestive of tissue specific sensitivity to VEGF-tareted therapy. Treatment related toxicity was signficiant with 23% discontinuing therapy due to adverse events. Responses to VEGF inhibition have been also been described in the context of metastatic disease outwith clinical trial setting [17, 18]. https://www.fda.gov/drugs/resources-information-approved-drugs/fda-approves-belzutifan-cancers-associated-von-hippel-lindau-disease.

Germline MET Variants: Hereditary Papillary Renal Cell Carcinoma (HPRC) Syndrome

Clinicopathological Hallmarks

HPRC is a rare autosomal dominant hereditary renal cancer syndrome characterised by the development of multifocal, bilateral type 1 papillary RCC. HPRC is highly penetrant (approaching 100%) although the age at onset varys widely (median 41 years (range, 19–66) [1, 19]. A single kidney may harbour over 3000 microscopic papillary tumours [20, 21]. There are no known extra renal manifestations [19, 22].

Genetics and Molecular Pathogenesis

Germline missence mutations [23, 24] in the tyrosine kinase domain of *MET* (7q31) result in ligand independent MET activation [23–25] and downstream signalling associated with cell proliferation, survival and motility [26]. Specific missence *MET* mutation might influence the age of onset [19]. Altered *MET* gene status or increased chromosome 7 copy number is seen in 81% of sporadic type 1 pRCC in the TCGA dataset [27].

Clinical Management and Therapeutic Approaches

HPRC related tumours have been reported to metastasise [21] however growth is typically indolent and patients are managed with active surveillance until the dominant lesion reaches 3 cm in size. When considering surgery, a nephron sparing approach is employed where possible [28].

The presence of activating *MET* mutations in patients with hereditary and sporadic papillary renal cancer has led to the evaluation of a targeted therapy approach. Foretinib, an oral multikinase inhibitor targeting *MET* and VEGFR, demonstrated a 100% disease control rate in patients with advanced disease and a germline *MET* mutation [29], leading to FDA approval for this indication. Clinical responses in patients with *MET* mutations have also been observed with *MET* kinase inhibitors crizotinib [30] and savolitinib [31] and a randomised study involving a number of *MET* targeting agents in papillary renal cancer is ongoing (NCT02761057).

Herediatry Leiomyomatosis and Renal Cell Carcinoma (HLRCC) Syndrome

Clinicopathological Hallmarks

HLRCC is an autosomal dominant familial cancer syndrome and affected individuals are at risk to develop benign cutaneous and uterine leiomyomas and an aggressive form of RCC: HLRCC-associated RCC (formally type 2 papillary renal cancer) [32]. The prevalence is unknown, although several hundred families have been described in the literature. Given its rarity, it is likely that HLRCC is an underdiagnosed clinical entity although establishment of HLRCC-associated RCC in the most recent WHO pathological classification and improved access to molecular diagnostics may increase diagnoses.

The most common manifestations of HLRCC are cutaneous leiomyomata, which occur in 76%–100% of patients [33–35] and present as multiple firm, flesh-colored nodules (10 to >100, <2.5 mm in size) that develop on the trunk and extremities [36]. Uterine leiomyomas are reported in over 80% of affected women and many experience frequent, severe irregular bleeding requiring hysterectomy [33]. Uterine leiomyomas have rarely been reported to transform to uterine leiomyosarcoma [37].

Lifetime risk of developing RCC is estimated 15–35% [33, 38, 39] with median age at presentation 41 years (range 10–90 years) and 5% of cases diagnosed under the age of 20 [38]. RCC lesions are typically solitary and have the potential for rapid primary tumour growth and early metastatic seeding, even when the primary tumour is small [40].

Germline Genetics and Molecular Pathogenesis

Pathogenic germline variants in the fumerate hydratase (*FH)* gene (1q43) [41, 42] are detected in affected individuals. No genotype-phenotype correlations have been described [42].

The FH enzyme plays an essential role in the Kreb's Cycle which enables hydration of fumerate to malate (Fig. 1). FH-deficient cells undergo a Warburg metabolic shift [43], characterised by a dependence on aerobic glycolysis, impaired oxidative phosphorylation and an intracellular accumulation of fumerate (see below *oncometabolites in RCC*). These changes give rise to a tumourigenic phenotype via stabilisation of HIFs, increased production of reactive oxygen species and histone hypermethylation (reviewed, [44, 45]).

Clinical Management and Therapeutic Considerations

Radiological surveillance screening for HLRCC-associated RCC is recommended from age 8 years [46]. Given the aggressive phenotype, prompt extirpation with wide resection margins is undertaken in individuals with a detectable renal mass. Lymphadenectomy may improve accuracy of staging given the frequency of lymph node metastasis [38].

Synthetic lethality occurs when the simultaneous perturbation of two genes results in cell death and this approach is being used to specifically target FH deficient cells. For example, the combination of bevacizumab and erlotinib (anti-VEGF-A and anti-EGFR, respectively) may constrain glucose delivery to tumour cells, exploiting reliance on aerobic glycolysis. This combination has demonstrated 100% disease control rate and median progression free survival of >24 months in HLRCC-associated RCC in one study [47]. Another strategy under clinical evaluation is the sensitisation of FH/SDH deficient RCCs to poly(ADP)-ribose polymerase (PARP) inhibition (see below *oncometabolites in RCC*).

Succinate Dehydrogenase Deficient RCC

Clinicopathological Hallmarks

Germline pathogenic *SDH* variants are associated with hereditary phaeochromocytoma (PCT) and paraganglioma (PGL) syndrome and at lower penetrance gastrointestinal stromal tuomurs (GIST) and RCCs [48]. The incidence is unknown.

The lifetime tumour risk exceeds 70% and clinical manifestations vary dependant on the mutated SDH subunit (reviewed [49]). The lifetime risk of developing a renal tumour has been estimated at approximately 5% for *SDHB* carriers but may be less in other affected subunits [48]. RCCs are typically solitary and unilateral. Median age of diagnosis was 37 years [50], although presentation with RCC as young as 14 has been reported [51]. Distant metastasis occurred in 9 of the 27 patients in one series and may be associated with sarcomatoid differentiation in the priamry [28].

Genetics and Molecular Pathogenesis

SDH is a tetrameric enzymatic complex consisting of four subunits (*SDHA, SDHB, SDHC, SDHD*) that localise to the inner mitochondrial membrane and are involved in both the Kreb's cycle and electron transport chain, catalysing the oxidation of succinate to fumerate (Fig. 1) [52].

SDH-deficient RCC was added to the WHO classification of renal tumours as a unique subtype in 2016 [32]. In patients with RCC, the most commonly mutated gene is *SDHB*, followed by *SDHC, SDHD*, and *SDHA* [50, 53]. Biallelic inactivation of SDH leads to a Warburg shift to aerobic glycolysis and impaired oxidative phosphorylation and intracellular accumulation of succinate (*see oncometabolites in RCC below*).

Clinical Management and Therapeutic Considerations

There are no specific clinical guidelines for the management of *SDH* deficient RCC. Proposed surveillance strategies [51, 54] reccomend lifelong radiological surveillance for metachronous RCCs and/or PCT/PGL. Upon detection of a renal mass, prompt extirapative surgery is performed given the risk of early metastatic seeding. SDH and HLRCC related RCCs are profoundly FDG PET avid which may be useful in identifying occult metastatic disease.

Disruption of the TCA Cycle: Oncometabolites in RCC

Loss of function of the SDH and FH enzymes leads to an accumulation of succinate and fumerate (so-called oncometabolites) that have pro-oncogenic functions [45]. Oncometabolites inhibit a family of enzymes known as α-ketoglutarate (αKG)-dependent dioxygenases, leading to epigenetic dysregulation and induction of a pseudohypoxic phenotype. Inhibition of specific αKG-dependent dioxegenases, KDM4A and KDM4B, leads to suppression of the homologous recombination DNA-repair pathway and a loss of genome integrity. Homologous recombination deficiency was shown to confer sensitivity to PARP inhibition in pre-clinical models and might offer a novel targeted therapy approach [55].

Birt-Hogg-Dube (BHD) Syndrome

Clinicopathological Hallmarks

BHD syndrome is an autosomal dominant cancer predisposition syndrome characterised by benign cutaenous fibrofolliculomas and cystic lung disease (occurring in >85% of kindred) that present in in young adulthood [56–58]. Lung cysts can predispose to spontaneous pneumothorax [59]. The exact prevalence is unknown but BHD has been reported in more than 200 families globally [12].

Bilateral and multifocal renal neoplasms occur in 15–29% of BHD patients; the median age at tumour diagnosis is 46–50 years although may occur as young as 20 years [58, 60]. The histological subtype can vary between and within patients (Table 1) with hybrid oncocytic tumours (50%) the most commonly seen followed by chromophobe RCC (chRCC) (34%) and oncocytoma (9%) [56, 57]. Macroscopically normal kidney contain scattered microscopic foci of oncocytic cells which may be precursor lesions [56].

Genetics and Molecular Pathogenesis

Pathogenic germline variants in the *FLCN gene* (17p11) are detected in affected kindred with [61, 62] no clear genotype/phenotype correlation [58, 60]. Inactivation of the *FLCN* gene promotes RCC tumourigenesis through dysregulation of the PI3K/AKT-mTOR pathway and activation of mitochondrial biogenesis leading to ROS production and activation of HIF transcriptional activity [52].

Clinical Management and Therapeutic Approaches

Life-long radiological surveillanve for renal tumours is reccomended [12, 46] and a nephron sparing surgical approach should be considered once the largest lesion reaches 3 cm in maximal diameter [63]. Metastasis can occur when patients are not receiving regular radiological surveillance [59] and are typically of clear cell histology and associated with a poor prognosis [56, 59]. There are no specific targeted therapy approaches for patients with BHD related RCC.

BRCA1-Associated Protein (BAP1) Tumour Predisposition Syndrome

Clinicopathological Hallmarks

This autosomal dominant tumour predisposition syndrome is characterised by an increased life-time risk of mesothelioma, uveal and cutaneous melanoma and RCC [64] with the full spectrum of associated tumours still to be defined. Penetrance is high with 85% of mutation carriers affected with a cancer [65]. The lifetime risk of RCC is approximately 10%, at a mean age of diagnosis for RCC 42 years (range 36–70). RCCs are typically solitary and of the clear cell subtype although other histologies have been described [66] and larger cohorts are needed to more clearly define the phenotype. Germline *BAP-1* mutation was detected in 0.8% of the TCGA ccRCC cohort, suggesting that *BAP1* tumour predisposition may be an underrecognised clinical entity [67].

Genomics and Molecular Pathogenesis

BAP1 (3p21) encodes a multifunctional deubiquitinating hydrolase enzyme that is involved in a number of biological processes including a key role in regulating chromatin dynamics, the DNA damage response and cell growth [68–70]. BAP1 alterations are seen in about 10–15% of patients with sporadic RCC, and are associated with a poor prognosis [67].

Pathogenic germline variants in *BAP1* (3p21) are detected in affected kindred with at least 46 unique mutations reported [65] and no clear genotype/phenotype correlations noted. Most families have at least two different tumour types diagnosed amongst kindred.

Clinical Management and Therapeutic Approaches

Evidence based guidelines have not been established but management involves regular examination/screening of affected organs to facilitate early diagnosis of tumours. Patients with a renal mass have have immediate surgery with wide surgical margins [65]. There are no approved targeted therapies for BAP1 driven malignancies.

Tuberous Sclerosis Complex (TSC) Syndrome

Clinicopathological Hallmarks

TSC is an autosomal dominant multiorgan tumour predisposition syndrome characterised by cutaneous lesions (hypopigmented macules, angiofibromas), CNS lesions (hamartomas, cortical dysplasia, subependymal giant cell astrocytoma), cardiac rhabdomyomas, retinal hamartomas and neurocognitive deficits and renal tumours [71]. The incidence of TSC is 1 in 6000–10,000 live births [72].

In the kidney, benign manifestations include angiomyolipomas (AMLs, present in up to 70%), oncocytomas and renal cysts. TSC associated RCCs occur in less than 5% of carriers and various histolopathological subtypes including ccRCC, pRCC and chRCC are seen (Table 1).

Genetics, Molecular Pathogenesis and Morphology

Pathogenic germline variants in either *TSC1* (chromosome 9p34; encoding hamartin) or *TSC2* (chromosome 16p13; encoding tuberin) are associated with TSC syndrome. Approximately 2/3 of carriers are new presentations with no family history. Hamartin and tuberin form part of a heterotrimeric complex with GTPase-activity involved in the negative regulation of the mTOR complex 1 (mTOR1), the key effector of the PI3K/AKT/mTOR pathway.

Clinical Management and Therapeutic Approaches

MRI surveillance to screen/monitor AMLs and/or RCCs is conducted and renal tumour biopsy may be necessary to differentiate between benign AMLs and RCC [73]. AMLs >3 cm in diameter are at risk of acute haemorrhage and should be treated with an mTOR inhibitor as the most effective first-line therapy [73–75]. This approach appears to be effective and well tolerated with surgery/ablation reserved as second line therapy [74]. Suspected malignant epithelial tumours are biopsied to confirm the diagnosis (if safe and practical to do so) and referred for nephron sparing surgery.

Cowden Syndrome

Clinicopathological Hallmarks

Cowden syndrome is an autosomal dominant tumour predisposition syndrome characterised by hamartomas, cutaneous manifestations (trichilemmomas, oral fibromas, and punctate palmoplantar keratoses), and an increased risk of breast, endometrial, thyroid, kidney and colorectal cancers [76]. There is an estimated incidence of 1 in 200,000 live births and nearly 100% of patients present in their 20s with mucocutaneous lesions.

Germline Genetics and Molecularpathogenesis

Pathogenic missense germline variants in *PTEN* (10q23) [77] are typically seen. *PTEN* is a negative regulator of the PI3K-AKT-mTOR signalling pathway. Heterogeneity of the genetic locus is observed in 20–34% of patients with clinical diagnosis of Cowden Syndrome, where germline variants are observed in related proteins such as *KLLN, PIK3CA* and *AKT1* [78, 79]. There are no clear genotype phenotype correlations. Estimated lifetime risk of renal cancer may be as high as 34% with increased risk from 40 years [80]. Histopathological subtype can vary, with case reports describing pRCC, chRCC, and ccRCC.

Conclusions

Hereditary RCC syndromes are caused by a number of pathogenic germline variants and each syndrome is associated with varying incidence of renal neoplasms and specific extrarenal manifestations. Management of such syndromes should be in the context of a bespoke specialist multidisciplinary team with underlined by principles of careful surveillance and patient centred management.

Identification of the culprit genes has given insight into the molecular drivers of the various RCC subtypes and highlights that an interconnected signalling network involving cellular sensing to oxygen, nutrients and/or energy production drive renal cancer growth. An improved understanding of these cellular processes can lead to rationally designed targeted therapeutic approaches to improve outcomes in both hereditary and sporadic manifestations of the disease.

Hereditary RCC syndromes are likely an under diagnosed clinical entitiy and this has implications for screening and surveillance of metachronous cancers and for identification of at risk family members. As manifestations of herediatary syndromes become clinically tractable, prompt diagnosis will optimise outcomes through use of novel targeted therapeutic strategies.

Key Points

1. Hereditary RCC syndromes account for 4–6% of all RCC diagnoses but some syndromes may be underecognised in the clinic.
2. Diagnosis may be suspected on the basis of family history, clinical features (multifocal or bilateral lesions; <46 years of age) or histopathological findings (e.g. HLRCC-associated RCC).
3. Management should be in the context of a multidisciplinary team, expert in the management of the renal and non-renal manifestations of the disease.
4. Active surveillance is the mainstay of management in asymptomatic patients with or suspected to have a pathogenic germline variant.
5. Wherever possible and clinically appropriate, imaging modalities such as MRI should be employed to minimise exposure to ionising radiation.
6. In syndromes where growth is likely to be indolent and the risk of metastasis is small, deferral of surgery until the solid component of the dominant lesion >3 cm is recommended.

7. In syndromes where risk of metastasis is high even when the primary tumour is small, immediate exiripative intervention with wide surgical margin is recommended.
8. A nephron sparing surgical approach (partial nephrectomy/enucleation) to preserve renal clearance is important in patients with a predisposition to bilateral and multifocal tumours that might require repeated surgical intervention.
9. An understanding of the consequences of the germline genetic event is leading to the development of targetetd therapeutic strategies in some syndromes and patients should be entered into clinical studies where possible.

References

1. Shuch B, et al. Defining early-onset kidney cancer: implications for germline and somatic mutation testing and clinical management. J Clin Oncol. 2014;32(5):431–7.
2. Hampel H, et al. A practice guideline from the American College of Medical Genetics and Genomics and the National Society of genetic counselors: referral indications for cancer predisposition assessment. Genet Med. 2015;17(1):70–87.
3. Maher ER, et al. Von Hippel-Lindau disease: a genetic study. J Med Genet. 1991;28(7):443–7.
4. Maddock IR, et al. A genetic register for von Hippel-Lindau disease. J Med Genet. 1996;33(2):120–7.
5. Chen F, et al. Germline mutations in the von Hippel-Lindau disease tumor suppressor gene: correlations with phenotype. Hum Mutat. 1995;5(1):66–75.
6. Maher ER, Webster AR, Moore AT. Clinical features and molecular genetics of Von Hippel-Lindau disease. Ophthalmic Genet. 1995;16(3):79–84.
7. Jilg CA, et al. Growth kinetics in von Hippel-Lindau-associated renal cell carcinoma. Urol Int. 2012;88(1):71–8.
8. Duffey BG, et al. The relationship between renal tumor size and metastases in patients with von Hippel-Lindau disease. J Urol. 2004;172(1):63–5.
9. Latif F, et al. Identification of the von Hippel-Lindau disease tumor suppressor gene. Science (New York, NY). 1993;260(5112):1317–20.
10. Nordstrom-O'Brien M, et al. Genetic analysis of von Hippel-Lindau disease. Hum Mutat. 2010;31(5):521–37.
11. Beroud C, et al. Software and database for the analysis of mutations in the VHL gene. Nucleic Acids Res. 1998;26(1):256–8.
12. Genetics of Kidney Cancer (Renal Cell Cancer) (PDQ(R)): Health Professional Version, in PDQ Cancer Information Summaries. 2002: Bethesda (MD).
13. Metwalli AR, Linehan WM. Nephron-sparing surgery for multifocal and hereditary renal tumors. Curr Opin Urol. 2014;24(5):466–73.
14. Goldfarb DA, et al. Results of renal transplantation in patients with renal cell carcinoma and von Hippel-Lindau disease. Transplantation. 1997;64(12):1726–9.
15. Jonasch E, et al. Pazopanib in patients with von Hippel-Lindau disease: a single-arm, single-Centre, phase 2 trial. Lancet Oncol. 2018;19(10):1351–9.
16. Jonasch E, et al. Pilot trial of sunitinib therapy in patients with von Hippel-Lindau disease. Ann Oncol. 2011;22(12):2661–6.
17. Kim HC, et al. Sunitinib treatment for metastatic renal cell carcinoma in patients with von hippel-Lindau disease. Cancer Res Treat. 2013;45(4):349–53.

18. Eric JF, et al. Belzutifan for Renal Cell Carcinoma in von Hippel–Lindau Disease. N Engl J Med. 2021;385(22):2036–46. https://doi.org/10.1056/NEJMoa2103425.
19. Schmidt LS, et al. Early onset hereditary papillary renal carcinoma: germline missense mutations in the tyrosine kinase domain of the met proto-oncogene. J Urol. 2004;172(4 Pt 1):1256–61.
20. Ornstein DK, et al. Prevalence of microscopic tumors in normal appearing renal parenchyma of patients with hereditary papillary renal cancer. J Urol. 2000;163(2):431–3.
21. Lubensky IA, et al. Hereditary and sporadic papillary renal carcinomas with c-met mutations share a distinct morphological phenotype. Am J Pathol. 1999;155(2):517–26.
22. Zbar B, et al. Hereditary papillary renal cell carcinoma. J Urol. 1994;151(3):561–6.
23. Schmidt L, et al. Germline and somatic mutations in the tyrosine kinase domain of the MET proto-oncogene in papillary renal carcinomas. Nat Genet. 1997;16(1):68–73.
24. Schmidt L, et al. Novel mutations of the MET proto-oncogene in papillary renal carcinomas. Oncogene. 1999;18(14):2343–50.
25. Dharmawardana PG, Giubellino A, Bottaro DP. Hereditary papillary renal carcinoma type I. Curr Mol Med. 2004;4(8):855–68.
26. Organ SL, Tsao MS. An overview of the c-MET signaling pathway. Ther Adv Med Oncol. 2011;3(1 Suppl):S7–S19.
27. Cancer Genome Atlas Research Network, et al. Comprehensive molecular characterization of papillary renal-cell carcinoma. N Engl J Med. 2016;374(2):135–45.
28. Walther MM, et al. Renal cancer in families with hereditary renal cancer: prospective analysis of a tumor size threshold for renal parenchymal sparing surgery. J Urol. 1999;161(5):1475–9.
29. Choueiri TK, et al. Phase II and biomarker study of the dual MET/VEGFR2 inhibitor foretinib in patients with papillary renal cell carcinoma. J Clin Oncol. 2013;31(2):181–6.
30. Schoffski P, et al. Crizotinib in patients with advanced, inoperable inflammatory myofibroblastic tumours with and without anaplastic lymphoma kinase gene alterations (European Organisation for Research and Treatment of Cancer 90101 CREATE): a multicentre, single-drug, prospective, non-randomised phase 2 trial. Lancet Respir Med. 2018;6(6):431–41.
31. Choueiri TK, et al. Biomarker-based phase II trial of Savolitinib in patients with advanced papillary renal cell Cancer. J Clin Oncol. 2017;35(26):2993–3001.
32. Moch H, et al. The 2016 WHO classification of Tumours of the urinary system and male genital organs-part a: renal, penile, and testicular Tumours. Eur Urol. 2016;70(1):93–105.
33. Toro JR, et al. Mutations in the fumarate hydratase gene cause hereditary leiomyomatosis and renal cell cancer in families in North America. Am J Hum Genet. 2003;73(1):95–106.
34. Wei MH, et al. Novel mutations in FH and expansion of the spectrum of phenotypes expressed in families with hereditary leiomyomatosis and renal cell cancer. J Med Genet. 2006;43(1):18–27.
35. Smit DL, et al. Hereditary leiomyomatosis and renal cell cancer in families referred for fumarate hydratase germline mutation analysis. Clin Genet. 2011;79(1):49–59.
36. Schmidt LS, Linehan WM. Hereditary leiomyomatosis and renal cell carcinoma. Int J Nephrol Renovasc Dis. 2014;7:253–60.
37. Ylisaukko-oja SK, et al. Analysis of fumarate hydratase mutations in a population-based series of early onset uterine leiomyosarcoma patients. Int J Cancer. 2006;119(2):283–7.
38. Menko FH, et al. Hereditary leiomyomatosis and renal cell cancer (HLRCC): renal cancer risk, surveillance and treatment. Familial Cancer. 2014;13(4):637–44.
39. Muller M, et al. Reassessing the clinical spectrum associated with hereditary leiomyomatosis and renal cell carcinoma syndrome in French FH mutation carriers. Clin Genet. 2017;92(6):606–15.
40. Grubb RL 3rd, et al. Hereditary leiomyomatosis and renal cell cancer: a syndrome associated with an aggressive form of inherited renal cancer. J Urol. 2007;177(6):2074–9. Discussion 2079–80
41. Alam NA, et al. Localization of a gene (MCUL1) for multiple cutaneous leiomyomata and uterine fibroids to chromosome 1q42.3-q43. Am J Hum Genet. 2001;68(5):1264–9.

42. Tomlinson IP, et al. Germline mutations in FH predispose to dominantly inherited uterine fibroids, skin leiomyomata and papillary renal cell cancer. Nat Genet. 2002;30(4):406–10.
43. Sudarshan S, et al. Fumarate hydratase deficiency in renal cancer induces glycolytic addiction and hypoxia-inducible transcription factor 1alpha stabilization by glucose-dependent generation of reactive oxygen species. Mol Cell Biol. 2009;29(15):4080–90.
44. Linehan WM, Rouault TA. Molecular pathways: fumarate hydratase-deficient kidney cancer--targeting the Warburg effect in cancer. Clin Cancer Res. 2013;19(13):3345–52.
45. Linehan WM, Ricketts CJ. The metabolic basis of kidney cancer. Semin Cancer Biol. 2013;23(1):46–55.
46. Board., P.C.G.E., Genetics of Kidney Cancer (Renal Cell Cancer) (PDQ®): Health Professional Version. 2019.
47. Srinivasan R, Su D, Stamatakis L, Siddiqui MM, Singer E, Shuch B, Nix J, Friend J, Hawks G, Shih J, Choyke P, Linehan WM. Mechanism based targeted therapy for hereditary leiomyomatosis and renal cell cancer (HLRCC) and sporadic papillary renal cell carcinoma: interim results from a phase 2 study of bevacizumab and erlotinib. Eur J Cancer. 2014;50(Supp 6):8.
48. Andrews KA, et al. Tumour risks and genotype-phenotype correlations associated with germline variants in succinate dehydrogenase subunit genes SDHB, SDHC and SDHD. J Med Genet. 2018;55(6):384–94.
49. Pasini B, Stratakis CA. SDH mutations in tumorigenesis and inherited endocrine tumours: lesson from the phaeochromocytoma-paraganglioma syndromes. J Intern Med. 2009;266(1):19–42.
50. Gill AJ, et al. Succinate dehydrogenase (SDH)-deficient renal carcinoma: a morphologically distinct entity: a clinicopathologic series of 36 tumors from 27 patients. Am J Surg Pathol. 2014;38(12):1588–602.
51. Ricketts CJ, et al. Succinate dehydrogenase kidney cancer: an aggressive example of the Warburg effect in cancer. J Urol. 2012;188(6):2063–71.
52. Linehan WM, et al. The metabolic basis of kidney Cancer. Cancer Discov. 2019;9(8):1006–21.
53. Yakirevich E, et al. A novel SDHA-deficient renal cell carcinoma revealed by comprehensive genomic profiling. Am J Surg Pathol. 2015;39(6):858–63.
54. Tufton N, Sahdev A, Akker SA. Radiological surveillance screening in asymptomatic succinate dehydrogenase mutation carriers. J Endocr Soc. 2017;1(7):897–907.
55. Sulkowski PL, et al. Krebs-cycle-deficient hereditary cancer syndromes are defined by defects in homologous-recombination DNA repair. Nat Genet. 2018;50(8):1086–92.
56. Pavlovich CP, et al. Renal tumors in the Birt-Hogg-Dube syndrome. Am J Surg Pathol. 2002;26(12):1542–52.
57. Schmidt LS, Linehan WM. Molecular genetics and clinical features of Birt-Hogg-Dube syndrome. Nat Rev Urol. 2015;12(10):558–69.
58. Toro JR, et al. BHD mutations, clinical and molecular genetic investigations of Birt-Hogg-Dube syndrome: a new series of 50 families and a review of published reports. J Med Genet. 2008;45(6):321–31.
59. Houweling AC, et al. Renal cancer and pneumothorax risk in Birt-Hogg-Dube syndrome; an analysis of 115 FLCN mutation carriers from 35 BHD families. Br J Cancer. 2011;105(12):1912–9.
60. Schmidt LS, et al. Germline BHD-mutation spectrum and phenotype analysis of a large cohort of families with Birt-Hogg-Dube syndrome. Am J Hum Genet. 2005;76(6):1023–33.
61. Nickerson ML, et al. Mutations in a novel gene lead to kidney tumors, lung wall defects, and benign tumors of the hair follicle in patients with the Birt-Hogg-Dube syndrome. Cancer Cell. 2002;2(2):157–64.
62. Lim DH, et al. A new locus-specific database (LSDB) for mutations in the folliculin (FLCN) gene. Hum Mutat. 2010;31(1):E1043–51.
63. Pavlovich CP, et al. Evaluation and management of renal tumors in the Birt-Hogg-Dube syndrome. J Urol. 2005;173(5):1482–6.
64. Popova T, et al. Germline BAP1 mutations predispose to renal cell carcinomas. Am J Hum Genet. 2013;92(6):974–80.

65. Rai K, et al. Comprehensive review of BAP1 tumor predisposition syndrome with report of two new cases. Clin Genet. 2016;89(3):285–94.
66. Carlo MI, et al. Prevalence of germline mutations in Cancer susceptibility genes in patients with advanced renal cell carcinoma. JAMA Oncol. 2018;4(9):1228–35.
67. Ricketts CJ, et al. The Cancer genome atlas comprehensive molecular characterization of renal cell carcinoma. Cell Rep. 2018;23(1):313–326 e5.
68. Jensen DE, et al. BAP1: a novel ubiquitin hydrolase which binds to the BRCA1 RING finger and enhances BRCA1-mediated cell growth suppression. Oncogene. 1998;16(9):1097–112.
69. White AE, Harper JW, Cancer. Emerging anatomy of the BAP1 tumor suppressor system. Science. 2012;337(6101):1463–4.
70. Scheuermann JC, et al. Histone H2A deubiquitinase activity of the Polycomb repressive complex PR-DUB. Nature. 2010;465(7295):243–7.
71. Randle SC. Tuberous sclerosis complex: a review. Pediatr Ann. 2017;46(4):e166–71.
72. Osborne JP, Fryer A, Webb D. Epidemiology of tuberous sclerosis. Ann N Y Acad Sci. 1991;615:125–7.
73. Krueger DA, Northrup H, G. International tuberous sclerosis complex consensus, tuberous sclerosis complex surveillance and management: recommendations of the 2012 international tuberous sclerosis complex consensus conference. Pediatr Neurol. 2013;49(4):255–65.
74. Bissler JJ, et al. Everolimus for renal angiomyolipoma in patients with tuberous sclerosis complex or sporadic lymphangioleiomyomatosis: extension of a randomized controlled trial. Nephrol Dial Transplant. 2016;31(1):111–9.
75. McCormack FX, et al. Efficacy and safety of sirolimus in lymphangioleiomyomatosis. N Engl J Med. 2011;364(17):1595–606.
76. Pilarski R. Cowden syndrome: a critical review of the clinical literature. J Genet Couns. 2009;18(1):13–27.
77. Nelen MR, et al. Localization of the gene for Cowden disease to chromosome 10q22-23. Nat Genet. 1996;13(1):114–6.
78. Orloff MS, et al. Germline PIK3CA and AKT1 mutations in Cowden and Cowden-like syndromes. Am J Hum Genet. 2013;92(1):76–80.
79. Pilarski R, et al. Predicting PTEN mutations: an evaluation of Cowden syndrome and Bannayan-Riley-Ruvalcaba syndrome clinical features. J Med Genet. 2011;48(8):505–12.
80. Mester JL, et al. Papillary renal cell carcinoma is associated with PTEN hamartoma tumor syndrome. Urology. 2012;79(5):1187. e1-7

Imaging in Renal Cancer

Vincenzo Ficarra, Simona Caloggero, Marta Rossanese, Silvio Mazziotti, Giuseppe Mucciardi, Giuseppe Cicero, Giuseppina Anastasi, and Giorgio Ascenti

Introduction

Imaging plays a pivotal role in the detection, characterization, volumetric assessment, staging and evaluation of response to the medical and surgical therapies of renal masses. Moreover, in the last decade, imaging features were also used to assign the nephrometry scores and to predict perioperative outcomes and risk of complications in patient candidates for partial nephrectomy [1, 2].

Abdominal ultrasonography (US), computed tomography (CT) and magnetic resonance imaging (MRI) represent the most common imaging investigations used in the management of parenchymal renal masses.

Abdominal US commonly represents the first step in the radiological framework of renal lesions due to its widespread availability, lack of ionizing radiation and high spatial resolution [3]. Indeed, most of renal tumors are incidentally diagnosed by an abdominal US performed for the suspicious of other medical conditions. Renal ultrasound can distinguish cystic from solid masses, may assist in identifying angiomyolipoma (AML), and can show vascularity with the additional use of ultrasound contrast agents, including microbubbles. The dynamic contrast enhanced ultrasound (CEUS) is performed through the injection of an intravenous contrast agent made of gas microbubbles, considered safe for allergic subjects and patients with renal failure [4–6]. Moreover, a quantitative assessment of the enhancement characteristics can be obtained through the automatic calculation of specific parameters (i.e. intensity curves, time to peak, peak intensity, etc.). Furthermore, US can also be employed

V. Ficarra (✉) · M. Rossanese · G. Mucciardi · G. Anastasi
Department of Human and Pediatric Pathology "Gaetano Barresi", Urologic Section, University of Messina, Messina, Italy
e-mail: vficarra@unime.it

S. Caloggero · S. Mazziotti · G. Cicero · G. Ascenti
Department of Biomedical Sciences and Morphological and Functional Imaging, Section of Radiological Sciences, University of Messina, Messina, Italy

C. Anderson, M. Afshar (eds.), *Renal Cancer*,
https://doi.org/10.1007/978-3-030-84756-2_4

as a useful guide for renal masses biopsy [7]. Because it is both less accurate than CT or MRI and user-dependent, US has a limited role in preoperative surgical planning.

Abdominal contrast enhanced computed tomography (CECT) is the reference standard for primary imaging and staging of renal masses [8]. Multiphasic protocol, including non-contrast (basal), corticomedullary (CM), nephrographic (NG) and urographic phases, is recommended for a correct renal masses assessment. Low accuracy on thin septa appraisal, frequent unclear differentiation among solid masses, radiation exposure and the nephrotoxic contrast media used are considered its main limitations [3, 6, 9].

More recent techniques, such as Dual-Energy CT (DECT), which is based on two simultaneous acquisitions at different energy levels, and perfusion contrast-enhanced CT (pCECT), consisting in fast scan repetition after contrast medium administration, can be associated with a significant reduction of radiation exposure by approximately 50% [10]. If iodine is removed from the postcontrast image, a virtual non-contrast image is acquired. For characterization of renal masses, DECT has similar accuracy to conventional two-phase CT examinations with a true non-contrast phase [11]. Although initial data are convincing, DECT technology is not yet broadly available and further data are required.

The lack of ionizing radiations and the high soft tissue contrast make abdominal MRI a suitable technique when US or CT findings are not conclusive [12]. Moreover, MRI is strongly recommended in patients who are allergic to intravenous CT contrast medium and in pregnancy without renal failure [8]. Its high soft tissue contrast resolution allows to detect fat or hemorrhagic components and to emphasize contrast-enhancement. Diffusion-weighted imaging (DWI), with related ADC (apparent diffusion coefficient) values, is a particular sequence based on the random "Brownian" motion of extracellular water molecules, and its performance lead to the assessment of cellular density. Highly cellular tissues, such as malignancies, demonstrate lower diffusion coefficients. Vascular supply of renal lesions can be appreciated after the intravenous administration of Gadolinium or through unenhanced acquisitions obtained with arterial spin labelling (ASP), a technique that exploits inflow blood as an endogenous contrast agent [13]. However, the main limitations of MRI include low sensitivity for calcium deposits, lower scanner availability, high healthcare costs and general contraindications to MR (i.e. metal implants, pacemakers, etc.) [6].

Other investigations such as renal arteriography and inferior vena cavography have a limited role in the management of renal masses and can be considered also in very selected cases. Positron-emission tomography (PET) is still not recommended by the international guidelines in the work-up of parenchymal renal tumors.

Detection and Characterization

On the basis of their morphological and structural features, lesions affecting the kidneys are generally distinguished into cystic or solid.

Cystic Renal Lesions

Bosniak classification is the most widely used and accepted system to distinguish renal cysts on the basis of the imaging findings [14, 15]. This classification is able to predict the different risk of malignancy and each category is associated with a well-defined treatment modality (Table 1). According to the Bosniak classification the risk of malignancy for complex renal cyst lesions is 2–3% for category I; 6–11% for category II; 7–27% for category IIF, 54-55% for category III and 88-91% for category IV [16, 17]. Therefore, categories I and II are considered benign lesions, category 2F required a follow-up. These lesions can be followed performing an abdominal CT scan after 6 months. In absence of any sign of progression, patients can be further followed using abdominal ultrasound examination every 6 months and abdominal CT scan every 2 years for a minimum follow-up period of 5 years [18]. Categories III and IV cystic lesions require standard surgical treatment, according to RCC guidelines [8].

Although initially based on CT findings, the use of Bosniak classification was extended to other imaging modalities, such as CEUS and MRI [19].

CT-scan performed after injection of intravenous contrast agent is considered a landmark in the diagnostic evaluation of cystic renal lesions. However, a current problem on CT-scan is represented by pseudo-enhancement, an artificial attenuation increase (10–20 HU) of a simple cyst on contrast-enhanced images caused by beam-hardening artifact and partial volume average from the surrounding parenchyma, mimicking an enhancing solid mass. This phenomenon results to be more evident for small size (<10 mm) and centrally displaced cysts. DECT, through iodine overlay maps, virtual non-contrast (VNC) and low-energy virtual monoenergetic images (VMI) reconstructions, has demonstrated capability in overcoming this artifact and in highlighting the real contrast enhancement [20, 21].

The high contrast resolution of US and the dynamic enhancement evaluation of CEUS provide detailed information about number and thickness of septa, solid components and the related contrast distribution.

Several studies revealed at least the same accuracy of CT and higher sensitivity and specificity than MRI in differentiating complex renal cysts and malignancies [6, 19, 22].

On the other hand, MRI takes advantage from a more accurate distinction between fluid from solid components that can lead to discrepancies with CT-scan in Bosniak classification of renal cysts. DWI and contrast-enhanced images, obtained with multiphasic or dynamic protocol, can respectively provide further information in terms of cellular density and vascularization [15].

The lack of ionizing radiation makes MRI more suitable in case of long-term follow-up patients [19, 23]. Notably, it is important to keep in mind that also hypovascular or necrotic solid renal masses fall within the differential diagnosis of cystic lesions [3].

The sequential use of CEUS, CT and MRI can be needed to better define the characteristics of cystic lesions and specifically to identify categories III-IV, candidate for surgical treatment. Figure 1 shows the evolution of a category IIF renal cyst in a category III after a follow-up of 24 months (Fig. 1).

Table 1 Work-up of renal cystic lesions classified according to Bosniak classification

Categories	Bosniak [a,b]	Proposed Bosniak Classification, Version 2019[c]	Outcome and Work-up
I	Simple benign cyst with a hairline-thin wall without septa, calcification, or solid components. Same density as water and does not enhance with contrast medium	**CT-scan**: Well-defined, thin (≤2 mm) smooth wall; homogeneous simple fluid (29 to 20 HU); no septa or calcifications; the wall may enhance **MRI**: Well-defined, thin (≤2 mm) smooth wall; homogeneous simple fluid (signal intensity similar to CSF); no septa or calcifications; the wall may enhance	Benign. No follow-up needed.
II	Cyst that may contain a few hairline-thin septa with or without perceived (not measurable) enhancement. Fine calcification may be present in the wall or septa. Uniformly high-attenuation lesions <3 cm in size, with sharp margins without enhancement.	**CT-scan**: • Cystic masses with thin (≤2 mm) and few (1–3) septa; septa and wall may enhance; may have calcification of any type. • Homogeneous hyperattenuating (≥ 70 HU) masses at noncontrast CT. • Homogeneous nonenhancing masses >20 HU at renal mass protocol CT, may have calcification of any type • Homogeneous masses −9 to 20 HU at noncontrast CT. • Homogeneous masses 21 to 30 HU at portal venous phase CT. • Homogeneous low-attenuation masses that are too small to characterize **MRI**: • Cystic masses with thin (≤2 mm) and few (1–3) enhancing septa; any nonenhancing septa; may have calcification of any type. • Homogeneous masses markedly hyperintense at T2-weighted imaging (similar to CSF) at noncontrast MRI. • Homogeneous masses markedly hyperintense at T1-weighted imaging (approximately x2.5 normal parenchymal signal intensity) at noncontrast MRI	Benign. No follow-up needed.

(continued)

Table 1 (continued)

Categories	Bosniak [a,b]	Proposed Bosniak Classification, Version 2019[c]	Outcome and Work-up
IIF	Cysts contain more hairline-thin septa. Minimal thickening and enhancement (perceived, not measurable) enhancement) of septa or wall: Minimal thickening of the septa or wall. The cyst may contain calcification, which may be nodular and thick, with no contrast enhancement. No enhancing soft-tissu elements. This category also includes totally intra-renal, non-enhancing, high attenuation renal lesions ≥3 cm. Generally well-marginated	**CT-scan**: Cystic masses with a smooth minimally thickened (3 mm) enhancing wall, or smooth minimal thickening (3 mm) of one or more enhancing septa, or many (≥4) smooth thin (≤2 mm) enhancing septa **MRI**: Cystic masses with a smooth minimally thickened (3 mm) enhancing wall, or smooth minimal thickening (3 mm) of one or more enhancing septa, or many (>4) smooth thin (≤2 mm) enhancing septa. Cystic masses that are heterogeneously hyperintense at unenhanced fat-saturated T1-weighted imaging	Generally benign. Follow-up including abdominal ultrasound and/or computed tomography.
III	These are indeterminate cystic masses with thickened irregular walls or septa with measurable enhancement	**CT-scan:** One or more enhancing thick (≥4 mm width) or enhancing irregular (displaying ≤3-mm obtusely margined convex protrusion[s]) walls or septa **MRI:** One or more enhancing thick (≥4 mm width) or enhancing irregular (displaying ≤3-mm obtusely margined convex protrusion[s]) walls or septa	Intermediate probability of Malignancy. Surgery or active surveillance according to treatment of solid tumors
IV	Clearly malignant containing soft-tissue components with measurable enhancement.	**CT-scan:** One or more enhancing nodule(s) (≥4-mm convex protrusion with obtuse margins, or a convex protrusion of any size that has acute margins) **MRI:** One or more enhancing nodule(s) (≥4-mm convex protrusion with obtuse margins, or a convex protrusion of any size that has acute margins)	Mainly malignant. Surgery according to treatment of solid tumors

[a]Silverman SG, Israel GM, Herts BR, Richie JP. Management of the incidental renal mass. Radiology. 2008;249(1):16-31
[b]Bosniak MA. The Bosniak renal cyst classification: 25 years later. Radiology 2012;262(3):781–785
[c]Silverman SG, et al. Bosniak Classification of Cystic Renal Masses, Version 2019: An Update Proposal and Needs Assessment. Radiology. 2019 Aug;292(2):475-488. doi: https://doi.org/10.1148/radiol.2019182646. Epub 2019 Jun 18

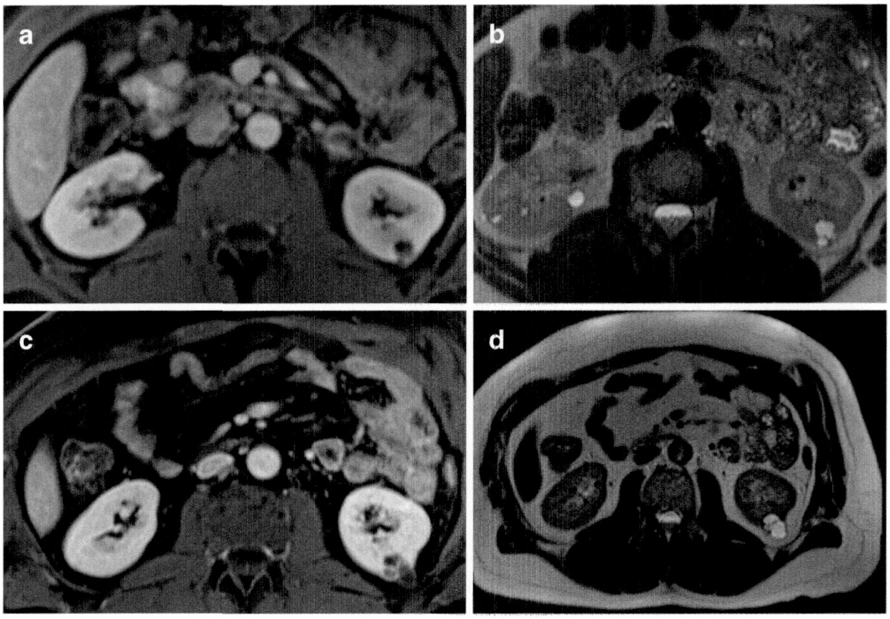

Fig. 1 Axial GE T1-weighted fat-suppressed (**a**) and axial TSE T2-w (**b**) images showing a well-circumscribed cystic lesion with thin septa located in the left kidney, consistent with Bosniak IIF lesion. The same acquisitions (**c**, **d**), obtained 1 year later, showed an increase of lesion size and number of septa, now configuring a Bosniak type III cyst

Solid Renal Masses

Parenchymal renal masses include a wide spectrum of different histopathological entities recently described in the 2016 World Health Organization (WHO) classification [24]. The most common benign histologic subtypes are represented by angiomyolipoma (AML) and oncocytoma. The three most frequent malignant renal tumors are represented by clear cell renal cell carcinoma (ccRCC), papillary renal cell carcinoma (pRCC) and chromophobe renal cell carcinoma (chRCC). However, very aggressive histologic subtypes such as renal medullary carcinoma, collecting duct carcinoma and renal carcinoma associated with Xp11.2 translocations/TFE3 gene fusions, can represent the remaining 10% of parenchyma renal tumors [25].

Although the correct characterization of malignant histologic subtypes remains a controversial issue, CT and MRI features should be considered by urologists mainly to differentiate tumor with more favorable histologic subtypes (oncocytoma and chRCC) from those with unfavorable prognosis (high-grade RCC, type 2 papillary RCC, collecting duct and medullary carcinomas).

The only ultrasound assessment does not allow a clear distinction among different solid renal lesions. Although, AML can be strongly suspected during US examination, a large amount of hyperechoic masses cannot be appropriately distinguished from other malignant masses [26]. Vascular supply information related to angiogenesis phenomenon can be provided by color-Doppler US and CEUS. While the former can solely show intralesional blood flow signals, CEUS provide a dynamic appraisal of contrast medium distribution and quantification of the related parameters. CEUS has demonstrated high degree of accuracy in tumor detection and correct identification of "pseudolesions" (i.e. prominent columns of Bertin, persistent fetal lobulation, or dromedary hump), showing a strong correlation with CT and MRI [9, 27, 28]. Features suspicious for a malignant behavior are heterogeneous enhancement, presence of pseudocapsule, and perilesional rim-like enhancement as well as hemorrhagic, necrotic, and cystic foci in large masses [27, 29–31].

The enhancement evaluation during the multiphase, abdominal CECT is essential for the characterization of parenchymal renal masses. An enhancement of >15–20 Hounsfield Units (HU) is considered the most important indicator of malignancy. The CM phase is used to assess the arterial system (number of renal arteries, feeding mass arteries) and the urographic phase to assess proximity to and involvement of the renal collecting system. Three-dimensional CT reconstruction depicts the vascular and renal mass anatomy in a format familiar to surgeons and serves to guide PN surgery, especially in complex cases.

Macroscopic fat (less than −20 HU) can generally be observed on CT scans of AMLs, so these can be differentiated from other renal tumors. Notably, the fat content may be difficult to diagnose in small AMLs because of the volume averaging effect and a proportion of AMLs are fat-poor. Oncocytomas are typically hypervascular and homogeneous and may have a characteristic central stellate scar; however, CT features cannot reliably distinguish an oncocytoma from other renal tumors. The ccRCCs usually show an early peak, higher than the renal cortex, while pRCCs commonly exhibit a delayed and lower enhancement. On the other hand, chRCCs is usually characterized by intermediate enhancement patterns [32, 33].

CT-scan is provided with a great sensitivity in detecting solid renal lesions (>90% if larger than 2 cm) [3, 13]. Owing to their pronounced vascularization, ccRCCs usually show high enhancement during the corticomedullary phase and rapid wash-out on the nephrogenic one (Fig. 2). Backwards, pCCRs are characterized by a subtle enhancement that can be absent in up to 25%. Both the two sub-types, especially when of large dimensions, can show an inhomogeneous appearance due to degenerative phenomenon [9, 13]. Considering the different energy level acquisitions, DECT can rely on post-processing algorithms, such as virtual monoenergetic images (VMI) and iodine overlay map, helpful in depicting and quantifying the real iodine content (Fig. 3) [34–36]. Although several attempts have been made for correlating iodine content and histological subtypes of RCCs, a univocal iodine density cut-off has not been yet established mainly due to the differences existing among scanners of different vendors [37]. Limits of DECT are a drop of sensitivity for lesions smaller than 1.5 cm and an underestimation of calcifications on Virtual non-contrast reconstructions [38]. As regard the histologic subtype correlation and the post-therapy assessment, also perfusion-CT parameters, such as blood flow (BF), blood volume (BV), mean transit time (MTT) and permeability (PMB), have been evaluated [10, 39, 40].

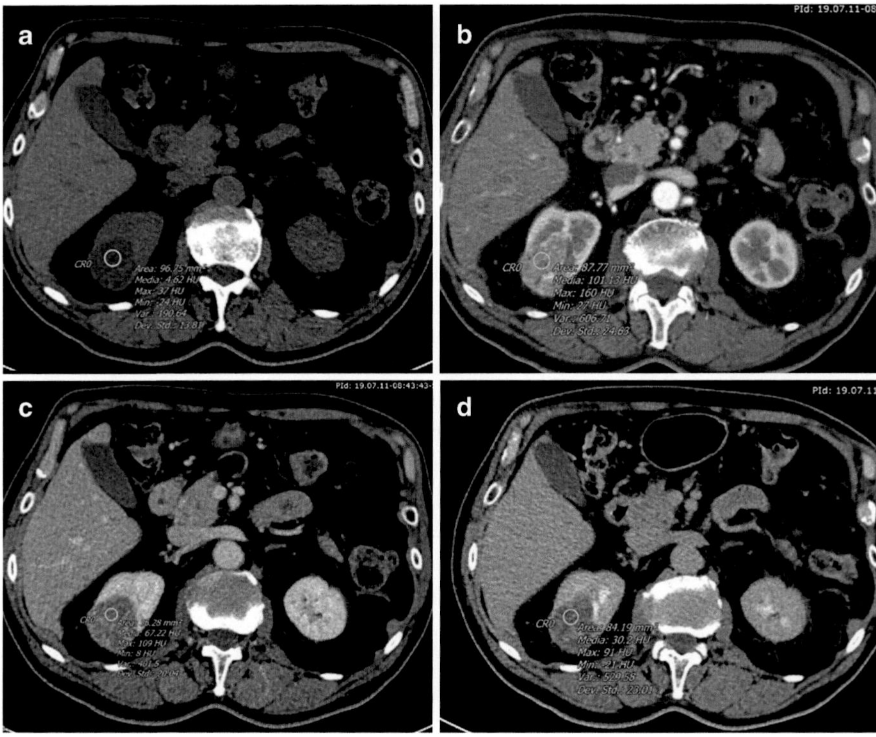

Fig. 2 Axial CT-scans obtained before (**a**) and after intravenous contrast medium injection (corticomedullary phase, **b**; nephrographic phase, **c**; excretory phase, **d**). The ovalar-shaped endophitic right renal mass is characterized by low HU values at non-enhanced CT with strong and inhomogeneous enhancement during the corticomedullary phase. Gradual and slow contrast-enhancement wash-out is detectable in the following acquisition phases. The lesion was consistent with cc-RCC

Magnetic resonance imaging (MRI) is an alternative imaging procedure and is commonly used as a problem solving tool in patients with indeterminate CT scans (eg, for complex cystic lesions, very small masses, enhancement of 10–20 HU) or contrast medium allergies. The ccRCCs are usually characterized by signal intensity similar to the adjacent renal parenchyma on T1-weighted sequences and higher on T2 images, with inhomogeneous areas in large lesions. In a significant percentage (60%) of ccRCCs a share of intracytoplasmic fat that can be detected as a drop of signal in out-of-phase T1-weighted chemical-shift sequences. Due to their hypervascularity, greater contrast enhancement, especially on corticomedullary phase, can be appreciated.

In contrast, pRCC are usually detected as hypointense masses on T2-weighted scans, with much lower and delayed enhancement than ccRCCs. Compared to the two previous types, chRCC has intermediate signal intensity characteristics on T2-weighted as well as on contrast-enhanced acquisitions [9, 39, 41, 42]. Vascularization patterns have been also confirmed by perfusion MRI and non-contrast-enhanced ASP technique [9, 13, 43]. DWI and related ADC map can be helpful in providing information about cellular density, although a clear correlation

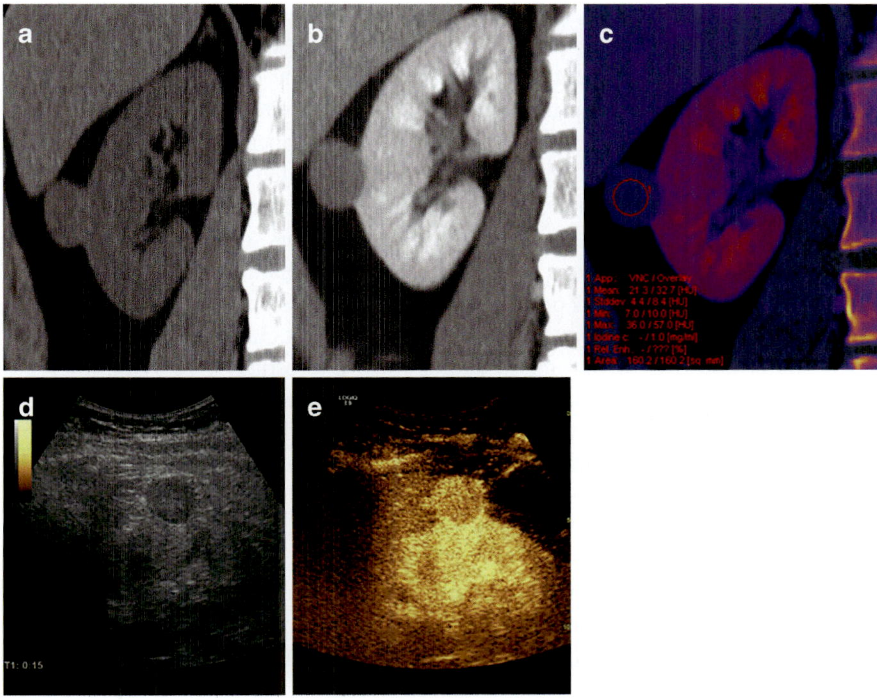

Fig. 3 Coronal CT image before (**a**) and after (**b**) contrast medium administration showed a 2 cm well-circumscribed exophitic right kidney mass with uncertain enhancement (HU values: unenhenced scan 21; nephrographic 39). This features could represent both cystic or solid mass. Coronal DECT color-coded iodine overlay image (**c**) showed iodine content (1 mgI/ml on ROI), thus demonstrating a hypo-vascularized lesion. Gray-scale US image (**d**) demonstrates a solid hypoechoic mass and CEUS (**e**) clearly shows a mild and homogeneous enhancement. The final diagnosis was a p-RCC

with histologic findings has not been achieved so far. In fact, while higher ADC values have been reported in oncocytomas rather than malignant lesions and in pCCR rather than ccRCC, a wide overlap is still observed between benign and malignant lesions [9, 13, 44, 45].

Anatomic and Topographic Features

The European Association of Urology (EAU) guidelines on renal cell carcinoma (RCC) suggest the use of nephrometry systems to predict objectively the potential morbidity of nephron-sparing surgery and tumor ablation techniques for renal masses [8]. These tools provide important information for treatment planning, patient counseling and comparison between different partial nephrectomy (PN) and ablative technique series [8].

RENAL nephrometry and PADUA classification were proposed in 2009 and widely used thereafter [1, 2]. Several studies externally validated both systems as predictors of overall complications, warm ischemia time (WIT), estimated blood loss (EBL) and renal function impairment [46]. Tumor size, exophytic/endophytic rate, medial/lateral location, polar location, distance to upper collecting system and/or renal sinus represent the imaging parameters included in the first-generation nephrometry systems. Moreover, tumors are classified according to axial plan location in anterior or posterior [1, 2]. Although in the last years some second-generation nephrometry systems have been proposed such as the Diameter-axial-polar (DAP) nephrometry systems, the Zonal Nephro scoring system, the Arterial Based Complexity (ABC) scoring system, RENAL and PADUA classifications are still the most popular and used nephrometry scores [46]. Interestingly, 10 years after the publication of the original PADUA classification, Ficarra et al. proposed an update and simplified version (Simplified PAdua REnal—SPARE) including only 4 parameters: tumor size, rime location, exophytic/endophytic rate and renal sinus involvement [47]. Table 2 summarizes the imaging features included in the first-generation nephrometry systems (Table 2). Figure 4 shows the features included in the SPARE system [47] (Fig. 4).

Other important parameters for surgery planning can be characterized by the description of renal arteries and perirenal fat tissue. In approximately 75% of cases a single artery arises bilaterally from the abdominal aorta. To plan adequately surgery, duplication of renal arteries or accessory renal arteries must be appropriately described. Interestingly, CT scan reconstruction should show appropriately the relationship between the arterial vascularization and renal mass. The description and

Table 2 First-generation of nephrometry systems: RENAL nephrometry [1], PADUA classification [2]

	R.E.N.A.L. Nephrometry Score	PADUA score
Variables included		
Tumor size (cm)	≤4, 4-7, >7	≤4, 4-7, >7
Exophytic rate (%)	≥50%, <50%, endophytic	≥50%, <50%, endophytic
Polar location	Superior vs inferior vs middle	Superior/inferior vs middle
Medial/lateral location	Not evaluated	Lateral vs medial
Anterior/posterior location	Included (a/p)	Included (a/p)
Renal sinus involvement	≥7 mm, 4-7 mm, <4 mm	Not involved vs involved
Collecting system involvement		Not involved vs dislocated/infiltrated

Table 2 (continued)

	R.E.N.A.L. Nephrometry Score	PADUA score
Definition of anatomical landmarks		
Anterior/ posterior face (D)	"This plane is best assessed on axial imaging by drawing a line paralleling the direction of hilar structures that bisects the renal parenchyma as shown in Fig. 3, B and C.14 the letter a is ascribed to tumors that lie primarily anterior to this axial midline while the letter p designates those in a more posterior location. When the mass grows from the tips of the renal poles or arises from the kidney so that a meaningful anterior or posterior designation is not possible (eg transverses the kidney or lies directly on the coronal plane), the suffix x is assigned to the tumor."	Anterior or posterior faces of the kidney were defined as those covered by the anterior or posterior layers of the renal fascia, respectively
Polar location (D)	Polar line d defined as the portion of the kidney where the concentric rim of the renal parenchyma is interrupted by the renal hilar vessels, pelvis, or fat on axial imaging	The upper part of the kidney (upper pole) extends from the upper extremity to the first CT image in which the renal hypodense sinus appears (upper sinus line). The middle part of the kidney (middle pole) corresponds to the extent of the renal sinus. The lower part of the kidney (inferior pole) extends from the first CT image in which the renal hypodense sinus disappears (inferior sinus line) to the lower extremity
Renal sinus (D)	Not defined	The spacious cavity surrounded by the kidney parenchyma, lined by the renal capsule, and almost filled by the renal pelvis and vessels, with the remaining space being filled by fat [Standring S, Borley NR, Collins P, et al., eds. Gray's anatomy. 40th ed.Spain: Churchill Livingstone; 2008. p. 1225–9]. On CT images the low attenuation fat outlines the collecting system and the blood vessels and differentiates the renal sinus from the parenchyma [Lockhart ME, Smith JK, Kenney PJ. The kidney and ureter. In: Lee JKT, Sagel SS, Stanley RJ, Heiken JP, eds. Computed body tomography with MRI correlation. Fourth ed. New York, NY: Lippincott William &Wilkins; 2005. p. 1234].
Subgroup stratification	4-6 vs 7-9 vs 10-12 (no criteria specified)	6-7 vs 8-9 vs $\geq$10 based on multivariate analysis

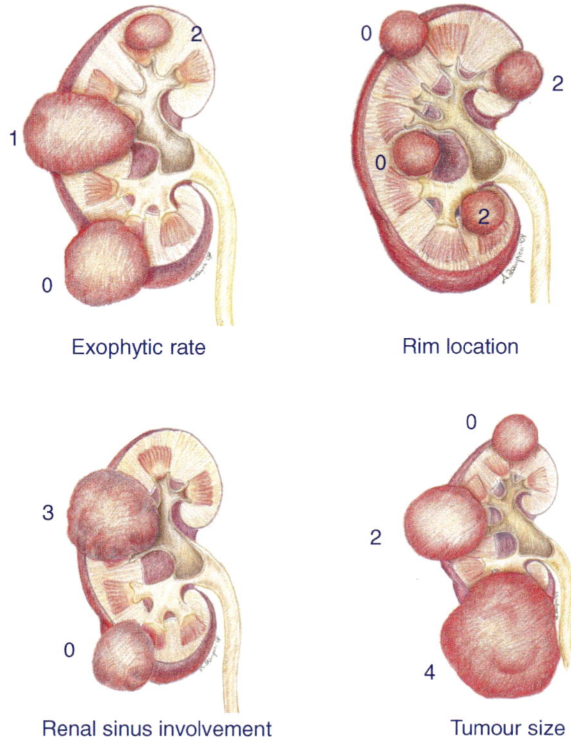

Fig. 4 The figure shows the 4 parameters included in the Simplified Padua Renal (SPARE) nephrometry system. Exophyitic rate distinguish three categories: (**a**) ≥ 50% (score 0); (**b**) <50% (score 1) and (**c**) entirely endophytic (score 2). Rim location: (**a**) lateral (score 0); medial (score 2). Renal sinus involvement: (**a**) absent (score 0); (**b**) present (score 3). Tumor size: (**a**) ≤ 4 cm (score 0); (**b**) 4.1-7 cm (score 2) and (**c**) > 4 cm (score 3)

visualization of the segmental arteries is really important in the planning of selective clamping technique when a partial nephrectomy is scheduled (Fig. 5).

Interestingly, in 2014 Davidiuk et al. proposed the Mayo Adhesive Probability (MAP) Score, an accurate image-based scoring system to predict the adherent perirenal fat tissue in patients suitable for partial nephrectomy [48]. The score was based on lateral and posterior perirenal fat thickness measured at level of the renal veins and on grading of the perinephric stranding.

Staging

The use of multi-phasic contrast-enhanced CT of abdomen and chest is strongly recommended for the staging of suspicious malignant renal tumors. MRI should be considered in patients in whom the use of intravenous CT contrast medium

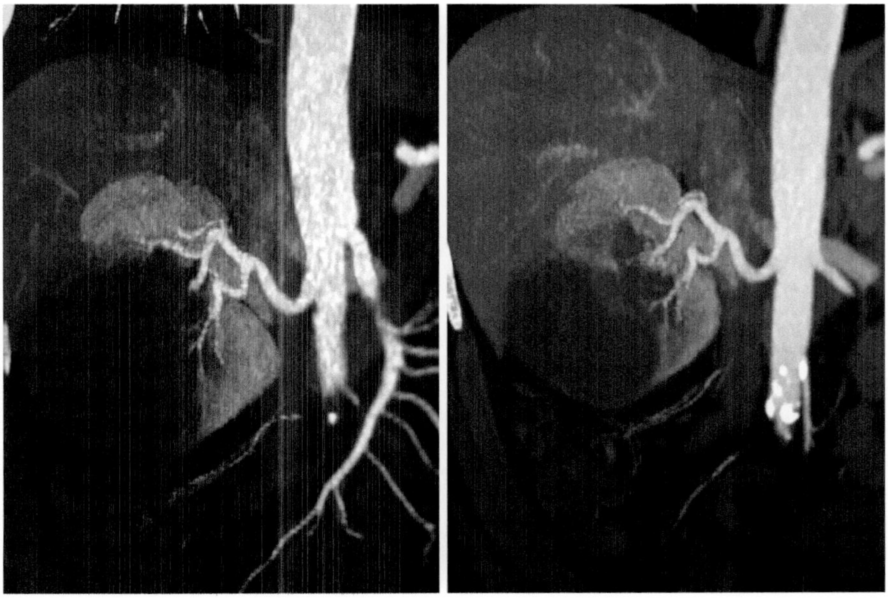

Fig. 5 Coronal CT-scan Maximum Intensity Projection (MIP) reconstructions obtained during corticomedullary phase. The figure shows the relationship between the renal mass and arterial vascolature of the kidney. Main renal artery and segmental arteries are well visible

should be avoided. Moreover, bone scan and/or PET are not routinely indicated for staging of renal tumors. The bone scan as well as brain CT or MRI should be considered only in presence of specific clinical or laboratory signs or symptoms suggestive of metastases. Table 3 summarizes the 2017 TNM classification system (Table 3).

Current Nuances

Three-dimensional (HA3D) reconstruction of the anatomical structures from CT-scan images represents an interesting new tool to plan surgical treatment. The process consisted of the rendering of a 3D virtual model of the affected kidney, on the basis of high-resolution CT scans. It was focused on the renal vasculature (both arterial and venous), collecting system, kidney shape, and tumor characteristics. The 3D images allow us to reconstruct the renal pedicle, the extra- and the intrarenal arteries with the possibility to see the segmental arteries and their relationship with the renal tumor (Fig. 6).

"Radiomics" is a recently developed technology that involves imaging modalities. This technique is based on the principle that radiological images obtained with CT-scan, MRI or PET are primarily numerical data and its aim is to elaborate and

Table 3 2017 TNM classification of parenchymal renal tumors

T- Primary tumor	
T1 – T1a – T1b	Tumor ≤7 cm limited to the kidney Tumor ≤4 cm Tumor 4.1–7 cm
T2 – T2a – T2b	Tumor >7 cm, limited to the kidney Tumor 7.1–10 cm Tumor >10 cm
T3 – T3a – T3b – T3c	Tumor extends into major veins or perinephric tissues but not into the ipsilateral adrenal gland and not beyond Gerota fascia Tumor grossly extends into renal vein or its segmental branches, or tumor invades perirenal and/or renal sinus fat, but not beyond Gerota fascia Tumor grossly extends into vena cava below diaphragm Tumor grossly extends into vena cava above the diaphragm or invades the wall of the vena cava
T4	Tumor invades beyond Gerota fascia (including contiguous extension into the ipsilateral adrenal fland)
N—Regional lymph nodes	
Nx	Regional lymph nodes cannot be assessed
N0	No regional lymph node metastasis
N1	Metastasis in regional lymph nodes
M—Distant metastasis	
M0	No distant metastasis
M1	Distant metastasis

correlate these quantitative raw datasets with external information, such as genomic patterns. In this specific case, it can also take the name of "radiogenomics".

The technique requires some mandatory steps. The first one include the acquisition of the images, which need the performance of strictly standardized protocol within the same imaging modality, in order to avoid bias or confounders for the following analysis.

The second is the identification of a body volume of interest and a sharp segmentation, which can be manually or automatically performed. At this point, the data achieved can be extracted and correlated to histopathologic findings. Once that a certain correlation is clearly established, artificial intelligence, machine algorithms, or statistical methods can extend the analysis on a large scale data [49, 50].

Oncology is naturally the main field of application of this technology and tumor renal lesions have been evaluated as well.

Encouraging results have been pointed out on CT-scan and MR images analysis in terms of benign vs malignant distinction and grade differentiation within the same tumor sub-type [51–54].

Nevertheless, this technology has also the potential to offer important information about quantitative assessment of treatment response [50].

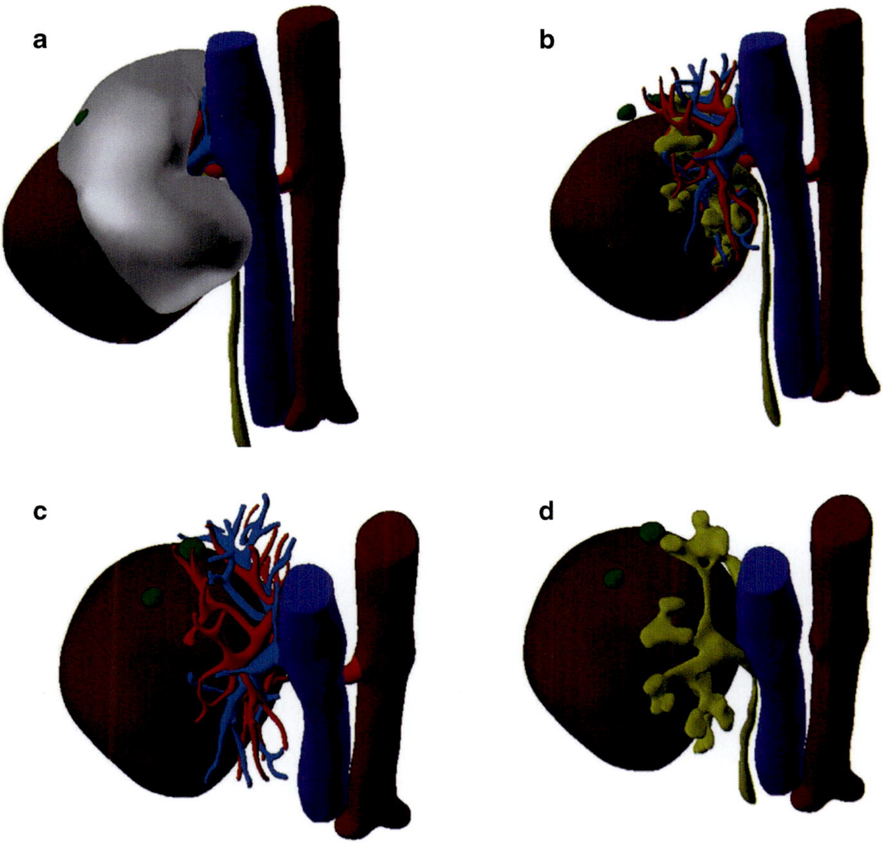

Fig. 6 Three-dimensional (HA3D) reconstruction of the right kidney and parenchymal renal tumor from CT-scan images (**a**). 3D model after removal of healthy renal parenchyma (**b**). 3D model focusing the relationship between the renal tumor and renal vasculature (both arterial and venous) (**c**). 3D model focusing the relationship between the renal mass and the upper collecting system (**d**)

Key Points

1. US is generally performed for preliminary characterization of renal lesions (fluid or solid) content.
2. CEUS is a more sensitive technique in the enhancement assessment, particularly useful for complex cysts and pRCC appraisal.
3. Contrast-enhanced CT-scan is currently the gold standard imaging, owing to its wide availability, spatial and contrast resolution, and the number of renal and extra-renal information useful in cancer staging.
4. DECT can distinguish different molecules with similar density, thus allowing material decomposition and iodine quantification.

5. MRI is a multiparametric imaging modality that allow providing internal content, cellular density and contrast enhancement information about renal lesions.
6. Vascular patterns can guide in the radiological diagnosis and can be assessed through US, CT or MRI performing multiphasic or dynamic protocols.
7. Radiomics is a promising technology that allow quantitative analysis of CT-scan, MRI and PET data and correlation with histological information.

References

1. Kutikov A, Uzzo RG. The R.E.N.a.L. nephrometry score: a comprehensive standardized system for quantitating renal tumor size, location and depth. J Urol. 2009;182:844–53.
2. Ficarra V, Novara G, Secco S, et al. Preoperative aspects and dimensions used for an anatomical (PADUA) classification of renal tumours in patients who are candidates for nephron-sparing surgery. Eur Urol. 2009;56:786–93.
3. Hindman NM. Imaging of cystic renal masses. Radiol Clin N Am. 2017 Mar;55(2):259–77.
4. Ascenti G, Mazziotti S, Zimbaro G, Settineri N, Magno C, Melloni D, Caruso R, Scribano E. Complex cystic renal masses: characterization with contrast-enhanced US. Radiology. 2007 Apr;243(1):158–65.
5. Albrecht T, Blomley M, Bolondi L, et al. Guidelines for the use of contrast agents in ultrasound: January 2004. Ultraschall Med. 2004;25:249–56.
6. Rossi SH, Prezzi D, Kelly-Morland C, Goh V. Imaging for the diagnosis and response assessment of renal tumours. World J Urol. 2018;36(12):1927–42. https://doi.org/10.1007/s00345-018-2342-3.
7. Sutherland EL, Choromanska A, Al-Katib S, Coffey M. Outcomes of ultrasound guided renal mass biopsies. J Ultrasound. 2018;21(2):99–104. https://doi.org/10.1007/s40477-018-0299-0.
8. Ljungberg B, Albiges L, Abu-Ghanem Y, et al. European Association of Urology guidelines on renal cell carcinoma: the 2019 update. Eur Urol. 2019;75:799–810.
9. van Oostenbrugge TJ, Fütterer JJ, Mulders PFA. Diagnostic imaging for solid renal tumors: a pictorial review. Kidney Cancer. 2018 Aug 1;2(2):79–93.
10. Das CJ, Thingujam U, Panda A, Sharma S, Gupta AK. Perfusion computed tomography in renal cell carcinoma. World J Radiol. 2015 Jul 28;7(7):170–9. https://doi.org/10.4329/wjr.v7.i7.170.
11. Chandarana H, Megibow AJ, Cohen BA, et al. Iodine quantification with dual-energy CT: phantom study and preliminary experience with renal masses. Am J Roentgenol. 2011;196:693–700.
12. Kwon T, Jeong IG, Yoo S, Lee J, Hong S, You D, Hong JH, Ahn H, Kim CS. Role of MRI in indeterminate renal mass: diagnostic accuracy and impact on clinical decision making. Int Urol Nephrol. 2015 Apr;47(4):585–93.
13. Kay FU, Pedrosa I. Imaging of solid renal masses. Radiol Clin N Am. 2017 Mar;55(2):243–58.
14. Bosniak MA. The current radiological approach to renal cysts. Radiology. 1986;158(1):1–10.
15. Bosniak MA. The Bosniak renal cyst classification: 25 years later. Radiology. 2012 Mar;262(3):781–5.
16. Richard PO, Violette PD, Jewett MA, et al. CUA guideline on the management of cystic renal lesions. Can Urol Assoc J. 2017;11:E66–73.
17. Sevcenco S, Spick C, Helbich TH, et al. Malignancy rates and diagnostic performance of the Bosniak classification for the diagnosis of cystic renal lesions in computed tomography–a systematic review and meta-analysis. Eur Radiol. 2017;27:2239–47.

18. Weibl P, Hora M, Kollarik B, et al. Management, pathology and outcomes of Bosniak category IIF and III cystic renal lesions. World J Urol. 2015;33:295–300.
19. Graumann O, Osther SS, Karstoft J, Hørlyck A, Osther PJ. Bosniak classification system: a prospective comparison of CT, contrast-enhanced US, and MR for categorizing complex renal cystic masses. Acta Radiol. 2016 Nov;57(11):1409–17.
20. Tappouni R, Kissane J, Sarwani N, Lehman EB. Pseudoenhancement of renal cysts: influence of lesion size, lesion location, slice thickness, and number of MDCT detectors. Am J Roentgenol. 2012;198(1):133–7.
21. Song KD, Kim CK, Park BK, Kim B. Utility of iodine overlay technique and virtual unenhanced images for the characterization of renal masses by dual-energy CT. Am J Roentgenol. 2011;197:6.
22. Xue LY, Lu Q, Huang BJ, Ma JJ, Yan LX, Wen JX, Wang WP. Contrast-enhanced ultrasonography for evaluation of cystic renal mass: in comparison to contrast-enhanced CT and conventional ultrasound. Abdom Imaging. 2014 Dec;39(6):1274–83.
23. Ferreira AM, Reis RB, Kajiwara PP, Silva GE, Elias J Jr, Muglia VF. MRI evaluation of complex renal cysts using the Bosniak classification: a comparison to CT. Abdom Radiol (NY). 2016 Oct;41(10):2011–9.
24. Moch H, Cubilla AL, Humphrey PA, et al. The 2016 WHO classification of tumours of the urinary system and male genital organs. Part a: renal, penile and testicular tumors. Eur Urol. 2016;70:93–105.
25. Ficarra V, Brunelli M, Cheng L, et al. Prognostic and therapeutic impact of the histopathologic definition of parenchymal epithelial renal tumors. Eur Urol. 2010;58:655–68.
26. Jinzaki M, Silverman SG, Akita H, Nagashima Y, Mikami S, Oya M. Renal angiomyolipoma: a radiological classification and update on recent developments in diagnosis and management. Abdom Imaging. 2014;39(3):588–604.
27. Ignee A, Straub B, Schuessler G, Dietrich CF. Contrast enhanced ultrasound of renal masses. World J Radiol. 2010 Jan 28;2(1):15–31.
28. Mazziotti S, Zimbaro F, Pandolfo A, Racchiusa S, Settineri N, Ascenti G. Usefulness of contrast-enhanced ultrasonography in the diagnosis of renal pseudotumors. Abdom Imaging. 2010 Apr;35(2):241–5.
29. Oh TH, Lee YH, Seo IY. Diagnostic efficacy of contrast-enhanced ultrasound for small renal masses. Korean J Urol. 2014 Sep;55(9):587–92.
30. Li F, Bai M, Wu Y, He Y, Gu J, Xing J, Du L. Comparative diagnostic performance of contrast-enhanced ultrasound versus baseline ultrasound for renal pelvis lesions. Ultrasound Med Biol. 2015 Dec;41(12):3109–19.
31. Xue LY, Lu Q, Huang BJ, Li Z, Li CX, Wen JX, Wang WP. Papillary renal cell carcinoma and clear cell renal cell carcinoma: differentiation of distinct histological types with contrast - enhanced ultrasonography. Eur J Radiol. 2015 Oct;84(10):1849–56.
32. King KG, Gulati M, Malhi H, Hwang D, Gill IS, Cheng PM, Grant EG, Duddalwar VA. Quantitative assessment of solid renal masses by contrast-enhanced ultrasound with time-intensity curves: how we do it. Abdom Imaging. 2015 Oct;40(7):2461–71.
33. Gerst S, Hann LE, Li D, Gonen M, Tickoo S, Sohn MJ, Russo P. Evaluation of renal masses with contrast-enhanced ultrasound: initial experience. AJR Am J Roentgenol. 2011 Oct;197(4):897–906.
34. Salameh JP, McInnes MDF, McGrath TA, Salameh G, Schieda N. Diagnostic accuracy of dual-energy CT for evaluation of renal masses: systematic review and meta-analysis. Am J Roentgenol. 2019;212(4):W100–5.
35. Schabel C, Patel B, Harring S, Duvnjak P, Ramírez-Giraldo JC, Nikolaou K, Nelson RC, Farjat AE, Marin D. Renal lesion characterization with spectral CT: determining the optimal energy for virtual Monoenergetic reconstruction. Radiology. 2018;287(3):874–83.
36. Wortman JR, Shyu JY, Fulwadhva UP, Sodickson AD. Impact analysis of the routine use of dual-energy computed tomography for characterization of incidental renal lesions. J Comput Assist Tomogr. 2019 Mar/Apr;43(2):176–82.

37. Zarzour JG, Milner D, Valentin R, Jackson BE, Gordetsky J, West J, Rais-Bahrami S, Morgan DE. Quantitative iodine content threshold for discrimination of renal cell carcinomas using rapid kV-switching dual-energy CT. Abdom Radiol. 2017 Mar;42(3):727–34.
38. Kaza RK, Ananthakrishnan L, Kambadakone A, Platt JF. Update of dual-energy CT applications in the genitourinary tract. AJR. 2017;208(6):1185–92.
39. Low G, Huang G, Fu W, Moloo Z, Girgis S. Review of renal cell carcinoma and its common subtypes in radiology. World J Radiol. 2016 May 28;8(5):484–500.
40. Mazzei FG, Mazzei MA, Cioffi Squitieri N, Pozzessere C, Righi L, Cirigliano A, Guerrini S, D'Elia D, Ambrosio MR, Barone A, del Vecchio MT, Volterrani L. CT perfusion in the characterisation of renal lesions: an added value to multiphasic CT. Biomed Res Int. 2014;2014:135013.
41. Cornelis F, Grenier N. Multiparametric magnetic resonance imaging of solid renal tumors: a practical algorithm. Semin Ultrasound CT MR. 2017 Feb;38(1):47–58.
42. Lopes Vendrami C, Parada Villavicencio C, DeJulio TJ, Chatterjee A, Casalino DD, Horowitz JM, Oberlin DT, Yang GY, Nikolaidis P, Miller FH. Differentiation of solid renal tumors with multiparametric MR imaging. Radiographics. 2017;37(7):2026–42.
43. Lanzman RS, Robson PM, Sun MR, Patel AD, Mentore K, Wagner AA, Genega EM, Rofsky NM, Alsop DC, Pedrosa I. Arterial spin-labeling MR imaging of renal masses: correlation with histopathologic findings. Radiology. 2012 Dec;265(3):799–808.
44. Krajewski KM, Pedrosa I. Imaging advances in the Management of Kidney Cancer. J Clin Oncol. 2018 Oct 29;36:JCO2018791236.
45. Gillies RJ, Kinahan PE, Hricak H. Radiomics: images are more than pictures, they are data. Radiology. 2016 Feb;278(2):563–77.
46. Klatte T, Ficarra V, Gratzke C, et al. A literature review of renal surgical anatomy and surgical strategies for partial nephrectomy. Eur Urol. 2015;68:980–92.
47. Ficarra V, Porpiglia F, Crestani A, et al. The simplified PADUA renal nephrometry system: a novel classification of parenchymal renal tumors suitable for partial nephrectomy. BJU Int. 2019 Apr;9 https://doi.org/10.1111/bju.14772.
48. Davidiuk AJ, Parker AS, Thomas CS, et al. Mayo adhesive probability score: an accurate image-based scoring system to predict adherent perinephric fat in partial nephrectomy. Eur Urol. 2014;66:1165–71.
49. de Leon AD, Kapur P, Pedrosa I. Radiomics in kidney cancer: MR imaging. Magn Reson Imaging Clin N Am. 2019 Feb;27(1):1–13.
50. Kocak B, Yardimci AH, Bektas CT, Turkcanoglu MH, Erdim C, Yucetas U, Koca SB, Kilickesmez O. Textural differences between renal cell carcinoma subtypes: machine learning-based quantitative computed tomography texture analysis with independent external validation. Eur J Radiol. 2018 Oct;107:149–57.
51. Shu J, Tang Y, Cui J, Yang R, Meng X, Cai Z, Zhang J, Xu W, Wen D, Yin H. Clear cell renal cell carcinoma: CT-based radiomics features for the prediction of Fuhrman grade. Eur J Radiol. 2018 Dec;109:8–12.
52. Yu H, Scalera J, Khalid M, Touret AS, Bloch N, Li B, Qureshi MM, Soto JA, Anderson SW. Texture analysis as a radiomic marker for differentiating renal tumors. Abdom Radiol (NY). 2017 Oct;42(10):2470–8.
53. Vendrami CL, Velichko YS, Miller FH, Chatterjee A, Villavicencio CP, Yaghmai V, McCarthy RJ. Differentiation of papillary renal cell carcinoma subtypes on MRI: qualitative and texture analysis. AJR Am J Roentgenol. 2018 Dec;211(6):1234–45.
54. Ding J, Xing Z, Jiang Z, Chen J, Pan L, Qiu J, Xing W. CT-based radiomic model predicts high grade of clear cell renal cell carcinoma. Eur J Radiol. 2018 Jun;103:51–6.

Pathological Classification and Biomarkers

Nicholas Archard, Athanasia Vargiamidou, Caitlin Beggan, and Colan M. Ho-Yen

Introduction

The classification of malignant epithelial neoplasms of the kidney has expanded significantly over the last 25 years [1–3]. At the time of the Heidelberg and Rochester consensus conferences in 1996 and 1997, there were 5 main sub-types of renal cell carcinoma (RCC) [1, 2]. The current World Health Organisation (WHO) classification is composed of 14 sub-types [4]. A recent consultation conference discussed another 5 tumour groups associated with specific genetic alterations, currently regarded as 'emerging renal cancer types' which may be recognised as distinct entities in future editions of the classification [3].

Accurate sub-typing of RCC is important for several reasons. Firstly, it provides prognostic information, with the more common sub-types associated with different survival profiles [5, 6]. Secondly, the sub-type may inform the therapeutic approach [4] and thirdly, in the rare instance of an RCC diagnosis uncovering a hereditary syndrome, patients should be offered genetic counselling [4].

In this section, we describe the morphological and immunohistochemical features of the recognised RCC sub-types, with those associated with hereditary syndromes discussed under a separate heading. We outline the characteristics of 2 'emerging renal cancer types' likely to be included in a future WHO classification before briefly mentioning the potential role of biomarkers in the histological assessment of RCC.

N. Archard · A. Vargiamidou · C. Beggan · C. M. Ho-Yen (✉)
St Georges University NHS Foundation Trust, London, UK
e-mail: Nicholas.Archard@stgeorges.nhs.uk; Athanasia.Vargiamidou@stgeorges.nhs.uk; Caitlin.Beggan@stgeorges.nhs.uk; Colan.HoYen@stgeorges.nhs.uk

C. Anderson, M. Afshar (eds.), *Renal Cancer*,
https://doi.org/10.1007/978-3-030-84756-2_5

WHO Classification of Renal Cell Carcinoma

Clear Cell Renal Cell Carcinoma

Clear cell renal cell carcinoma (CCRCC) is the most common subtype of RCC accounting for 60–70% of adult renal cancer [4, 7].

Morphology

Most CCRCCs are well-defined exophytic renal cortical based lesions, some with a pseudocapsule. They typically show a golden yellow cut surface. The tumour cells are arranged in a mixture of solid, trabecular, alveolar and acinar patterns. The tumour is interspersed with a delicate thin walled vascular network. The tumour cells have a predominance of clear cytoplasm (Fig. 1), resulting from high lipid and glycogen content of the cells. The tumour nuclei should be graded on a scale of 1–4, according to the prominence of nucleoli (grades 1–3) and presence of marked nuclear pleomorphism/sarcomatoid or rhabdoid change (International society of urological pathology (ISUP) grading system) [8].

Sarcomatoid or rhabdoid morphology is seen in approximately 5% of tumours. Sarcomatoid differentiation is characterised by a spindle cell growth pattern and is indicative of dedifferentiation within the CCRCC [9]. Rhabdoid morphology is characterised by tumour cells with large irregular nuclei, prominent nucleoli and abundant eccentric eosinophilic cytoplasm [10].

Immunohistochemical Profile

CCRCCs show nuclear positivity for PAX8 in nearly all cases. They are usually positive for CAIX, AE1/3, CAM5.2, EMA, CD10 (membranous staining) and Vimentin [4] (Table 1).

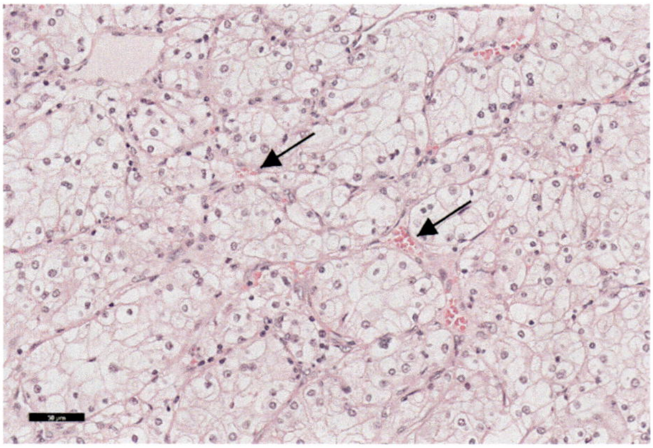

Fig. 1 Clear cell renal cell carcinoma, showing tumour cells with optically clear cytoplasm, prominent cell membranes and a well-defined vascular network (arrows)

Table 1 Immunohistochemical profiles of RCC subtypes, emerging entities in italics

RCC sub-type	Antibody															
	CAIX	CK7	CD117	Cathep-sin K	HMB45	AMACR	34BE12	KSP-Cadherin	Vimen-tin	Pax8	INI-1 / BAF47	Oct4	CD10	CK	EMA	Other
Clear cell [4, 11]	+ (mem)	–	–	–	–	–	–		+	+			+ (mem)	+	+	RCC antigen +
Papillary type 1 [4, 11, 12]	–	+	–	–	–	+	–		+	+			–	+	–	RCC antigen +
Papillary type 2 [4, 11, 12]	–	+/–	–	–	–	+	–		+	+			+	+	+	RCC antigen +
Chromophobe [4, 11, 12]	–	+	+ (mem)	–	–			+	–	+			–		+	Parvalbumin +
Clear cell paplillary [4, 11, 12]	+ (cup-like)	+	–	–	–	–	+			+			+/–	+	+	
MiT XP11 [11, 12]	+ (focal)	–	+/–	+	–	+	–			+			–	+/–	+/–	TFE3 +
MiT t(6;11) [4, 11, 12]	+ (focal)	–	–	+	+	+	–			+			–	+/–	+/–	TFEB +, Melan-A +
Medullary [4, 11]		+								+	–	+		+		p-CEA +, UEG-1 +
Collecting duct [4, 11, 12]	–	+	–	–		+/–			+/–	+	+	–	–	+	+	
Mucinous tubular/spindle cell [4, 11]		+				+				+						
Tubulocystic [11, 12]	–	–				+				+			–		–	

(continued)

Table 1 (continued)

RCC sub-type	Antibody															
	CAIX	CK7	CD117	Cathep-sin K	HMB45	AMACR	34BE12	KSP-Cadherin	Vimen-tin	Pax8	INI-1 / BAF47	Oct4	CD10	CK	EMA	Other
Acquired cystic disease-associated [4, 11, 12]	–	+/–				+/–				+			+		+	RCC antigen +
Multilocular cystic renal neoplasm [11, 12]	+	+				+/–				+			+		+	
Unclassified [4, 11]										+			+			RCC antigen +
SDH-deficient [4, 11]		–	–					+		+				+/–		SDHB -
HLRCC-RCC [4, 11]										+						FH -
Eosinophilic solid/cystic [13]		–	–		–	+/–			+	+			+/–			CK20 +
TFEB-amplified [14, 15]		+/–		+	+/–					+				+		Melan-A +, TFEB +

Abbreviations: *CAIX* Carbonic anhydrase IX, *CK* cytokeratin, *EMA* epithelial membrane antigen, *p-CEA* polyclonal carcinoembryonic antigen, *UEG-1* Ulex europaeus agglutinin-1, *SDHB* Succinate dehydrogenase-B, *FH* Fumarate hydratase

Papillary Renal Cell Carcinoma

Papillary renal cell carcinoma (PRCC) is the second most common subtype of RCC.

Morphology

PRCCs are discrete masses located within the renal cortex and tumours may be multifocal. The tumour is typically well circumscribed with a pseudocapsule. Cut sections vary from grey to yellow, tan or dark brown in colour. PRCCs are characterised by a papillary architecture with papillae showing delicate fibrovascular cores. The cores often contain foamy macrophages or psammoma bodies (Fig. 2). Less commonly they can show a more tubular morphology. Haemorrhage within the tumour is a typical finding and extensive necrosis is common. Sarcomatoid and rhabdoid morphology are observed in approximately 5% of PRCCs.

PRCC has traditionally been subdivided into type 1 and type 2 tumours with type 1 tumours characterised by papillae covered by cells with nuclei arranged in a single layer on the papillary core with scant pale cytoplasm. Type 2 tumours, in contrast, show nuclear pseudostratification and are often higher grade. The cells in type 2 tumour characteristically show more abundant eosinophilic cytoplasm.

Immunohistochemical Profile

PRCC characteristically shows positive staining for AE1/3, CAM5.2, high molecular weight cytokeratins (HMWCK), AMACR, RCC antigen and Vimentin. CK7 expression is variable with positive staining seen more commonly in type 1 tumours than in type 2 tumours. EMA and CD10 are positive in type 2 tumours (Table 1).

Chromophobe Renal Cell Carcinoma

Chromophobe renal cell carcinoma (ChRCC) accounts for 5–7% of all RCCs [4, 7]. Most tumours are sporadic.

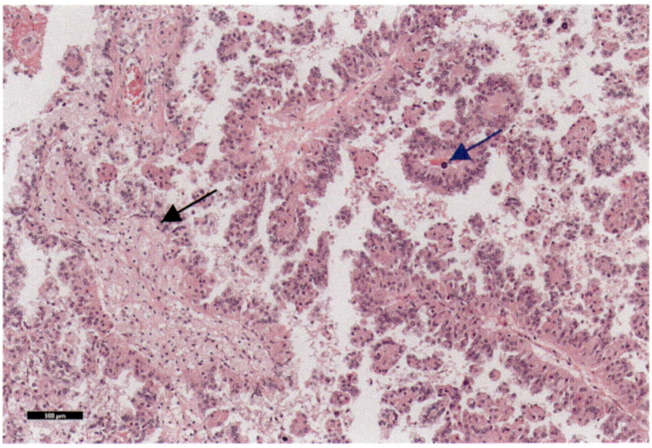

Fig. 2 Papillary renal cell carcinoma (type 1), showing papillary fibrovascular cores (some of which contain foamy histiocytes, black arrow) and basophilic concretions (psammoma bodies, blue arrow)

Morphology

ChRCC is characteristically a well-circumscribed unencapsulated renal cortical tumour with light tan to brown solid cut surface. A central scar can sometimes be seen. The tumour cells are arranged in solid sheet-like patterns. Less common patterns include small nests, tubular, microcystic, trabecular and rarely focal papillary areas [4]. The tumour cells are commonly a mixed population of large pale cells and eosinophilic cells. Cell membranes are prominent. The nuclei have distinct wrinkled irregular nuclear membranes imparting a so-called 'raisinoid' appearance (Fig. 3). The chromatin texture is coarse, binucleation is common and perinuclear halos are characteristic. Sarcomatoid change occurs in 2–8% of tumours [4].

The WHO/ISUP grading system is not recommended for use for ChRCC [8].

Immunohistochemical Profile

ChRCC is positive for KIT (CD117), parvalbumin and kidney specific cadherin. Hale colloidal iron often shows diffuse cytoplasmic staining. CK7 is often diffusely positive. Vimentin is generally negative (Table 1).

MiT Family Translocation-Associated Renal Cell Carcinoma

MiT family translocation-associated renal cell carcinomas harbour gene fusions involving members of the MiT subfamily of transcription factors, predominantly TFE3 and TFEB. Xp11 translocation RCC harbour gene fusions involving TFE3. t(6,11) renal cell carcinomas harbour a MALAT1-TFEB gene fusion. These tumours usually present in childhood and at a younger age than other subtypes of renal cell carcinoma.

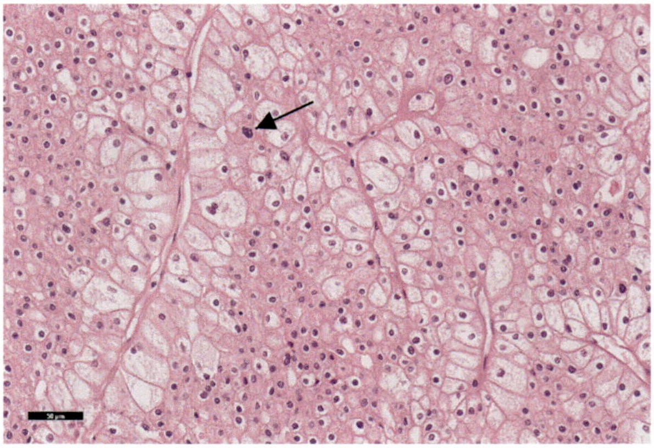

Fig. 3 Chromophobe renal cell carcinoma, showing eosinophilic cells with prominent cell membranes, widespread perinuclear clearing and occasional raisinoid nuclei (arrow)

Morphology

The most recognisable pattern of Xp11 translocation RCC is that of a papillary neoplasm with epithelioid clear cells and scattered psammoma bodies [7]. There is considerable heterogeneity in the morphology and these tumours can mimic almost any other renal cell carcinoma subtype.

The most distinctive histologic pattern of t(6,11) renal cell carcinoma is a biphasic neoplasm composed of nests of larger epithelioid cells and smaller cell clusters around basement membrane material. They entrap single native renal tubules at their periphery [4]. The larger cells have clear to eosinophilic cytoplasm, and their nested architecture is similar to clear cell RCC. The smaller cells cluster around basement membrane material resembling the Call-Exner bodies of adult granulosa cell tumour [16].

Immunohistochemical Profile

MiT family translocation RCCs under express epithelial markers such as cytokeratins and EMA, but they do consistently express PAX8 (Table 1).

Xp11 translocation RCCs express TFE3 (nuclear staining) and approximately 60% stain with cathepsin K [4].

Tumours with the t(6,11) translocation consistently express the melanoma markers Melan A and HMB45 and cathepsin K [4]. Nuclear immunoreactivity for TFEB protein is highly specific for the t(6;11) RCCs.

Renal Medullary Carcinoma

Renal Medullary Carcinoma (RMC) is a rare highly aggressive renal tumour with a predilection for young males in the second to third decade. The tumour is more common in Africans than Caucasians [4, 17]. Patients with RMC suffer from sickle cell trait, disease or other hemoglobinopathies, which are important diagnostic criteria when making the diagnosis [7].

Morphology

RMC is a poorly defined tumour centered on the medulla. The tumour adopts several patterns such as solid sheets and cords, nests, papillae, tubulopapillary structures, infiltrating small and medium sized glandular structures resting in a desmoplastic fibromyxoid stroma. The tumour exhibits high grade cytological atypia with rhabdoid morphology frequently encountered [4, 17].

Immunohistochemical Profile

The tumour is positive for CK7, CAM5.2, PAX8, S100A, Ulex europaeus agglutinin-1. RMC exhibits loss of nuclear INI1 staining (due to *SMARCB1* gene loss expression) and may show positive OCT3/4 immunolabelling (Table 1).

Renal Collecting Duct Carcinoma

Collecting duct carcinoma (CDC) is a rare and highly aggressive adenocarcinoma. The tumour is more common men than women (2:1). CDC is not associated with sickle cell disorders or hemoglobinopathies.

Morphology

This is a medullary based adenocarcinoma which resembles closely RMC. The tumour shows infiltrating glands, tubules, tubulopapillary and tubulocystic structures resting on a desmoplastic stroma [4, 17]. The kidney adjacent can show intratubular dysplasia.

Immunohistochemical Profile

The tumour shows positive immunolabelling for 34BE12, CK19, CK7, PAX8, S100A1 and negative staining for OCT3/4 (Table 1). CDC is important to differentiate from primary urothelial carcinomas, other aggressive renal adenocarcinomas and metastasis and thus wide spectrum immunohistochemistry is advised.

Clear Cell Papillary Renal Cell Carcinoma

Clear Cell Papillary Renal Cell Carcinoma (CCP RCC) is an indolent, rare (1–4% of renal neoplasms) [4] tumour recently added to the WHO classification as a distinct entity. It has no sex predilection and a mean age of 60 years. The tumour arises mostly sporadically, but it can also be associated with end stage renal disease and Von-Hippel-Lindau syndrome [4, 18].

Morphology

The tumour arising in the renal cortex, is generally small, well defined and encapsulated. It can show predominant cystic change. Microscopically the tumour comprises tubules, papillae, acini and cysts. These are lined by cells with clear cytoplasm, low grade nuclei which are aligned away from the basement membrane (reverse polarity) [18].

Immunohistochemical Profile

The tumour shows positive immunolabelling for CK7, 34BE12, CAIX (cup-like staining), PAX2, PAX8, vimentin, e-cadherin, beta-catenin and negative for AMACR, TFE3 (Table 1).

Mucinous Tubular and Spindle Cell Renal Cell Carcinoma

Mucinous tubular and spindle cell renal cell carcinoma (MTS RCC) is a rare, indolent, low grade renal tumour originating from the proximal nephron. It has a predilection for females with a female to male ratio 3:1 [4, 19].

Morphology

This a well-defined and partly encapsulated tumour based in the renal cortex. The tumour comprises variably sized tightly packed tubules. The tubules consist of bland cells with scanty cytoplasm. The second major feature is that of bland looking spindle cells. A transition between tubules to spindle cells is commonly identified the tumour. The tumour also comprises myxoid or mucinous stroma in between the tubules [4, 19, 20].

Immunohistochemical Profile

The tumour shows positive immunolabelling for CK7, AMACR and PAX8 [4, 11] (Table 1).

Multilocular Cystic Renal Cell Neoplasm of Low Malignant Potential

Multilocular cystic renal cell neoplasm (MLCRCN) has a predilection for middle-aged adults. It is more common in men with a ratio 2:1 to women. It is a rare tumour with an incidence of 1%. It has excellent prognosis with no recurrence or metastasis.

Morphology

The tumour is well defined and encapsulated. It comprises variably sized cysts separated by thin fibrous septae. The cysts are lined by low grade (ISUP1, ISUP2) atypical cells with mostly clear but also granular cytoplasm. Nests of these atypical cells are also identified within the septae. These nests do not form expansile nodules as in the case of CCRCC (with cystic change), and this in fact is their defining feature. The cysts can contain clear serous, gelatinous for haemorrhagic fluid.

Immunohistochemical Profile

MLCRCN is positive for PAX8, EMA, CD10, CAIX and CK7 [11, 12] (Table 1).

Tubulocystic Renal Cell Carcinoma

Tubulocystic RCC is rare, accounting for less than 1% of RCCs. These tumours show a male predominance, are often discovered incidentally, and occur more frequently in the left kidney. Tubulocystic RCC is typically an indolent neoplasm and only rarely metastasizes [4, 21].

Morphology

On macroscopic examination, they are typically well circumscribed, with a spongey cut surface. Histologically, the tumour is composed of multiple, variably sized tubules lined by a single layer of cells which vary from flat or cuboidal to columnar. Nucleoli are usually prominent. The stroma between the tubules is fibrotic.

Immunohistochemical Profile

The tumour cells express PAX8 and AMACR and are negative for CAIX, CK7, CD10 and EMA [11, 12] (Table 1).

Acquired Cystic Disease Associated Renal Cell Carcinoma

Acquired cystic disease associated RCC (ACD RCC) occurs in patients with acquired cystic disease, typically in those receiving haemodialysis [4, 22, 23]. The tumours may be multifocal and bilateral and may appear to arise from cysts. ACD RCC is typically indolent, although high grade transformation may occur and may be associated with aggressive behaviour [4, 22].

Morphology

Macroscopically, they are well circumscribed, with a yellow to tan cut surface. Histologically, they are composed of cells with abundant eosinophilic cytoplasm and prominent nucleoli. A wide range of architectural patterns may be seen but there is usually prominent microcystic or cribriform architecture with numerous calcium oxalate crystals.

Immunohistochemical Profile

ACD RCC shows reactivity for PAX8, CD10, EMA and may be positive for CK7 and AMACR; CAIX is negative [11, 12] (Table 1).

Unclassified Renal Cell Carcinoma

Unclassified RCC is not a distinct entity but a category used to describe tumours either without typical features of a recognised subtype or showing a combination of features of different subtypes. As such, it comprises a heterogenous group, including both low grade and high grade tumours [4]. This category is used infrequently, with unclassified RCC typically representing up to around 5% of RCC diagnoses and the main predictors of prognosis are grade and stage at presentation [24].

Immunohistochemical Profile

Unclassified RCCs should express RCC marker, CD10 and PAX8 [4, 11] (Table 1).

Hereditary Renal Cancer Syndromes

RCC is usually a sporadic malignancy but may occur in the context of several inherited tumour syndromes. Such syndromes are typically inherited as autosomal dominant disorders and may be associated with extrarenal neoplasms and other manifestations. Two syndromes are associated with rare, specific subtypes of RCC: hereditary leiomyomatosis and renal cell carcinoma (HLRCC) and germline *SDH* mutations. Other syndromes are associated with subtypes of RCC which also occur sporadically.

HLRCC is a tumour syndrome associated with a syndrome-specific subtype of RCC, hereditary leiomyomatosis-associated renal cell carcinoma (HLRCC-RCC). HLRCC results from mutation of the *FH* gene (1q42), which encodes fumarate hydratase and, in addition to HLRCC-RCC, is characterised by multiple leiomyomas of the skin and uterus. Histologically, HLRCC-RCC demonstrates papillary morphology, large cells with abundant eosinophilic cytoplasm, large nuclei, and prominent, inclusion-like nucleoli. Immunohistochemistry shows tumour cell loss of fumarate hydratase (Table 1). Prognosis is generally poor, with metastases often occurring early [4, 25, 26].

Germline *SDH* mutations are associated with paragangliomas, phaeochromocytomas, gastrointestinal stromal tumours and a rare sub-type of RCC, succinate dehydrogenase-deficient renal cell carcinoma (SD-RCC). SD-RCC almost always occurs in the context of such a syndrome. Mutations may occur in any of the four *SDH* genes, which encode the proteins of mitochondrial complex II. Mutations occur most commonly in *SDHB* and less frequently in *SDHA*, *SDHC* and *SDHD*. SDH-RCC shows distinctive morphology with a solid, nested, or tubular arrangement of cells with cytoplasmic vacuolation. Immunohistochemical staining shows loss of SDHB. Most tumours are low grade and have a favourable prognosis but occasionally high grade features are seen, in which case prognosis is less favourable [4, 27].

Of the tumour syndromes associated with sub-types of RCC which also occur sporadically, Von Hippel-Lindau disease (VHL) and Birt-Hogg-Dubé syndrome (BHD) are possibly the best characterised. VHL is caused by mutation of the *VHL* gene (3p25), which encodes the VHL protein. It is associated with clear cell RCC, which may be multiple and bilateral, and renal cysts. Extrarenal tumours include retinal and cerebellar haemangioblastoma, phaeochromocytoma, pancreatic cysts and neuroendocrine tumours. BHD is caused by mutation of the *FCLN* gene (17p11), which encodes the protein folliculin. Associated renal tumours include chromophobe RCC, hybrid chromophobe RCC/oncocytoma and papillary RCC. Extrarenal manifestations include pulmonary cysts, pneumothorax and facial fibrofolliculomas [4].

Emerging Renal Cancer Types

In addition to the established sub-types, there is growing evidence for the existence of several new entities [3].

TFEB-Amplified RCC

RCC associated with amplification of the 6p21.1 region that includes *TFEB* shares some features with t(6;11) RCC such as immunohistochemical expression of TFEB, melanocytic markers (Melan-A and HMB45) and Cathepsin K [14, 15, 28]. Compared with t(6;11) RCC, 6p21.1 amplified tumours have a more heterogenous morphology with eosinophilic cells containing high grade nuclei, arranged in pseudopapillary, papillary, nested and tubulopapillary patterns [14, 15, 28]. Furthermore, 6p21.1 amplified tumours behave more aggressively than their translocated counterparts, possibly due to co-amplified genes at this locus [29].

Eosinophilic Solid and Cystic RCC

Originally described as one of 3 patterns of Tuberous Sclerosis (TS)-associated RCC [30], eosinophilic solid and cystic RCC (ESC-RCC) has subsequently been shown to exist in sporadic form in patients without clinical features of TS, predominantly in females [13, 31].

Microscopically, ESC-RCC shows a solid (nested), microcystic and macrocystic architecture composed of eosinophilic cells with abundant cytoplasm, often demonstrating a hob-nail appearance. Features unusual in other RCCs include cytoplasmic stippling with basophilic granules and positive immunolabelling for CK20 [13, 31].

Mutations in *TSC1/2* have been identified in most ESC-RCCs studies [32].

The evidence for other potential new entities such as *ALK*-rearranged RCC and *TCEB1*-mutated RCC is weaker, but they are possible candidates for future classifications [3].

Biomarkers in RCC

In addition to histological sub-type, several established parameters have prognostic significance in RCC, such as tumour grade, pathological stage, the presence of sarcomatoid differentiation and necrosis [5, 6].

With widespread utilisation of molecular techniques, further potential biomarkers have emerged, that may refine prognostication in RCC. The tumour suppressor genes *PBRM1, BAP1* and *SETD2* are mutated in a proportion of clear cell RCC and correlate with loss of protein expression on immunohistochemistry [33]. Loss of protein expression of PBRM1, BAP1 and H3K36me3 (a surrogate for SETD2 activity) were associated with high tumour grade/stage and necrosis, although no biomarker added independent prognostic information at multivariate analysis [33].

The emergence of novel therapies targeting the immune checkpoint proteins programmed cell death 1 (PD-1) and programmed death—ligand 1 (PDL-1) in advanced RCC has led several groups to evaluate these proteins as potential predictive/prognostic biomarkers [34–36]. PD-1/PDL-1 expression has been correlated with adverse clinicopathological factors, including sarcomatoid morphology [34]. This latter finding is supported by a meta-analysis showing sarcomatoid histology is associated with improved response to anti PD-1/PDL-1 therapy [35].

Although immunohistochemical PD-1/PDL-1 expression has potential as a biomarker, practical application is currently limited by tumour heterogeneity, variable concordance between different assays, a lack of standardised scoring methods and inter-observer variation [34, 36, 37].

Conclusion

Our understanding of the biology of RCC has advanced substantially in recent years and the classification continues to evolve. Although most RCCs can be diagnosed by recognising characteristic features on conventional histochemical stains, the use of a broad immunohistochemical panel is necessary in more challenging cases. Unusual morphological or immunohistochemical features should alert the pathologist to the possibility of an underlying hereditary syndrome or an 'emerging' sub-type. In the future, the classification of RCC and the application of novel biomarkers may become more relevant as patients are stratified for new therapies.

Key Points

1. The pathological classification of RCC is essentially based on tumour morphology (cytological and architectural features) and the immunohistochemical expression profile.
2. Accurate classification is important for prognostication, directing treatment and identifying the need for genetic counselling.
3. The WHO classification is reviewed periodically, partly to consider whether newer entities should be formally recognised.
4. The most common sub-types of RCC are clear cell RCC (60–70% of RCCs), followed by papillary RCC and then chromophobe RCC.
5. Sub-types associated with a good prognosis include multilocular cystic renal neoplasm of low malignant potential, tubulocystic RCC, acquired cystic disease-associated RCC, mucinous tubular and spindle cell RCC and clear cell papillary RCC.
6. Collecting duct carcinoma and renal medullary carcinoma are aggressive RCCs.
7. A broad immunohistochemical panel is necessary for diagnosing tumours with unusual features or rarer sub-types, including those associated with hereditary syndromes.
8. Succinate dehydrogenase-deficient RCC and fumarate hydratase-deficient RCC are associated with germline mutations in *SDH* genes and the *FH* gene respectively.
9. In addition to sub-typing RCC, several other pathological features yield important prognostic information, such as grade (clear cell and papillary RCC only), stage, sarcomatoid differentiation and the presence of necrosis.
10. Pathological analysis of novel biomarker expression may help select patients for targeted therapies in the future, but further work is necessary to establish standardised protocols for the reliable assessment of PD-1/PDL-1 expression.

References

1. Kovacs G, Akhtar M, Beckwith BJ, Bugert P, Cooper CS, Delahunt B, et al. The Heidelberg classification of renal cell tumours. J Pathol. 1997 Oct;183(2):131–3.
2. Störkel S, Eble JN, Adlakha K, Amin M, Blute ML, Bostwick DG, et al. Classification of renal cell carcinoma: workgroup no. 1. Union Internationale Contre le cancer (UICC) and the American joint committee on cancer (AJCC). Cancer. 1997 Sep 1;80(5):987–9.
3. Williamson SR, Gill AJ, Argani P, Chen Y, Egevad L, Kristiansen G, et al. Report from the International Society of Urological Pathology (ISUP) consultation conference on molecular pathology of urogenital cancers: III: molecular pathology of kidney cancer. Am J Surg Pathol. 2020 Jul;44(7):e47–65.

4. Moch H, Humphrey PA, Ulbright TM, Reuter VE, editors. WHO classification of tumours of the urinary system and male genital organs (4th edition). Lyon: IARC; 2016.
5. Moch H, Gasser T, Amin MB, Torhorst J, Sauter G, Mihatsch MJ. Prognostic utility of the recently recommended histologic classification and revised TNM staging system of renal cell carcinoma: a Swiss experience with 588 tumors. Cancer. 2000 Aug 1;89(3):604–14.
6. Amin MB, Amin MB, Tamboli P, Javidan J, Stricker H, Venturina M, et al. Prognostic impact of histologic subtyping of adult renal epithelial neoplasms: an experience of 405 cases. Am J Surg Pathol. 2002 Mar;26(3):281–91. https://doi.org/10.1097/00000478-200203000-00001.
7. Trpkov K, Hes O, Williamson SR, Adeniran AJ, Agaimy A, Alaghehbandan R, et al. New developments in existing WHO entities and evolving molecular concepts: the genitourinary pathology society (GUPS) update on renal neoplasia. Mod Pathol. 2021 Mar 4;34(7):1392–424.
8. Delahunt B, Cheville JC, Martignoni G, Humphrey PA, MagiGalluzzi C, McKenney J, et al. The International Society of Urological Pathology (ISUP) grading system for renal cell carcinoma and other prognostic parameters. Am J Surg Pathol. 2013;37:1490–504.
9. Thomas JO, Tawfik O. Recent advances in the diagnosis of renal cell carcinoma. Diagn Histopathol. 2008;14(4):157–63.
10. Delahunt B. Advances and controversies in grading and staging of renal cell carcinoma. Mod Pathol. 2009 Jun;22(Suppl 2):S24–36.
11. Reuter VE, Argani P, Zhou M, Delahunt B. Members of the ISUP immunohistochemistry in diagnostic urologic pathology group. Best practices recommendations in the application of immunohistochemistry in the kidney tumors: report from the International Society of Urologic Pathology consensus conference. Am J Surg Pathol. 2014 Aug;38(8):e35–49.
12. Kim M, Joo JW, Lee SJ, Cho YA, Park CK, Cho NH. Comprehensive Immunoprofiles of renal cell carcinoma subtypes. Cancers (Basel). 2020 Mar 5;12(3):602.
13. Trpkov K, Hes O, Bonert M, Lopez JI, Bonsib SM, Nesi G, et al. Eosinophilic, solid, and cystic renal cell carcinoma: Clinicopathologic study of 16 unique, sporadic neoplasms occurring in women. Am J Surg Pathol. 2016 Jan;40(1):60–71.
14. Argani P, Reuter VE, Zhang L, Sung Y, Ning Y, Epstein JI, et al. TFEB-amplified renal cell carcinomas: an aggressive molecular subset demonstrating variable melanocytic marker expression and morphologic heterogeneity. Am J Surg Pathol. 2016 Nov;40(11):1484–95.
15. Gupta S, Johnson SH, Vasmatzis G, Porath B, Rustin JG, Rao P, et al. TFEB-VEGFA (6p21.1) co-amplified renal cell carcinoma: a distinct entity with potential implications for clinical management. Mod Pathol. 2017 Jul;30(7):998–1012. https://doi.org/10.1038/modpathol.2017.24.
16. Argani P, Lae M, Hutchinson B, Reuter VE, Collins MH, Perentesis J, et al. Renal carcinomas with the t(6;11)(p21;q12): clinicopathologic features and demonstration of the specific alpha-TFEB gene fusion by immunohistochemistry, RT-PCR, and DNA PCR. Am J Surg Pathol. 2005;29:230–40.
17. Ohe C, Smith S, Sirohi D, Divatia M, De Peralta-Venturina M, Paner GP, et al. Reappraisal of morphological differences between renal medullary carcinoma, collecting duct carcinoma, and fumarate hydratase-deficient renal cell carcinoma. Am J Surg Pathol. 2018;42(3):279–92.
18. Zao J, Eyzaguirre E. Clear cell papillary renal cell carcinoma. Arch Pathol Lab Med. 2019;143:1154–8.
19. Nathany S, Monnapa V. Mucinous and spindle cell carcinoma: a review of histopathology and clinical and prognostic implications. Arch Pathol Lab Med. 2020;144(1):115–8.
20. Zhao M, He X, Teng X. Mucinous tubular and spindle cell renal cell carcinoma: a review of clinicopathologic aspects. Diagn Pathol. 2015;10:168.
21. Amin MB, Maclennan GT, Gupta R, Grignon D, Paraf F, Viellefond A, et al. Tubulocystic carcinoma of the kidney: clinicopathologic analysis of 31 cases of a distinctive rare subtype of renal cell carcinoma. Am J Surg Pathol. 2009;33:384–92.
22. Tickoo SK, deParalta-Venturina MN, Harik LR, Worcester HD, Salama ME, Young AN, et al. Spectrum of epithelial neoplasms in end-stage renal disease: an experience from 66 tumor-bearing kidneys with emphasis on histologic patterns distinct from those in sporadic adult renal neoplasia. Am J Surg Pathol. 2006;30:141–53.

23. Enoki Y, Katoh G, Okabe H, Yanagisawa A. Clinicopathological features and CD57 expression in renal cell carcinoma in acquired cystic disease of the kidneys: with special emphasis on a relation to the duration of haemodialysis, the degree of calcium oxalate deposition, histological type, and possible tumorigenesis. Histopathology. 2010;56:384–94.
24. Lopez-Beltran A, Kirkali Z, Montironi R, Blancan A, Algaba F, Scarpelli M, et al. Unclassified renal cell carcinoma: a report of 56 cases. BJU Int. 2012;110:786–93.
25. Kiuru M, Launonen V, Hietala AK, Vierimaa O, Salovaara R, Arola J, Pukkala E, Sistonen P, Herva R, Aaltonen LA. Familial cutaneous leiomyomatosis is a two-hit condition associated with renal cell cancer of characteristic histopathology. Am J Pathol. 2001;159:825–9.
26. Launonen V, Vierimaa O, Kiuru M, Isola J, Roth S, Pukkala E, Sistonen P, Herva R, Aaltonen LA. Inherited susceptibility to uterine leiomyomas and renal cell cancer. Proc Natl Can Sci USA. 2001;13(98):3387–92.
27. Gill AJ, Hes O, Papathomas T, Sedivcova M, Tan PH, Agaimy A, et al. Succinate dehydrogenase (SDH)-deficient renal cell carcinoma: a morphologically distinct entity: a clinicopathologic series of 36 tumors from 27 patients. Am J Surg Pathol. 2014;38:1588–602.
28. Skala SL, Xiao H, Udager AM, Dhanasekaran SM, Shukla S, Zhang Y, et al. Detection of 6 TFEB-amplified renal cell carcinomas and 25 renal cell carcinomas with MITF translocations: systematic morphologic analysis of 85 cases evaluated by clinical TFE3 and TFEB FISH assays. Mod Pathol. 2018 Jan;31(1):179–97. https://doi.org/10.1038/modpathol.2017.99.
29. Gupta S, Argani P, Jungbluth AA, Chen Y, Tickoo SK, Fine SW, et al. TFEB expression profiling in renal cell carcinomas: Clinicopathologic correlations. Am J Surg Pathol. 2019 Nov;43(11):1445–61.
30. Guo J, Tretiakova MS, Troxell ML, Osunkoya AO, Fadare O, Sangoi AR, et al. Tuberous sclerosis-associated renal cell carcinoma: a clinicopathologic study of 57 separate carcinomas in 18 patients multicenter study. Am J Surg Pathol. 2014 Nov;38(11):1457–67.
31. Li Y, Reuter VE, Matoso A, Netto GJ, Epstein JI, Argani P. Re-evaluation of 33 'unclassified' eosinophilic renal cell carcinomas in young patients. Histopathology. 2018 Mar;72(4):588–600. https://doi.org/10.1111/his.13395.
32. Palsgrove DN, Li Y, Pratilas CA, Lin M, Pallavajjalla A, Gocke C, et al. Eosinophilic solid and cystic (ESC) renal cell Carcinomas Harbor TSC mutations: molecular analysis supports an expanding Clinicopathologic Spectrum. Am J Surg Pathol. 2018 Sep;42(9):1166–81.
33. Bihr S, Ohashi R, Moore AL, Rüschoff JH, Beisel C, Hermanns T, et al. Expression and mutation patterns of PBRM1, BAP1 and SETD2 Mirror specific evolutionary subtypes in clear cell renal cell carcinoma. Neoplasia. 2019 Feb;21(2):247–56.
34. Ueda K, Suekane S, Kurose H, Chikui K, Nakiri M, Nishihara K, et al. Prognostic value of PD-1 and PD-L1 expression in patients with metastatic clear cell renal cell carcinoma. Urol Oncol. 2018 Nov;36(11):499.e9–499.e16. https://doi.org/10.1016/j.urolonc.2018.07.003.
35. Buonerba C, Dolce P, Iaccarino S, Scafuri L, Verde A, Costabile F, et al. Outcomes associated with first-line anti-PD-1/PD-L1 agents vs. Sunitinib in patients with Sarcomatoid renal cell carcinoma. A Systematic Review and Meta-Analysis Cancers (Basel). 2020 Feb 10;12(2):408.
36. Sommer U, Eckstein M, Ammann J, Braunschweig T, Macher-Göppinger S, Schwamborn K, et al. Multicentric analytical and inter-observer comparability of four clinically developed programmed death-ligand 1 immunohistochemistry assays in advanced clear-cell renal cell carcinoma. Clin Genitourin Cancer. 2020 Oct;18(5):e629–42.
37. Kim KS, Sekar RR, Patil D, Dimarco MA, Kissick HT, Bilen MA, et al. Evaluation of programmed cell death protein 1 (PD-1) expression as a prognostic biomarker in patients with clear cell renal cell carcinoma. Onco Targets Ther. 2018 Jan 10;7(4):e1413519.

Biomarkers, Early Detection and Biomarker Based Treatment of Renal Cancer

Sashi S. Kommu

Introduction

The lifetime risk of being diagnosed with kidney cancer in men is estimated to be around 2%. The lifetime risk for women is around 1%) [1]. It remains among the 10 most common cancers in both males and females. Renal Cell Cancer (RCC) remains the most common form of renal cancer. There has been a general pattern over the last 20 years an increase in the annual incidence of renal cancer approximating to 2% worldwide [2, 3]. The management of kidney cancer imparts a huge health burden on healthcare systems. When detected early, often incidentally with increased use of imaging tools, the prognosis remains generally favorable. When detected late, survival despite treatment, remains poor.

A major challenge in managing renal cancer stems from the heterogenous nature of the disease. There is a diverse range in terms of tumour phenotypes and histological profiles. Furthermore, a renal tumour can range from the benign end of the spectrum e.g. oncocytoma to clinically less aggressive variants e.g. chromophobe renal cell caners to poor prognostic variants such as high-grade clear cell and papillary type 2 renal cell cancers. To add complexity, some of these cancer types have their own genetic variants adding a somewhat unpredictable and uncomfortable aura in deciphering long-term prognosis.

The increase in incidence and evolving burden on healthcare coupled with recent advances in biomarker evaluation and imaging modalities has ushered a renewed interest in biomarker and other early detection strategies. Herein, this chapter will outline the current existing and future perspectives on biomarkers and early detection strategies. Some of the biomarkers have helped individualize and specialize a

S. S. Kommu (✉)
School of Biosciences, Kent & Medway Medical School, University of Kent, Canterbury, UK

Department of Urology, Kent & Canterbury Hospital, Canterbury, UK
e-mail: s.kommu@nhs.net

C. Anderson, M. Afshar (eds.), *Renal Cancer*,
https://doi.org/10.1007/978-3-030-84756-2_6

signatured approach to oncological management either in conjunction with surgical extirpation or on their own.

Biomarkers and Imaging Modalities

Molecular biomarkers can be broadly stratified based on their individual physiologic location. Of these, circulating biomarkers include VEGF and VEGF-related proteins, cytokine and angiogenic factors (CAF), lactate dehydrogenase (LDH) and circulating endothelial cells (CEC). Tissue Based Biomarkers (TBMs) include biomarkers related to the von Hippel–Lindau (VHL) single-nucleotide, mammalian target of rapamycin (mTOR) pathways and polymorphisms (SNP). The role of imaging biomarkers is two-fold. The main role is to ideally apply a non-invasive platform to identify and predict the likely histological profile of a renal lesion. Thus, stratifying and timing the treatment of the more aggressive subtypes and at the same time deferring or conservatively managing the more indolent types [4]. The second role is in the prediction of treatment responses with a view to tailoring second and third-line oncological treatment.

Serum Biomarkers

VEGF

Vascular endothelial growth factor (VEGF) is a homodimeric glycoprotein and is a key mediator of angiogenesis in cancer, in which it is up-regulated by oncogene expression, a variety of growth factors and also hypoxia. It plays a key role in the angiogenesis of RCC and the VEGF pathway is a major are of interest in research. The role of serum levels of VEGF as a biomarker for prognostication and prediction of response to treatment has been studied. The TARGET (Treatment Approach in Renal cancer Global Evaluation Trial) Study looked at the role of sorafenib versus placebo in the second line treatment of RCC and explored the utility of VEGF levels as a biomarker of Sorafenib treatment response [5]. VEGF baseline levels were found to correlate inversely with progression free survival and overall survival. Multivariate analysis showed that baseline VEGF was an independent prognostic prediction factor for progression free survival in patients receiving placebo. This was not the case in the Sorafenib administered group. Those patients with high-VEGF levels were noted to have more benefit from sorafenib than the low-VEGF group [5].

Interleukin 6

Although it is known that inflammatory cytokines are detected in the plasma of patients with RCC and are associated with poor prognosis, the primary cell type involved is unknown. Interleukin 6 (IL-6) has been identified as a potential biomarker with evidence that it is secreted by RCC cells when they are exposed to hypoxia [6]. Fitzgerald et al. identified that interleukin-6 and interleukin-8 (IL-6 and IL-8) are secreted solely from RCC cells exposed to hypoxia and demonstrated that the NADPH oxidase isoform, Nox4, play a key role in hypoxia-induced IL-6 and IL-8 production in RCC. They also demonstrated enhanced levels of IL-6 and IL-8 result in RCC cell invasion and that activation of AMPK reduces Nox4 expression, IL-6 and IL-8 production, and RCC cell invasion.

Furthermore, we demonstrate that the NADPH oxidase isoform, Nox4, play a key role in hypoxia-induced IL-6 and IL-8 production in RCC. Finally, we have characterized that enhanced levels of IL-6 and IL-8 result in RCC cell invasion and that activation of AMPK reduces Nox4 expression, IL-6 and IL-8 production, and RCC cell invasion [6].

Tran et al. showed that serum levels of hepatocyte growth factor (HGF), IL-6, and IL-8 correlated with greater tumour size reduction with pazopanib therapy [7]. Zurita et al. found that low IL-6 and high E-selectin were associated with prolonged PFS. Considering the results of the previously discussed sorafenib study [8]. In patients treated with pazopanib, low levels of IL-8, HGF, osteopontin and TIMP-1 all correlated with significantly longer PFS [7]. In patients receiving placebo, IL-6, IL-8 and osteopontin were noted to have prognostic correlation with PFS. Whereas IL-6 shows promise as a predictive biomarker, robust prospective studies validating its role are lacking. A systematic review by Funakoshi et al. of the predictive and prognostic biomarkers for VEGF-targeted therapy in renal cell carcinoma found no level 1 evidence for a biomarker predictive of survival with VEGF-directed therapy [9].

LDH and mTOR

Mammalian Target 0f Rapamycin (mTOR) and Lactate Dehydrogenase (LDH) have also been explored for potential biomarker-based applications in renal cancer. LDH with its inherent role in anaerobic glycolysis is known to be regulated by the PI3-K/AKT/mTOR pathway [10]. LDH is embedded in the MSKCC Risk Score as a prognostic factor for RCC in which a high serum LDH is an established poor prognostic factor. Armstrong et al. showed that high serum LDH is a poor prognostic marker with a HR for death of 2.8 for patients with LDH greater than the upper limit of normal and that elevated LDH predicted OS benefit with Temsirolimus as compared to Interferon Therapy [10]. Voss et al. identified 5 biomarkers (CSF1, ICAM1, IL-18BP, KIM1, TNFRII) with the strongest association for everolimus (an mTOR inhibitor) PFS and created a composite biomarker score (CBS) [11]. It was shown that everolimus-treated patients with high starting CBS had significantly better PFS than those with low CBS. The composite biomarker score showed no correlation with PFS in sunitinib patients. This led to the prospect that everolimus-specific set of biomarkers and the potential of serum biomarkers for prediction of treatment outcome [12].

Non-CAF Prognostic Serum Biomarkers

Several non-cytokine and angiogenic factors (CAF) serum biomarkers have been studied as prognostic models to predict survival of metastatic Renal Cell Cancer (mRCC) patients.

Heng et al. studied the prognostic factors for overall survival in mRCC patients treated with vascular endothelial growth factor-targeted agents. The subsequent Heng score was described based on the findings and is now a validated platform used to aid in prediction of median OS in mRCC patients receiving VEGF TT [13]. Motzer et al. published the findings of survival and prognostic stratification of 670 patients with advanced renal cell carcinoma. The resultant Motzer Score (MSKCC Score) utilizes haemoglobin, calcium, and LDH to predict median OS in mRCC patients [14]. Additional non-CAF prognostic serum biomarkers of recent interest are those related to systemic inflammation, as chronic inflammation may suppress anti-tumoral immune system activity. The neutrophil-lymphocyte ratio (NLR) was also studied as a biomarker related to the tumour-inflammation dynamics associated with RCC. Boissier et al. identified seven studies looking at the potential role of NLR in mRCC or locally advanced RCC. They found that a high NLR independently predicted worse OS [15].

Ohno et al. in a study looking at clinical variables for predicting metastatic renal cell carcinoma patients who might not benefit from cytoreductive nephrectomy found that NLR independently predicts OS in patients with mRCC undergoing cytoreductive nephrectomy [16].

Urinary Biomarkers

Urine biomarkers have been the focus of attention for urological cancers. The current advances in urine proteomic and genomic evaluation have revamped the prospect of seeking both diagnostic and prognostic biomarkers in urological cancers particularly renal cancer [17, 18]. Despite several studies looking at urine as a portal for biomarker discovery, there has been little in applicable biomarkers discovery. Morrissey et al. analysed urine samples in patients with RCC and compared these with controls and found that RCC patients had a 23-fold increase in aquaporin-1 (AQP-1). They also found a four-fold increase in another exosomal protein called perilipin-2 (PLIN2). Both proteins were shown to decrease significantly following nephrectomy [19]. Gatto et al. studied the prognostic value of glycosaminoglycans (GAGs) in urine. GAGs are transcriptionally upregulated in mRCC. They collected GAG levels in both urine and serum in a relatively small study involving patients with metastatic ccRCC and urine GAG score independently predicted both PFS and OS [20].

Urine as a readily accessible and non-invasive medium continues to be of significant interest among biomarker discovery groups.

ctDNA (Liquid Biopsy)

Liquid biopsies involve the capture of tumour based or derived biomarkers in a fluid (liquid) sample rather than actual tissue. Recent advances in high throughput analysis of samples and the minimally invasive means by which the samples can be acquired, make liquid biopsy a popular and evolving area of interest [21–23]. Circulating tumour DNA (ctDNA) from blood samples has been of immense recent interest. Pal et al., collected ctDNA in patients with mRCC and GAs were compared in patients receiving first or second-line therapy and found that second-line patients who previously underwent first-line VEGF-directed therapy had significant differences in p53 and mTOR GAs compared to first-line cohorts [24]. Other studies looking at circulating tumour cells have found interesting correlations but were all retrospective [25]. The current consensus in biomarker liquid biopsy discovery is to emphasize on high volume prospective studies.

Tissue Based Biomarkers

The classification of renal tumours is complex and is riddled with the inherent heterogeneous nature of the disease with further layers of difficulty in stratification based on histology, morphology and genetic variations. Some tumours require immunohistochemical and chromosomal characterisation. The classification process continues to evolve. Biomarker discovery is thus a challenge, particularly when tissue-based biomarkers are sought.

Immunohistochemistry

PAX8 and PAX2 transcription factors are expressed by both normal and cancerous renal parenchyma. They can thus act as biomarkers to guide management towards identification of potential metastatic renal cancer foci. They are negative in angiomyolipoma [26].

Cytokeratins and Vimentin, though it is less specific and less sensitive than PAX8 or PAX2, are raised in the most common types of RCC. Clear and Papillary RCC express both and particularly useful to aid in differentiation of chRCC and oncocytomas [27, 28]. CK7 is a cytokeratin that stains cytoplasm and is useful for differentiation of multiple types of RCC. Martignoni et al. validated the use of 34βE12 in identifying pRCC and to aid in distinguishing it from ccRCC [29]. Cathepsin K was shown to be a marker for angiomyolipoma and translocation RCC. Alpha- SMA and desmin are muscle markers and help in diagnosis of angiomyolipomas. P53 is a tumour suppressor gene that shows positivity in epithelioid angiomyolipoma. It may stain in classic angiolipoma, but it stains much stronger in epithelioid angiolipoma. Other immunohistochemical markers include α-methylacyl coenzyme A racemase (AMACR), epithelial membrane antigen (EMA), CD10 and CA-IX. Immunohistochemical markers continue to be developed but their robust role beyond deciphering tumour characteristics in early detection remains to be established further.

Genetic Based Biomarkers

VHL Gene

von Hippel-Lindau (VHL) disease is an autosomal dominant tumour syndrome which predisposes patients to development of benign and malignant tumours including the nervous system and internal organs. The molecular basis of von Hippel-Lindau disease is the loss of function of the VHL protein. This leads to accumulation of hypoxia-inducible factor with downstream effects on cellular function and differentiation. Whereas the large majority of RCCs are sporadic, some are associated have hereditary associations. The most common RCC, ccRCC usually involves the VHL gene. Clinically, patients can be divided into VHL type 1 mainly without pheochromocytoma, and VHL type 2 mainly with pheochromocytoma. VHL type 2 is further stratified into type 2A and type 2B the former, with renal cancer and the latter without. Cytogenetically, there is loss of heterozygosity (LOH) of chromosome 3p, and biallelic inactivation of VHLgene (3p25), as well as gain of 5q22, loss of 6q, 8p, 9p and 14q. A screening platform with biomarker use and targeted treatment of lesions are of paramount importance in patients affected by VHL disease.

Other Genetic Based RCCs

Birt-Hogg-Dubé (BHD) syndrome is an inherited renal cancer syndrome caused by germline mutations in the *FLCN* gene on chromosome 17. Patients are at risk of developing cutaneous fibrofolliculomas, pulmonary cysts, spontaneous pneumothoraces, and kidney tumours. Emerging evidence links FLCN with a number of other molecular pathways and cellular processes including regulation of TFE3/TFEB transcriptional activity, amino acid-dependent mTOR activation through Rag GTPases, TGF-β signalling and PGC1α-driven mitochondrial activity. The potential role of biomarkers and surveillance with imaging modalities is evident. There is a need for biomarker discovery in these patients.

Imaging Modalities for Early Detection

Quantitative MRI and PET scan acquisitions and radiomic analysis provides an additional method to help decipher heterogeneity and better tumour characterization. Radiogenomics, radio metabolomics and coupling of these with clinical and tissue-based large data, can potentially improve diagnosis and tailored treatment of renal tumours.

MRI

Magnetic Resonance Imaging (MRI) represents a useful imaging biomarker for aiding in prediction of tumour subtype and for follow-up of patients to monitor treatment response.

Perfusion MRI (pMRI) detects tissue perfusion at the microcapillary level and involves dynamic contrast enhanced (DCE), dynamic susceptibility contrast (DSC) and arterial spin labelling (ASL). All three have been validated in the assessment of renal masses in terms of histology and grade. Lanzman et al. studied the diagnostic accuracy of ASL pMRI in predicting final histology of extirpated renal tumours. Correlating pre-procedural MRI with final histology, they found that ASL perfusion levels reliably allowed for differentiation between papillary RCC from other types of RCC. They also found reliable differentiation between oncocytomas and RCC. They also found reliability of ASL pMRI in monitoring response to systemic treatment in mRCC [30].

De Bezelaire et al. looked at the role of MRI in measured blood flow change after antiangiogenic therapy with PTK787/ZK 222584 and found that it correlates with clinical outcome in metastatic renal cell carcinoma. Patients with ASL pMRI at 1 and 4 months after tyrosine kinase inhibitor therapy were found to have early tumour blood flow changes that predicted clinical outcome [31]. The challenge with pMRI in terms of widespread and general application remain the technical challenges, cost and consistent expertise required to run a routine high-volume service. Diffusion MRI also has a role. The images exploit the observed differences in water movement in different tissue interfaces which aids in tumour histological prediction. Kang et al. did a systematic review and meta-analysis of diffusion-weighted imaging (DWI) studies in renal mass characterisation and found reasonable accuracy in distinguishing benign vs. malignant lesions (86% sensitivity and 78% specificity) and low-vs. high-grade ccRCC (AUC of 0.83) but could not reliably discriminate ccRCC from other renal tumours [32].

PET

Positron Emission Tomography (PET) scan is a form of functional and dynamic imaging that exploits molecular biology and tumour location and provides quantitative information about alterations in metabolism, cell proliferation, cell membrane metabolism, or the receptor expression using the standardized uptake value (SUV) [33–36]. While ^{18}F-fluoro-2-deoxy-2-d-glucose (FDG) PET is the most commonly used radiotracer in PET scanning. The National Comprehensive Cancer Network (NCCN) guidelines of 2020 and the European Association of Urology (EAU) guidelines of 2019 do not recommend the use of FDG PET scan in the staging of RCC [37, 38]. One must recall that the older studies on PET scans used for the previous studies did not utilize the modern PET scanners which are hybrid scanners, using multidetector row CT (MDCT) scan systems along with the PET scan to couple both anatomical and functional scanning.

Tracers targeting prostate specific membrane antigen (PSMA) and Carbonic Anhydrase (CA) IX which are expressed in RCC have evolved bring prospects of better imaging channels using PET. Large scale studies are pending. Modern PET/

CT scanners have the ability to potentially decipher the primary renal, predict grade and guide prognostication based on the intensity of FDG uptake. They are sensitive in detection of extrarenal synchronous or metachronous metastases. This aids optimisation of primary treatment and follow-up planning. The coupling of PET/CT with MRI has a role in tailoring the signatured treatment of specific cases e.g. the combined use of PET/CT or MRI picks up the changes indicating response to TKI therapy earlier than conventional imaging modalities. This is because of the ability to pick up alterations in the tumour microvascularity. Another role of PET is the ability to provide clinician with an image of the whole body in a single session. Apart from diagnosis, newer agents such as $^{Ga}68$ PSMA-labelled could have theragnostic applications in the treatment of metastatic RCC refractory to first- and second-line therapy.

The role of imaging modalities as biomarkers in diagnosis and treatment of renal tumours is an area of intense focus at present among research groups.

Newer Imaging Platforms

Novel imaging and radiomic analysis include texture quantification. This is a technique whereby automated image analysis is used to acquire a huge spectrum of imaging data to make quantitative decisions about defined tumour regions [39]. This can be used to aid in prediction of tumour phenotype and characteristics. Several groups are assessing the role of various modalities such as fractional water content (FWC) texture analysis (TA) to generate biologically relevant information from routine PET/MRI acquisitions for renal cancer patients.

Conclusions

Early diagnosis and treatment of disease processes is the remit of modern medicine. Renal cancer is no exception. However, renal cancer with its inherent heterogeneity, and often unpredictable nature, coupled with genetic variants add challenges to clinicians in deciphering optimal treatment regimens and predicting long-term prognosis. Renal tumours would benefit immensely from early diagnosis through optimal biomarker discovery and tailored treatment. Cross specialty research using high throughput data analysis and multicentre collaborative efforts through bioinformatics are clearly needed [40]. The present, near exponential development of novel tools both in the laboratory and at the bedside coupled with propulsion in advanced data analysis ushers with it an exciting time that could see paradigms in biomarker discovery.

Key Points

1. Renal cancer continues to impose a huge health burden on healthcare systems.
2. Despite the rapid developments in serum and urinary fluid analysis with high throughput diagnostic platforms, there is a dearth of optimal biomarkers in renal cancer.

3. More investment in research geared to biomarker discovery is needed.
4. Novel Imaging modalities will play a key area in the image-based stratification of renal tumours.
5. Multicentered high volume center collaboratives with robust tissue banking and evaluation will play a key role in the future of biomarker discovery.
6. Proteomics, genomics, metabolomics and radiomics and the combination of these platforms with high throughput real-time prospective evaluation will play a future key role in biomarker discovery.

References

1. https://www.cancer.org/cancer/kidney-cancer/about/key-statistics.html
2. Ferlay J, et al. Cancer incidence and mortality patterns in Europe: estimates for 40 countries and 25 major cancers in 2018. Eur J Cancer. 2018;103:356.
3. Capitanio U, et al. Epidemiology of renal cell carcinoma. Eur Urol. 2019;75:74.
4. Finelli A, Ismaila N, Bro B, et al. Management of small renal masses: american society of clinical oncology clinical practice guideline. J Clin Oncol. 2017;35:668–80.
5. Escudier B, Eisen T, Stadler WM, et al. Sorafenib for treatment of renal cell carcinoma: final efficacy and safety results of the phase III treatment approaches in renal cancer global evaluation trial. J Clin Oncol. 2009;27:3312–8.
6. Fitzgerald JP, Nayak B, Shanmugasundaram K, et al. Nox4 mediates renal cell carcinoma cell invasion through hypoxia-induced interleukin 6- and 8- production. PLoS One. 2012;7:e30712.
7. Tran HT, Liu Y, Zurita AJ, et al. Prognostic or predictive plasma cytokines and angiogenic factors for patients treated with pazopanib for metastatic renal-cell cancer: a retrospective analysis of phase 2 and phase 3 trials. Lancet Oncol. 2012;13:827–37.
8. Zurita AJ, Jonasch E, Wang X, et al. A cytokine and angiogenic factor (CAF) analysis in plasma for selection of sorafenib therapy in patients with metastatic renal cell carcinoma. Ann Oncol. 2012;23:46–52.
9. Funakoshi T, Lee CH, Hsieh JJ. A systematic review of predictive and prognostic biomarkers for VEGF-targeted therapy in renal cell carcinoma. Cancer Treat Rev. 2014;40:533–47.
10. Armstrong AJ, George DJ, Halabi S. Serum lactate dehydrogenase predicts for overall survival benefit in patients with metastatic renal cell carcinoma treated with inhibition of mammalian target of rapamycin. J Clin Oncol. 2012;30:3402–7.
11. Voss MH, Chen D, Marker M, et al. Circulating biomarkers and outcome from a randomised phase II trial of sunitinib vs everolimus for patients with metastatic renal cell carcinoma. Br J Cancer. 2016;114:642–9.
12. Modi PK, Farber NJ, Singer EA. Precision oncology: identifying predictive biomarkers for the treatment of metastatic renal cell carcinoma. Transl Cancer Res. 2016;5:S76–80.
13. Heng DY, Xie W, Regan MM, et al. Prognostic factors for overall survival in patients with metastatic renal cell carcinoma treated with vascular endothelial growth factor-targeted agents: results from a large, multicenter study. J Clin Oncol. 2009;27:5794–9.
14. Motzer RJ, Mazumdar M, Bacik J, et al. Survival and prognostic stratification of 670 patients with advanced renal cell carcinoma. J Clin Oncol. 1999;17:2530–40.
15. Boissier R, Campagna J, Branger N, et al. The prognostic value of the neutrophil-lymphocyte ratio in renal oncology: a review. Urol Oncol. 2017;35:135–41.
16. Ohno Y, Nakashima J, Ohori M, et al. Clinical variables for predicting metastatic renal cell carcinoma patients who might not benefit from cytoreductive nephrectomy: neutrophil-tolymphocyte ratio and performance status. Int J Clin Oncol. 2014;19:139–45.
17. Kommu S, Sharifi R, Edwards S, Eeles R. Proteomics and urine analysis: a potential promising new tool in urology. BJU Int. 2004 Jun;93(9):1172–3.

18. Kommu S, Sharifi R, Eeles RA. The proteomic approach to urological biomarkers. BJU Int. 2004 Dec;94(9):1215–6.
19. Morrissey JJ, London AN, Luo J, Kharasch ED. Urinary biomarkers for the early diagnosis of kidney cancer. Mayo Clin Proc. 2010 May;85(5):413–21.
20. Gatto F, Maruzzo M, Magro C, et al. Prognostic value of plasma and urine glycosaminoglycan scores in clear cell renal cell carcinoma. Front Oncol. 2016;6(253)
21. Wan JCM, Massie C, Garcia-Corbacho J, Mouliere F, Brenton JD, Caldas C, Pacey S, Baird R, Rosenfeld N. Liquid biopsies come of age: towards implementation of circulating tumour DNA. Nat Rev Cancer. 2017;17(4):223–38.
22. Quandt D, Zucht HD, Amann A, Wulf-goldenberg A, Borrebaeck C, Cannarile M, Lambrechts D, Oberacher H, Garrett J, Nayak T, Kazinski M, Massie C. Implementing liquid biopsies into clinical decision making for cancer immunotherapy. Oncotarget. 2017 Jul 18;8(29):48507–20.
23. Perakis S, Speicher MR. Emerging concepts in liquid biopsies. BMC Med. 2017;15(1):75.
24. Pal SK, Sonpavde G, Agarwal N, et al. Evolution of circulating tumor DNA (ctDNA) profile from first-line (1L) to second-line (2L) therapy in metastatic renal cell carcinoma (mRCC). J Clin Oncol. 2017;35. Abstract 434
25. Ball MW, Gorin MA, Guner G, et al. Circulating tumor DNA as a Marker of therapeutic response in patients with renal cell carcinoma: a pilot study. Clin Genitourin Cancer. 2016;14:e515–e20.
26. Shen SS, Truong LD, Scarpelli M, et al. Role of immunohistochemistry in diagnosing renal neoplasms: when is it really useful? Arch Pathol Lab Med. 2012;136:410–7.
27. Tan PH, Cheng L, Rioux-Leclercq N, et al. Renal tumors: diagnostic and prognostic biomarkers. Am J Surg Pathol. 2013;37:1518–31.
28. Kryvenko ON, Jorda M, Argani P, et al. Diagnostic approach to eosinophilic renal neoplasms. Arch Pathol Lab Med. 2014;138:1531–41.
29. Martignoni G, Brunelli M, Segala D, et al. Validation of 34betaE12 immunoexpression in clear cell papillary renal cell carcinoma as a sensitive biomarker. Pathology. 2017;49:10–8.
30. Lanzman RS, Robson PM, Sun MR, et al. Arterial spin-labeling MR imaging of renal masses: correlation with histopathologic findings. Radiology. 2012;265:799–808.
31. Bazelaire C, Alsop DC, George D, et al. Magnetic resonance imaging-measured blood flow change after antiangiogenic therapy with PTK787/ZK 222584 correlates with clinical outcome in metastatic renal cell carcinoma. Clin Cancer Res. 2008;14:5548–54.
32. Kang SK, Zhang A, Pandharipande PV, et al. DWI for renal mass characterization: systematic review and meta-analysis of diagnostic test performance. AJR Am J Roentgenol. 2015;205:317–24.
33. Haberkorn U, Strauss LG, Dimitrakopoulou A, Engenhart R, Oberdorfer F, Ostertag H, et al. PET studies of fluorodeoxyglucose metabolism in patients with recurrent colorectal tumors receiving radiotherapy. J Nucl Med. 1991;32:1485–90.
34. Kapoor V, BM MC, Torok FS. An introduction to PET-CT imaging. Radiographics. 2004;24:523–43.
35. Delbeke D, Martin WH. Positron emission tomography imaging in oncology. Radiol Clin N Am. 2001;39:883–917.
36. Liu Y, Ghesani NV, Zuckier LS. Physiology and pathophysiology of incidental findings detected on FDG-PET scintigraphy. Semin Nucl Med. 2010;40:294–315.
37. Comprehensive Cancer Network. Kidney Cancer NCCN Clinical Practice Guidelines in Oncology. Version 1.2021. [Last accessed on 22/08/2020]. https://www.nccn.org/professionals/physician_gls/pdf/kidney.pdf
38. Ljungberg B, Albiges L, Abu-Ghanem Y, Bensalah K, Dabestani S, Fernández-Pello S, et al. European Association of Urology guidelines on renal cell carcinoma: the 2019 update. Eur Urol. 2019;75:799–810.
39. Farber NJ, Wu Y, Zou L, et al. Challenges in RCC imaging: renal insufficiency, post-operative surveillance, and the role of Radiomics. Kidney Cancer J. 2015;13:84–90.
40. Kommu SS, Campbell C. The impact of recent developments in bioinformatics in uro-oncological research. BJU Int. 2006 Aug;98(2):249–51.

The Role of Biopsy in RCC

Nicholas Campain and Ravi Barod

Introduction

Small renal masses SRMs account for an increasing proportion of diagnosed RCCs [1]. Currently partial nephrectomy remains the 'gold standard' treatment for localised cT1a SRMs according to current guidelines [2, 3], aiming to preserve renal function and offer long term oncological control. With the increased detection of incidental SRMs, more widespread use of ablative treatments, increasing adoption of active surveillance strategies and ongoing developments in the management of metastatic disease, the indication for renal mass biopsy (RMB) has evolved significantly in recent years across all aspects of kidney cancer diagnosis and management. We describe the current role of RMB with a focus on aspects most relevant to patient management and clinical pathways.

Why Perform Renal Mass Biopsy

Increasing numbers of renal lesions are diagnosed as incidental findings due to the widespread utilisation of abdominal imaging, the majority of which are small renal masses (SRMs) defined as cT1a tumours <4 cm limited to the kidney [4]. Management strategies for cT1a SRMs include active surveillance, ablation or surgical excision with partial or radical nephrectomy. The choice between these options depends on patient and tumour factors as well as institution and surgeon experience. Although the majority of SRMs are malignant, up to 30% can be benign lesions [5, 6]. Imaging alone cannot reliably distinguish between benign and malignant renal masses. In the British Association of Urological Surgeons (BAUS) national partial

N. Campain · R. Barod (✉)
Specialist Centre for Kidney Cancer, Royal Free Hospital, London, UK
e-mail: r.barod@nhs.net

C. Anderson, M. Afshar (eds.), *Renal Cancer*,
https://doi.org/10.1007/978-3-030-84756-2_7

nephrectomy audit in 2012, 18% of surgically resected tumours were benign. The rate of benign histology increased to 36% in those under 40 years of age [7]. Likelihood of benign histology was also demonstrated with smaller tumour size (29% if tumour size <2.5 cm) and these findings have been replicated elsewhere [8]. Similarly in a large study of 18,060 patients who underwent partial nephrectomy over a 7 year period found consistently high rates of benign pathology of >30% were found for nearly every year of the study period [6].

Since partial or radical nephrectomy is associated with a 5% risk of ≥ Clavien 3 complication and a 0.5% mortality rate [9], efforts to minimise overtreatment of SRMs should be considered so patients who undergo potentially avoidable surgery for benign tumours are not exposed to unnecessary risks.

Historically the role of RMB was limited due to concerns regarding safety and accuracy [10], however contemporary studies have shown high diagnostic rates and a low side effect profile [10, 11]. RMB can therefore allow more informed patient decision making by differentiating between benign and malignant disease, which may affect treatment choice between surveillance, ablation, surgery, or follow up frequency. It may also allow differentiation between low and high grade kidney cancer, which can influence treatment choice and even type of surgery (partial vs radical nephrectomy).

Despite this, contemporary national datasets still provide evidence of low utilisation of RMB. In the 2013 to 2016 BAUS nephrectomy register 32,130 renal surgical cases were recorded. An analysis of the management of patients with a final histological diagnosis of oncocytoma (n = 1202), a benign renal lesion, demonstrated that only 2.9% of patients had preoperative RMB [12]. 683 patients (56.8%) underwent radical nephrectomy and 20.2% of the cohort had in-hospital complications, 48 of which were Clavien–Dindo grade ≥ III (4% of the total cohort), including five surgery related deaths. This clearly highlights the potential risks of surgery for benign disease, which may have potentially been avoided by use of RMB.

Current Trends

There remains significant variation in utilisation of RMB, with known differences in practice across the UK regarding if patients are offered a biopsy [13]. A survey of Canadian urologists in 2016 similarly highlighted low usage of RMB (53% of respondents never perform or perform RMB in <25% cases) [14].

The American Urological Association (AUA) guidelines state that renal mass biopsy should be considered when a mass is suspected to be hematologic, metastatic, inflammatory, or infectious [3]. In the setting of a solid renal mass, RMB is not required for young or healthy patients who are unwilling to accept the uncertainties associated with RMB. This is reflected in an analysis of the Surveillance, Epidemiology and End Results-Medicare (SEER) database of over 24,000 patients with RCC. Only 20% of patients underwent biopsy, although there was an increase in uptake with time this was mainly in patients having ablative treatment or with metastatic disease [15].

Doubt amongst urologists about the ability of RMB to change clinical practice appears to be one of the barriers to more widespread adoption. However evidence from high volume centres demonstrates that academic institutions are more likely to use active surveillance protocols for SRMs or residents with urological oncology fellowship training are more likely to request RMB to aid patient management [14].

The utility of RMB is not just limited to the management of SRMs. With the advent of immunotherapy and advances in targeted therapy for metastatic RCC, RMBs are increasingly used to obtain histological diagnosis prior to starting systemic therapy. Knowledge of histological sub-type can guide type of systemic treatment and also further inform decision-making when upfront cytoreductive nephrectomy is not indicated. Knowledge of histological sub-type in the metastatic setting also permits patient entry into novel clinical trials or may steer oncologists to consider immunotherapy rather than tyrosine-kinase inhibitors if biopsies indicate high degree of sarcomatoid differentiation.

How to Perform RMB

Percutaneous biopsies can be performed with either USS or CT guidance depending on local availability and expertise [16]. The EAU guidelines [2] recommend use of an eighteen gauge needle [17] to provide enough tissue for diagnosis and minimise morbidity, using a co-axial technique to allow multiple biopsies and minimise risk of seeding.

Non-diagnostic results are more likely with smaller masses, cystic masses and in early years of study, likely related to experience [8]. A retrospective analysis from our institution found a non-diagnostic rate of 42% when <2 cm in size [18]. For this reason the policy in the authors' institution is to avoid biopsy for lesions < 2cm in size and recommend active surveillance after appropriate counselling.

Needle core biopsies have been shown to have better sensitivity and specificity when compared with fine-needle aspiration technique in a meta-analysis of 57 studies with 5228 patients, with an overall median diagnostic rate of 92% [10]. A good agreement for histological subtype (K = 0.683) and surgical specimen was demonstrated with fair agreement for Furhrman grade and a low rate of CD > 2 complications. Most included studies were case series from single institutions and reported on patients who underwent surgery, with only 5 prospective studies. The CB non-diagnostic rate was 0–22.6% (8% in meta-analysis), however repeat biopsies are known to be diagnostic in majority of cases (83%) [19]. Another systematic review of 2979 patients from 20 studies also showed high diagnostic accuracy of RMB with sensitivity of 97.5% and specificity of 96.2%, again with good concordance for histological sub-type [11].

Practicalities to maximise diagnostic yield include:

- Two good quality core biopsies
- Avoid necrotic areas

- Peripheral biopsies preferable for larger tumours (to avoid necrotic areas)
- Multiple quadrant technique from four separate solid enhancing areas (for cT2a lesions—0% non-diagnostic yield with improved sensitivity (>85%) for detecting sarcomatoid features) [20].
- Avoid RMB of cystic masses

RMB have low morbidity. In the meta-analysis of 5228 patients spontaneously resolving haematoma were reported in 4.3% of cases but clinically significant bleeding was only 0.7% in the pooled analysis [10]. In a large retrospective series of 529 patients adverse events were low (8.5%) and self-limiting in all but one case [21]. RMB has also been shown to be safe for larger renal masses (no complications with n = 78 patients with multi-quadrant technique in T2 tumours) [20].

Common side effects that patients should be warned about include: discomfort at biopsy site, skin bruising, requirement for multiple puncture sites, no guarantee of definitive diagnosis, need for further/repeat procedures and 2% risk of bleeding from biopsy site.

Due to the well known tumour heterogeneity seen in RCC, grade concordance on RMB has been challenging, with sub-optimal levels using the 4-stage Fuhrman grading system. However by grouping Fuhrman grade into 'low' and 'high' grade good prognostic value has been demonstrated [22]. Biopsies of cystic masses have a lower diagnostic yield, but can still be used when solid areas are present (for example in Bosniak IV cysts) [21, 23].

Controversies in Renal Biopsy

Concerns have previously been raised about the false negative rate of RMB. Most false negative biopsies are due to sampling error, with the biopsy yielding normal renal tissue. In this situation, patients should be offered a repeat biopsy [18] or a period of initial surveillance, unless they have a clear preference for an intervention to treat their renal mass. True false negatives, where an inaccurate misdiagnosis of pathological tissue is made, is becoming increasingly rare with more sophisticated immunohistochemical characterization of the biopsy sample. The frequency of this is unquantified but there is currently no evidence to suggest that this is significant.

Tumour seeding in the biopsy tract has also been a concern of urologists and is another barrier to the use of RMB. The occurrence of microscopic tumour seeding is thought to be under reported but is quoted at <1%. A recent report highlighted tumour seeding on histological examination of the resection specimen after surgical treatment for RCC and found 7 cases of tumour seeding [23]. Six of these 7 cases were papillary RCC subtype and 6 of the patients remained recurrence free at last follow up [13]. Therefore, even though microscopic tumour cell seeding is rare, subsequent clinical consequence is even rarer.

The effect of RMB on subsequent surgery has also been questioned, with a perception that it leads to increased complexity. A review of patients undergoing nephrectomy after renal mass biopsy from the Ontario Cancer Registry found that although operative times were slightly higher, there was no difference in complications when compared with those who had not had a prior biopsy. Those that were biopsied had a decreased likelihood of undergoing surgery for benign disease [24].

How RMB Can Change Clinical Management

Routine use of RMB is associated with lower rates of histologically benign tumours after surgery, as demonstrated in a multi-centre study comparing centres that routinely use RMB compared to those with selective use of RMB (5% vs 16%). This suggests that biopsies may reduce surgery and associated risks for benign tumours [14].

Histological confirmation of SRM grade and sub-type also allows more informed patient decision making and may help identify tumours at lower risk of progression. This may identify patients who can be safely managed with active surveillance or delayed intervention.

EAU guidelines make a 'strong' recommendation to perform RMB before ablative therapy to avoid potential overtreatment. A recent study comparing RMB biopsy before vs during thermal ablation (TA) demonstrated that 80% of those patients with a benign biopsy chose not to undergo intervention [25]. Historically many reported series of ablative treatment outcomes have included large numbers of numbers of patients undergoing treatment for SRMs identified on imaging alone. Since the likelihood of benign histology is greater with smaller tumour size [8, 21, 26], it is likely that a high proportion of patients may have had unnecessary treatment. Patients without biopsy undergoing ablative therapy are often then subsequently submitted to potentially unnecessary and costly radiological follow up.

In addition to the benefits of RMB to better inform urologists and patients to assist with treatment decision making, RMB has also been shown to be cost-effective when integrated into the diagnostic pathway. Using a decision-analytic Markov model, RMB and upfront surgery demonstrated similar quality adjusted life expectancy but at lower lifetime cost for RMB, highlighting the use of RMB as a cost-effective strategy to triage patients for surgery and avoiding unnecessary treatment [27].

Conclusions

Modern management of the small renal mass involves surgery, ablation and surveillance. RMB is safe, accurate and does not significantly complicate surgery. It can increase diagnostic certainty of radiologically identified enhancing renal masses and can be used intelligently to guide the management of renal cancer.

Key Points

1. RMB is a safe diagnostic test with low complication rates
2. RMB provides more detailed histological information to inform treatment choice
3. Surgical treatment and risk can be avoided if benign histology confirmed
4. RMB can stratify patients to active surveillance +/− delayed intervention
5. RMB prior to ablative therapy for SRMs can avoid unnecessary treatment and cross-sectional imaging follow up
6. RMB can change operative decision making (radical rather than partial nephrectomy if aggressive sub-type identified)
7. RMB prior to surgery is not associated with adverse perioperative or oncological outcomes
8. Seeding from RMB is rare and of uncertain clinical significance
9. RMB facilitates appropriate systemic therapy in the metastatic setting
10. RMB is cost-effective when used to avoid surgery (and its complications) in patients with benign disease

References

1. Hollingsworth JM, Miller DC, Daignault S, Hollenbeck BK. Rising incidence of small renal masses: a need to reassess treatment effect. J Natl Cancer Inst. 2006;98(18):1331–4. Available from: https://pubmed.ncbi.nlm.nih.gov/16985252/
2. EAU Guidelines: Renal Cell Carcinoma|Uroweb [Internet]. [cited 2021 May 7]. Available from: https://uroweb.org/guideline/renal-cell-carcinoma/
3. Renal Cancer: Renal Mass & Localized Renal Cancer Guideline–American Urological Association [Internet]. [cited 2021 May 7]. Available from: https://www.auanet.org/guidelines/guidelines/renal-cancer-renal-mass-and-localized-renal-cancer-guideline
4. Volpe A, Panzarella T, Rendon RA, Haider MA, Kondylis FI, MAS J. The natural history of incidentally detected small renal masses. Cancer. 2004;100(4):738–45. Available from: https://pubmed.ncbi.nlm.nih.gov/14770429/
5. Frank I, Blute ML, Cheville JC, Lohse CM, Weaver AL, Zincke H. Solid renal tumors: an analysis of pathological features related to tumor size. J Urol. 2003;170(6 I):2217–20. Available from: https://pubmed.ncbi.nlm.nih.gov/14634382/
6. Kim JH, Li S, Khandwala Y, Chung KJ, Park HK, Chung BI. Association of Prevalence of benign pathologic findings after partial nephrectomy with preoperative imaging patterns in the United States from 2007 to 2014. JAMA Surg. 2019;154:225–31. American Medical Association; Available from: /pmc/articles/PMC6439638/
7. Fernando A, Fowler S, O'Brien T, Abbasi Z, Adamson AS, Addla SK, et al. Nephron-sparing surgery across a nation–outcomes from the British Association of Urological Surgeons 2012 national partial nephrectomy audit. BJU Int. 2016;117(6):874–82. Available from: https://pubmed.ncbi.nlm.nih.gov/26469291/
8. Jeon HG, Seo SIL, Jeong BC, Jeon SS, Lee HM, Choi HY, et al. Percutaneous kidney biopsy for a small renal mass: a critical appraisal of results. J Urol. 2016;195(3):568–73. Available from: https://pubmed.ncbi.nlm.nih.gov/26410732/

9. Ljungberg B, Bensalah K, Canfield S, Dabestani S, Hofmann F, Hora M, et al. EAU guidelines on renal cell carcinoma: 2014 update. Eur Urol. 2015;67(5):913–24. Available from: https://pubmed.ncbi.nlm.nih.gov/25616710/
10. Marconi L, Dabestani S, Lam TB, Hofmann F, Stewart F, Norrie J, et al. Systematic review and meta-analysis of diagnostic accuracy of percutaneous renal tumour biopsy. Eur Urol. Elsevier B.V. 2016;69:660–73.
11. Patel HD, Johnson MH, Pierorazio PM, Sozio SM, Sharma R, Iyoha E, et al. Diagnostic accuracy and risks of biopsy in the diagnosis of a renal mass suspicious for localized renal cell carcinoma: systematic review of the literature. J Urol. 2016;195(5):1340–7. Available from: https://pubmed.ncbi.nlm.nih.gov/26901507/
12. Neves JB, Withington J, Fowler S, Patki P, Barod R, Mumtaz F, et al. Contemporary surgical management of renal oncocytoma: a nation's outcome. BJU Int. 2018;121(6):893–9. Available from: https://pubmed.ncbi.nlm.nih.gov/29397002/
13. Tran MGB, Barod R, Bex A, Macklin PS, Sullivan ME, Tapping CR, et al. Tumour seeding in the tract of percutaneous renal tumour biopsy: a report on seven cases from a UK tertiary referral Centre. Eur Urol. 2019;75:861–7. Vol. 75, European Urology. Elsevier B.V.; 2019 [cited 2021 May 5]. p. e181–2. Available from: https://pubmed.ncbi.nlm.nih.gov/30833137/
14. Richard PO, Martin L, Lavallée LT, Violette PD, Komisarenko M, Evans AJ, et al. Identifying the use and barriers to the adoption of renal tumour biopsy in the management of small renal masses. Can Urol Assoc J. 2018;12(8):260–6. Available from: https://pubmed.ncbi.nlm.nih.gov/29629862/
15. Leppert JT, Hanley J, Wagner TH, Chung BI, Srinivas S, Chertow GM, et al. Utilization of renal mass biopsy in patients with renal cell carcinoma. Urology. 2014;83(4):774–80. Available from: https://pubmed.ncbi.nlm.nih.gov/24529579/
16. Leveridge MJ, Finelli A, Kachura JR, Evans A, Chung H, Shiff DA, et al. Outcomes of small renal mass needle core biopsy, nondiagnostic percutaneous biopsy, and the role of repeat biopsy. Eur Urol. 2011;60(3):578–84.
17. Breda A, Treat EG, Haft-Candell L, Leppert JT, Harper JD, Said J, et al. Comparison of accuracy of 14-, 18- and 20-G needles in ex-vivo renal mass biopsy: a prospective, blinded study. BJU Int. 2010;105(7):940–5. Available from: https://pubmed.ncbi.nlm.nih.gov/19888984/
18. BAUS 2020 Abstracts, 2020 [Internet]. [cited 2021 May 11]. https://doi.org/10.1177/2051415820963006.
19. Richard PO, Jewett MAS, Tanguay S, Saarela O, Liu ZA, Pouliot F, et al. Safety, reliability and accuracy of small renal tumour biopsies: results from a multi-institution registry. BJU Int. 2017 Apr 1;119(4):543–9.
20. Abel EJ, Heckman JE, Hinshaw L, Best S, Lubner M, Jarrard DF, et al. Multi-quadrant biopsy technique improves diagnostic ability in large heterogeneous renal masses. J Urol. 2015;194(4):886–91. Available from: https://pubmed.ncbi.nlm.nih.gov/25837535/
21. Richard PO, Jewett MAS, Bhatt JR, Kachura JR, Evans AJ, Zlotta AR, et al. Renal tumor biopsy for small renal masses: a single-center 13-year experience. Eur Urol. 2015;68(6):1007–13.
22. Evans AJ, Delahunt B, Srigley JR. Issues and challenges associated with classifying neoplasms in percutaneous needle biopsies of incidentally found small renal masses. Semin Diagn Pathol. 2015;32(2):184–95. Available from: https://pubmed.ncbi.nlm.nih.gov/25769205/
23. Volpe A, Mattar K, Finelli A, Kachura JR, Evans AJ, Geddie WR, et al. Contemporary results of percutaneous biopsy of 100 small renal masses: a single center experience. J Urol. 2008;180(6):2333–7. Available from: https://pubmed.ncbi.nlm.nih.gov/18930274/
24. Wallis CJD, Garbens A, Klaassen Z, Kodama RT, Herschorn S, Nam RK. Effect of renal mass biopsy on subsequent nephrectomy outcomes: a population-based assessment. Eur Urol. Elsevier B.V. 2020;77:136–7. https://doi.org/10.1016/j.eururo.2019.09.025.
25. Widdershoven CV, Aarts BM, Zondervan PJ, Henderickx MMEL, Klompenhouwer EG, van Delden OM, et al. Renal biopsies performed before versus during ablation of T1 renal tumors:

implications for prevention of overtreatment and follow-up. Abdom Radiol. 2021;46(1):373–9. Available from: https://pubmed.ncbi.nlm.nih.gov/32564209/
26. Parks GE, Perkins LA, Zagoria RJ, Garvin AJ, Sirintrapun SJ, Geisinger KR. Benefits of a combined approach to sampling of renal neoplasms as demonstrated in a series of 351 cases. Am J Surg Pathol. 2011;35(6):827–35. Available from: https://pubmed.ncbi.nlm.nih.gov/21552112/
27. Pandharipande PV, Gervais DA, Hartman RI, Harisinghani MG, Feldman AS, Mueller PR, et al. Renal mass biopsy to guide treatment decisions for small incidental renal tumors: a cost-effectiveness analysis. Radiology. 2010;256(3):836–46. Available from: https://pubmed.ncbi.nlm.nih.gov/20720070/

Active Surveillance in Renal Cancer

Sonpreet Rai, Yaamini Premakumar, and Ben Challacombe

Introduction

The American Joint Committee on Cancer (AJCC) tumour-node-metastasis (TNM) staging for renal cancer defines a small renal mass (SRM) as stage T1a [1]; a solid renal cortical neoplasm that is less than or equal to 4 cm in greatest dimension and limited to the kidney [2].

The last few decades have seen the emergence of nephron sparing approaches to manage the SRM. The preferred surgical option and current standard of care is a partial nephrectomy which has been shown to provide excellent oncologic outcomes with preservation of renal function [3]. Non-surgical thermal ablative techniques including cryoablation and radiofrequency ablation have also been shown to have very low rates of local tumour progression and metastatic disease.

The emergence of Active Surveillance (AS) as an oncologically safe and effective management option for the SRM has also gained traction over the last decade. Approximately 20–40% of SRM's are benign [4] and a large proportion, 70% to 80% of malignant SRM's are low grade renal cell carcinomas. The rates of metastatic disease for tumours 3 cm or less are <1% and approximately 2% for 4 cm tumours [5, 6].

S. Rai (✉) · Y. Premakumar · B. Challacombe
Department of Urology, Guys and St. Thomas' NHS Foundation Trust, London, UK
e-mail: SRAI2@gstt.nhs.uk

C. Anderson, M. Afshar (eds.), *Renal Cancer*,
https://doi.org/10.1007/978-3-030-84756-2_8

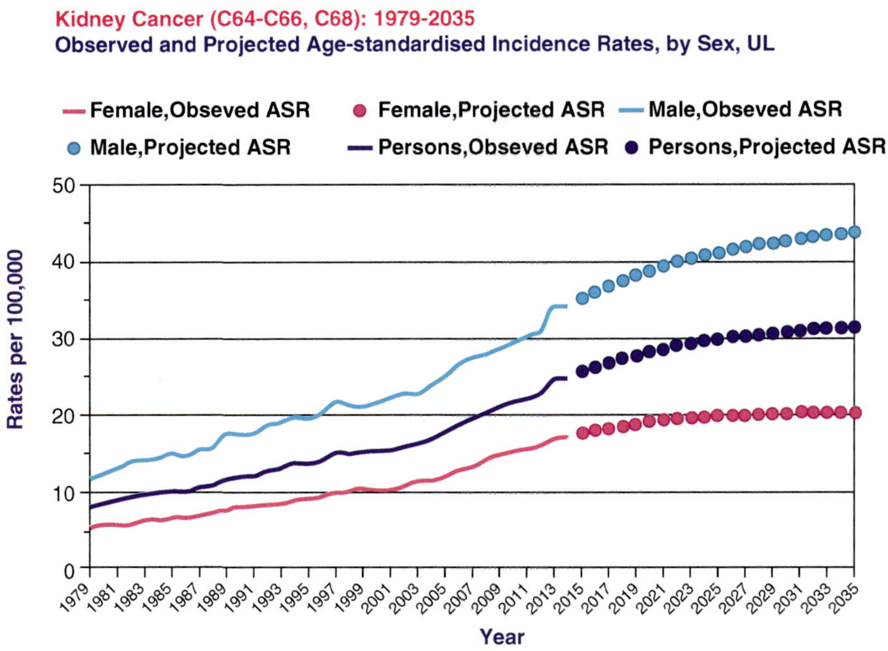

Fig. 1 The observed and projected age-standardised incidence rates, by gender, of renal cancer in the United Kingdom

Active Surveillance

Active surveillance (AS) is a form of expectant management defined as a scheduled serial assessment to evaluate tumour progression and growth rate with a view to initiating curative management once specified criteria are met. AS differs from 'watchful waiting' or 'observation' where serial assessment may be used for diagnostic and monitoring purposes without a specified schedule and may be based on subjective patient symptoms with a view to palliation if needed. AS offers a significant benefit of avoiding side effects from unnecessary treatment whilst providing clinicians and patients with a more proactive method of monitoring tumours [7].

AS of SRMs has evolved as a safe management option over the last few decades. AS may be used in conjunction with a delayed intervention as an option for patients who:

- Wish to avoid surgery
- Are willing to accept the risk of potential tumour progression compared to curative management
- Are considered high risk for surgical therapy [8].

Evaluation of AS as a management option requires thorough assessment of patient baseline/functional status, tumour, and treatments (see Table 1).

Table 1 Important factors when considering active surveillance [8–12]

Patient factors	Tumour factors	Treatment factors
Age	Imaging – Degree of infiltration – Endophytic/exophytic component – Degree and pattern of enhancement	Risk of tumour progression and/or metastasis and the subsequent effect on: – Renal function – Suitability for other management options – Patient's well-being
Co-morbidities	– Renal tumour biopsy – Histological subtype – Grade – Tumour biomarkers	Triggers for delayed intervention
Life expectancy	Progression and expected growth rate (e.g., compared to previous imaging)	Efficacy of intervention
Functional status		Availability of management options
Patient expectations		
Psychological outcomes		
Renal function		

Patient Selection

With the majority of SRMs now being diagnosed incidentally as result of widespread imaging, the incidence of real cancer is projected to rise (Fig. 1). It is important to consider the investigation and management of these often asymptomatic patients. Active surveillance is considered most useful for those whose tumour appears benign or likely to be indolent. In general, the advice is that larger tumours (>3–4 cm) and those with aggressive appearances (e.g., infiltrative growth patterns) should be managed in a proactive manner as they may be associated with increased risk of progression and metastasis [9].

There is no consensus regarding which patients are most appropriate for AS. The American Society of Clinical Oncology (ASCO) recommend active surveillance as an initial management option for those with significant comorbidities and limited life expectancy. They recommend absolute indications for AS consisting of patients with high risk for anaesthetic and intervention, or life expectancy <5 years. Relative indications include significant risk of end-stage renal disease if the SRM is treated, SRM <1 cm, or life expectancy <10 years.

The Delayed Intervention and Surveillance for Small Renal Masses (DISSRM) Registry (a multi-centre cohort study in United States of America following over 400 AS patients) do not recommend specific criteria for which patients should be managed with AS but found that patients opting for AS compared to intervention were older (70.8 years vs 61.8 years; $P < 0.001$), in worse health (based on performance status) and had smaller tumours (1.8 cm vs 2.5 cm; $P < 0.001$) [11]. The DISSRM registry acknowledges AS as an initial management option for all patients with SRM, encouraging shared decision-making between patients and clinicians. They also recommend it as a primary management option for patients with tumours <2 cm or those of 'advanced age with medical comorbidities' but do not specify definitions.

Role of Renal Tumour Biopsy

The role of percutaneous renal tumour biopsy (RTB) continues to remain a contentious area. There is no consensus as to whether every patient with a SRM should undergo a biopsy procedure or select cases only on an individualised basis. A diagnosis of malignancy ascertained by RTB is considered fairly accurate with the overall median diagnostic rate as 92%, with a sensitivity and specificity of 99.1% and 99.7% for core biopsy [6, 13].

The ASCO guidelines recommend all patients with a SRM should be considered for RTB, based on tumour-specific findings, competing risks of mortality, and when the results may alter management [12]. Specifically, they recommend RTB may be useful in patients with clinical findings suggesting lymphoma, abscess, or secondary renal metastasis. ASCO also recommend RTB should be considered for patients undergoing AS as the biopsy helps assess metastatic risk and therefore helps with patient counselling and managing patient expectations [12].

American Urological Association (AUA) guidelines recommend RTB in any mass not considered to be a primary solid renal tumour (e.g., haematological, metastatic, inflammatory, infectious appearances) as it will help confirm diagnosis and direct therapy. It does not recommend RTB for young or healthy patients unwilling to accept the uncertainty or who will elect for intervention regardless of the result. Nor does it recommend RTB for older or frail patients who will be managed conservatively. If proceeding with RTB, AUA recommends multiple core biopsies (2–3 cores with a 16–18-gauge needle under CT/US guidance rather than FNA) [8]. Finally, AUA recommends RTB in all patients undergoing thermal ablation as the tissue necrosis post-intervention hinders subsequent histological diagnosis.

European Association of Urology (EAU) guidelines recommend a RTB should be considered in patients who are candidates for AS of small masses, to obtain histology prior to ablative treatment and for the selection of the most suitable medical and surgical management in metastatic disease [10–12]. A RTB is not indicated in frail or comorbid patients that are planned for a watchful waiting approach and masses that are contrast enhancing or cystic, and in whom surgery in planned. RTB of cystic tumour masses are not recommended [14].

A renal tumour biopsy is not without its complications. The non-diagnostic rate has been reported as between 10–20% [5]. Common complications have been reported to include lumbar pain and haematoma (4.3%), of which the majority are self-resolving [15]. The risk of tumour seeding along the tract is relatively rare, especially with the co-axial technique. The Renal Cancer Group from Oxford have reported 7 cases where tumour seeding was identified on histological examination of the resection specimen after surgical resection of the renal cell carcinoma following diagnostic percutaneous biopsy [16]. Six of the seven cases were of papillary RCC type. The clinical significance of this remains uncertain, only one of the patients developed local tumour recurrence at the site of the previous biopsy.

A multicentre study has shown that in departments where renal tumour biopsies are performed frequently, the likelihood of benign findings at pathology is significantly lower (5% vs. 16%) suggesting renal tumour biopsies could reduce the incidence of surgery for benign tumours and the associated risk and morbidity that is involved [17].

Overall, it is important to consider the role of RTB in AS, as imaging alone cannot provide a definitive diagnosis of malignancy. Factors to take into account when deciding if RTB is appropriate would be whether patients are fit candidates for surgery, the suspected tumour aetiology and whether systemic and/or other non-cancer treatments are indicated.

Imaging Surveillance

Numerous imaging modalities may be used for serial assessment of SRMs. Ultrasound imaging (USS) tends to be low cost, avoids radiation exposure and relatively easily accessible; however, can be operator-dependent and may not provide the level of detail required to fully assess the tumour for signs of growth and/or progression. Thus, often the size/diameter is the key factor reported. Computed tomography (CT) offers detailed assessment of the tumour and is relatively accessible, however it exposes patients to radiation and/or contrast depending on the protocol used, which is not ideal in a population likely to have or to develop reduced kidney function. Finally magnetic resonance imaging (MRI) offers a very detailed assessment of the tumour however is costly, less accessible, and may be contraindicated in certain patients depending on their medical history.

There is no consensus regarding which imaging modality is ideal for AS. Different protocols exist and tend to incorporate a mix of modalities. AUA guidelines recommend cross-sectional imaging and/or USS every 3–6 months alongside assessment of renal function (serum creatinine level, proteinuria) and metabolism (liver function tests); and chest imaging [8]. The ASCO protocol is axial imaging (or USS) every 3 months for the first year, followed by every 6 months in the second and third years, and annually thereafter [12].

The DISSRM protocol consists of USS every 6 months for 2 years and then annually afterwards. They report alternating between cross-sectional imaging and USS for most patients alongside monitoring renal function annually [11]. Following this protocol, there was a 100% and 99% 5-year cancer-specific survival for patients undergoing AS compared to primary intervention. The 5-year overall survival was 75% and 92% respectively [18].

An important factor in deciding the frequency for serial imaging is tumour size and growth rate. Growth is often expressed as maximum tumour diameter over time (e.g., mm/year). Growth is considered the most objective factor to aid identifying sinister SRMs [6].

It is accepted that smaller tumours are often associated with reduced malignancy risk, with SRMs <1 cm considered benign in 50% of cases [8]. However the risk of malignancy increases to 75% in lesions 1–2.9 cm in size. In those lesions diagnosed as renal cell carcinomas, aggressive tumour behaviour has only been observed in 20–25% of cases of lesions <7 cm [8, 12, 13]. Given that a high propensity of SRMs are likely to be benign, there may be an argument for the least invasive and safest imaging modality of USS to be used.

Tumour growth rate and metastatic potential are also factors to consider when deciding frequency and imaging modality. SRMs are considered low metastatic risk as they have an annual metastatic potential of approximately 3%. SRMs tend to grow at a rate of roughly 2–3 mm per year [19]. However, it should be noted that the natural history of SMRs is difficult to ascertain as it was previously thought the gold standard of care was surgical removal soon after diagnosis, which resulted in a lack of long-term data [20]. There is an overall belief that SRMs experience variable growth each year, from positive growth to no growth, therefore deciding when to change to curative intervention should not be based on growth alone [21, 22]. Deciding on frequency of imaging in AS and criteria for when to change from AS to definitive management should incorporate growth alongside other clinical and biochemical factors. The benefit of using AS is that it allows for a personalised and dynamic approach to patients and their SRM.

Currently, there is no widely accepted protocol for optimal imaging modality and frequency in AS but USS is often recommended based on its safety profile allowing it to be used more regularly as needed. Published protocols and guidelines seem to suggest a range of frequencies for imaging from 3 months to annually.

Chest imaging is often considered as part of monitoring for SRMs to detect metachronous or synchronous metastatic disease. A recent study from the DISSRM registry analysed the chest imaging performed on initiation of AS and found that 19% (51/268) of patients had abnormal baseline chest radiographs. Of this, 22 (43%) had pathology which was acted upon (e.g., pulmonary nodules, thyroid nodules, mediastinal masses). Of the 217 who had normal initial chest radiographs, only 23 (11%) developed abnormal findings on subsequently yearly chest imaging with 10 having actionable pathology. No patient developed metastatic RCC [23]. From these findings, it may be recommended to perform chest radiograph or CT monitoring for patients who are high risk of metastatic RCC and/or patients who have abnormal findings on baseline chest imaging.

Parameters to Monitor in AS

There are no set criteria which should trigger a change in management for the SRM undergoing AS. Criteria which may be considered include: tumour size, rate of tumour growth, level of infiltration, surrounding structures infiltrated, clinical

Table 2 Triggers for intervention when on AS from ASCO, AUA and DISSRM guidelines

ASCO [12]	AUA Guidelines [8]	DISSRM [11]
Tumour size >4 cm	Tumour size >3 cm	Tumour size >4 cm
Tumour growth >5 mm/year	Tumour growth >5 mm/year	Tumour growth >5 mm/year
	Clinical changes in patient/tumour factors	Elective crossover (e.g., change in patient preference or improvement in patient health)
	Stage progression	Metastatic progression of disease
		Development of symptoms (e.g., haematuria without other cause)

AUA American Urological Association, *DISSRM* Delayed Intervention and Surveillance for Small Renal Masses.

changes in patient, change in patient preference. The Table 2 below summarises existing guidelines:

Risks and Benefits of AS

The risks and benefits of AS should be considered with every patient and a balanced discussion should take place prior to commencing AS.

Risks include a small but present risk of cancer progression and potential lack of curative therapies should the cancer metastasize [24, 25]. AS has been associated with relatively low rates of growth and metastatic progression of tumour in short-term follow-up (2–3 years) as it tends to be selected for smaller and more benign-appearing tumours [8]. The window for surgical management may also be missed either due to tumour progression and/or patients' overall health status deteriorating.

Benefits include avoiding overdiagnosis and overtreatment of potentially elderly and comorbid patients. A concern of initiating AS is whether it would have an effect on patients' psychology given that some may interpret it as a more passive form of management. However, it should be emphasized to patients and clinicians alike that AS consists of active monitoring with the view to changing management, if appropriate, when triggers are met. The only study to look at the effect of AS on patients' well-being was a multicentre study which assessed quality of life (QoL) of patients undergoing AS ($n = 101$) vs immediate intervention ($n = 226$) and they found that there was no adverse effect on mental health 1 year on [26].

What Do the Guidelines State?

A summary of association recommendations is as follows (Table 3):

Table 3 A summary of guidelines published regarding AS

	American Society of Clinical Oncology (ASCO) [12]	American Urological Association (AUA) [8]	Delayed Intervention and Surveillance for Small Renal Masses (DISSRM) Registry [11]	European Association of UrologY (EAU) [10]
Candidate for AS	Absolute indications High risk for anaesthetic and/or intervention Life expectancy <5 years Relative indications Significant risk of end-stage renal disease if treated SRM <1 cm Life expectancy <10 years	Any renal mass < 2 cm Significant comorbidities Significant life expectancy Risk of intervention outweighs potential benefits of active treatment	Did not recommend specific criteria however found patients opting for AS were: – Older – In worse health (based on performance status) – Smaller tumours (<2 cm)	Significant comorbidities Elderly
RTB	Suggests all patients with SRM should be considered for RTB based on tumour-specific findings, competing risks of mortality and when results may alter management (specifically in patients with clinical findings suggesting lymphoma, abscess or secondary renal metastasis). They recommend considering it in every patient as biopsy may help assess metastatic risk and guide patient counselling.	Suggests RTB for any mass not considered to be a primary solid tumour (e.g., haematological, metastatic, inflammatory, infectious appearances) to help confirm diagnosis and direct therapy. Does not recommend for young or healthy patients unwilling to accept the uncertainty or who elect for intervention regardless of the result. Does not recommend for older or frail patients who will be managed conservatively.	Suggests in patients for whom choice of AS or primary intervention is unclear Patient undergoing AS with growth >5 mm/year	Suggests RTB in patients who are candidates for AS with small masses Suggests RTB prior to ablative therapy Suggests RTB in SRMs to select most suitable medical/surgical management of metastatic disease. Does not recommend for frail or comorbid patients undergoing watchful waiting Does not recommend for masses that contrast-enhancing or cystic tumour masses Does not recommend for patients undergoing surgery

Table 3 (continued)

AS protocol suggested	Axial abdominal imaging (or USS) every 3 months in the first year, twice in the second and third years, and annually afterwards.	Cross-sectional imaging +/– USS every 3–6 months. Consider alternatives to contrast when possible or necessary (doppler, diffusion weighted images, etc). Consider renal function assessment (serum Cr, proteinuria), liver function tests and chest imaging.	USS every 6 months for 2 years and then annually afterwards. Recommend alternating between cross-sectional and USS. Monitor renal function annually. Recommend annual chest imaging if baseline chest radiograph is abnormal.	Does not specify
Triggers for intervention	Tumour size>4 cm Tumour growth >5 mm/year	Tumour size >3 cm Tumour growth >5 mm/year Clinical changes in patient/tumour factors Stage progression Benefits of treatment outweigh the risk	Tumour size >4 cm Tumour growth >5 mm/year Elective crossover (e.g., change in patient preference or improvement in patient health) Metastatic progression of disease Development of symptoms (e.g., haematuria without other cause)	Does not specify

AS Active surveillance, *SRM* small renal mass, *RTB* renal tumour biopsy, *USS* ultrasound scan, *cm* centimetre, *mm* millimetre, *Cr* Creatinine.

Key Points

- A Small Renal Mass (SRM) is classified as stage T1a - ≤4 cm
- 20–40% of SRM's are benign
- The risk of metastases from a SRM that is ≤3 cm is less than 1%
- Active surveillance consists of scheduled serial monitoring of the tumour with the view to changing the management approach should specified criteria be met (i.e., tumour growth, tumour progression, patient preference).
- The rationale for Active surveillance is that the slow-growth and low metastatic rates of SRMs could negate the beneficial effect of active management and avoid unnecessary procedures in poor surgical candidates: the elderly and/or comorbid patients with low life expectancy.
- There are patient factors, tumour factors and treatment factors that must be considered as part of the shared decision-making process with the patient
- Renal tumour biopsy should be considered when a histological diagnosis will change management, which ranges from confirming a benign diagnosis, preventing further surgery or to confirm metastatic disease from extrarenal malignancies.
- The non-diagnostic rate of renal tumour biopsy is approximately 10–20%, however, in centres where high numbers of renal mass biopsy is performed, the likelihood of benign surgical histopathology has dropped to ≤5%
- There is no ideal imaging modality type or schedule. Each patient must have an individualised plan based on their tumour characteristics and comorbidities.
- A combination of USS/CT/MRI imaging will provide the most detailed information to aid surveillance planning and protocol
- The patient may choose to come off Active Surveillance at any time with the knowledge that treatment with curative intent is available

Conclusion

The literature on SRMs is limited to case series, observational studies, and non-randomized comparative studies using statistical means to compensate for biases. Of this, most of the literature is based on open surgical approaches while few studies focus on AS [8]. Therefore, the evidence for and against AS ought to be considered in the context of this paucity of literature and could serve as a focus for future research.

Active surveillance proves to be a useful management option of small renal masses. It is particularly useful in elderly and comorbid patients, who are increasing in numbers given our ageing population, however, it should not be underestimated as a management option for others. AS is useful for SRMs, which are statistically likely to be benign and/or remain indolent, and could avoid unnecessary overtreatment.

The most important aspect of a patient's SRM management is the personalised multidisciplinary approach alongside patient preference. AS is a management option that facilitates shared decision-making between the clinician and patient. The highly selective group of elderly and comorbid patients should be offered an individualised AS plan as part of the standard discussion for their SRM management.

References

1. Amin MB, Edge SB, Greene FL, et al., editors. AJCC cancer staging manual. 8th ed. Switzerland: Springer; 2017.
2. Swami U, Nussenzveig RH, Haaland B, Agarwal N. Revisiting AJCC TNM staging for renal cell carcinoma: quest for improvement. Ann Transl Med. 2019 Mar;7(S1):S18.
3. Campbell SC, Lane BR. Malignant renal tumours. In: Wein AJ, Kavoussi LR, Partin AW, et al., editors. Campbell-Walsh Urology. 11th ed. Philadelphia: Elsevier; 2016. p. 1314–1364.e14.
4. Johnson DC, Vukina J, Smith AB, Meyer A-M, Wheeler SB, Kuo T-M, et al. Preoperatively misclassified, surgically removed benign renal masses: a systematic review of surgical series and United States population level burden estimate. J Urol. 2015 Jan;193(1):30–5.
5. Thompson RH, Hill JR, Babayev Y, Cronin A, Kaag M, Kundu S, et al. Metastatic renal cell carcinoma risk according to tumor size. J Urol. 2009 Jul;182(1):41–5.
6. Smaldone MC, Kutikov A, Egleston BL, Canter DJ, Viterbo R, Chen DYT, et al. Small renal masses progressing to metastases under active surveillance: a systematic review and pooled analysis. Cancer. 2012 Feb 15;118(4):997–1006.
7. National Cancer Institute. NCI dictionary of cancer terms. [online]. 2021. Available at: https://www.cancer.gov/publications/dictionaries/cancer-terms/def/active-surveillance. Accessed 20 May 2021.
8. Campbell S, Uzzo R, Allaf M., Bass, E. Cadeddu, J., Chang A, et al. Renal cancer: renal mass & localized renal cancer guideline–American urological association. [online] Auanet.org. 2017. Available at: https://www.auanet.org/guidelines/guidelines/renal-cancer-renal-mass-and-localized-renal-cancer-guideline. Accessed 21 May 2021.
9. Sowery RD, Siemens DR. Growth characteristics of renal cortical tumors in patients managed by watchful waiting. Can J Urol. 2004 Oct;11(5):2407–10.
10. Ljungberg B, Albiges L, Bedke J, Bex A, Capitanio U, Giles RH, et al. EAU guidelines: renal cell carcinoma. Edn. presented at the EAU Annual Congress Milan 2021.
11. Ray S, Cheaib JG, Pierorazio PM. Active surveillance for small renal masses. Rev Urol. 2020;22(1):9–16.
12. Finelli A, Ismaila N, Bro B, Durack J, Eggener S, Evans A, et al. Management of small renal masses: American society of clinical oncology clinical practice guideline. JCO. 2017 Feb 20;35(6):668–80.
13. Richard PO, Jewett MAS, Bhatt JR, Kachura JR, Evans AJ, Zlotta AR, et al. Renal tumor biopsy for small renal masses: a single-center 13-year experience. Eur Urol. 2015 Dec;68(6):1007–13.
14. Volpe A, Mattar K, Finelli A, Kachura JR, Evans AJ, Geddie WR, et al. Contemporary results of percutaneous biopsy of 100 small renal masses: a single center experience. J Urol. 2008 Dec;180(6):2333–7.
15. Marconi L, Dabestani S, Lam TB, Hofmann F, Stewart F, Norrie J, et al. Systematic review and meta-analysis of diagnostic accuracy of percutaneous renal tumour biopsy. Eur Urol. 2016 Apr;69(4):660–73.
16. Macklin PS, Sullivan ME, Tapping CR, Cranston DW, Webster GM, Roberts ISD, et al. Tumour seeding in the tract of percutaneous renal tumour biopsy: a report on seven cases from a UK tertiary referral Centre. Eur Urol. 2019 May;75(5):861–7.

17. Richard PO, Lavallée LT, Pouliot F, Komisarenko M, Martin L, Lattouf J-B, et al. Is routine renal tumor biopsy associated with lower rates of benign histology following nephrectomy for small renal masses? J Urol. 2018 Oct;200(4):731–6.
18. Pierorazio PM, Johnson MH, Ball MW, Gorin MA, Trock BJ, Chang P, et al. Five-year analysis of a multi-institutional prospective clinical trial of delayed intervention and surveillance for small renal masses: the DISSRM registry. Eur Urol. 2015 Sep;68(3):408–15.
19. McDermott K, Mehan N, Challacombe B. Modern management of small renal masses. Urology News. 2019 Oct;23(6)
20. Volpe A, Panzarella T, Rendon RA, Haider MA, Kondylis FI, Jewett MAS. The natural history of incidentally detected small renal masses. Cancer. 2004 Feb 15;100(4):738–45.
21. Uzosike AC, Patel HD, Alam R, Schwen ZR, Gupta M, Gorin MA, et al. Growth kinetics of small renal masses on active surveillance: variability and results from the DISSRM registry. J Urol. 2018 Mar;199(3):641–8.
22. Finelli A, Cheung DC, Al-Matar A, Evans AJ, Morash CG, Pautler SE, et al. Small renal mass surveillance: histology-specific growth rates in a biopsy-characterized cohort. Eur Urol. 2020 Sep;78(3):460–7.
23. Kassiri B, Cheaib JG, Pierorazio PM. Patients with small renal masses undergoing active surveillance–is yearly chest imaging necessary? J Urol. 2019 Jun;201(6):1061–3.
24. Chawla SN, Crispen PL, Hanlon AL, et al. The natural history of observed enhancing renal masses: meta-analysis and review of the world. J Urol. 2006;175:425.
25. Crispen PL, Viterbo R, Fox EB, et al. Delayed intervention of sporadic renal masses undergoing active surveillance. Cancer. 2008;112:1051.
26. Pierorazio P, McKiernan J, Allaf M. 633 quality of life on active surveillance for a small renal masses versus immediate intervention: interim analysis of the DISSRM (delayed intervention and surveillance for small renal masses) registry. J Urol 2013 Apr [cited 2021 May 26];189(4S). Available from: https://doi.org/10.1016/j.juro.2013.02.185.
27. Data were provided by the National Cancer Registration and Analysis Service (part of Public Health England), on request through the Office for Data Release, November 2019. Similar data can be found here: https://www.ons.gov.uk/peoplepopulationandcommunity/healthandsocialcare/conditionsanddiseases/bulletins/cancerregistrationstatisticsengland/previousReleases.
28. Cancer Research UK. https://www.cancerresearchuk.org/sites/default/files/cstream-node/proj_inc_asr_Kid.pdf. Accessed May 2021.

The Role of Ablative Therapies in Renal Cancer

Alaina Garbens and Jeffrey A. Cadeddu

Introduction

With the rising use of cross sectional imaging, the rate of incidentally found renal masses has increased [1, 2]. While the majority of these masses will be T1a (≤4 cm) lesions [3], most will be malignant (approx. 80%) and many will require treatment for cure [4–6].

Currently, the gold standard treatment for T1a renal masses is partial nephrectomy (PN) [5, 7]. However, as urologists continue to look for new techniques to preserve renal function while minimizing the morbidity of surgery, percutaneous focal ablative therapies have evolved and are an option for many patients with T1a renal masses [5, 7]. Ablative techniques have been shown to have low complication rates, low morbidity, comparable short-term oncological outcomes and lower costs [8]. Currently, there are four ablative treatments: radiofrequency ablation (RFA), cryoablation (CRA), microwave ablation (MWA) and irreversible electroporation (IRE).

In this chapter, we will discuss the role of ablative therapies for the treatment of renal masses.

Indications for Ablation Treatment

Urologists can refer to major guidelines, all which discuss ablative techniques in the management of T1a renal tumors. Current guideline recommendations are listed in Table 1. Recommendations range from offering ablative therapies as an option to most patients with T1a renal tumors (ASCO, AUA, NCCN), to only offering ablation to patients who are elderly or have significant comorbidities (EAU).

A. Garbens · J. A. Cadeddu (✉)
University of Texas Southwestern Department of Urology, Dallas, TX, USA
e-mail: Jeffrey.cadeddu@utsouthwestern.edu

C. Anderson, M. Afshar (eds.), *Renal Cancer*,
https://doi.org/10.1007/978-3-030-84756-2_9

Table 1 Major guideline recommendations for the use of ablative therapies in the management of renal tumors

Guideline	Year Published	Recommendation	Strength
ASCO [9]	2017	"Percutaneous thermal ablation should be considered an option for patients who possess tumors such that complete ablation will be achieved. A biopsy should be obtained before or at the time of ablation."	Evidence quality: Intermediate, strength of recommendation: Strong.
AUA [5]	2017	"Physicians should consider thermal ablation (TA) as an alternate approach for the management of cT1a renal masses <3 cm in size. A renal mass biopsy should be performed prior to ablation to provide pathologic diagnosis and guide subsequent surveillance."	Conditional recommendation, evidence level: Grade C.
EAU [7]	2018	"Offer active surveillance, radiofrequency ablation and cryoablation to elderly and/or comorbid patients with small renal masses."	Strength rating: Weak
NCCN [10]	2019	"Thermal ablation (cryosurgery, radiofrequency ablation) is an option for the management of patient with clinical stage T1 renal lesions."	Category of evidence: 2A

ASCO American Society of Clinical Oncology, *AUA* American Urological Association, *EAU* European Association of Urology, *NCCN* National Comprehensive Cancer Network

As mentioned previously, T1a tumors (≤4 cm) are most amenable to treatment [8]. However, there have been reports in the literature of treatment of cT1b tumors in select patients [11, 12]. The size criteria is important not only for oncologic outcomes, but also for bleeding risk as the risk of bleeding increases with tumor size [13]. Most guidelines recommend a renal mass biopsy prior to or at the time of ablation to confirm that the mass is malignant [5, 7, 9]. Finally, location within the kidney is important, as anterior tumors, tumors <5 mm from the collecting system and surrounding structures (colon, larger vessels, "heat sinks") are more difficult/contraindicated to treat [14].

While tumor factors play an important role in determining a patient's eligibility for treatment, there are patient factors to consider. The most important ones are patient's risk for multifocality (i.e. genetic conditions such as von Hippel-Lindau Syndrome), patients where renal preservation is important (i.e. patients with renal dysfunction or solitary kidney) and patients who are not medically fit to undergo a surgical operation (elderly, frail, multiple medical comorbidities) [15, 16]. Patients should not have an uncontrolled coagulopathy, and most clinicians recommend an internal normalized ratio (INR) of <1.5 and platelet count to be greater than 50,000/μL [16].

Technical Considerations for Treatment

All ablative technologies aim to achieve the same final outcome—a negative margin of at least 5–10 mm and to achieve a predictable and continuous lethal cell ablation zone. How each ablation type achieves this is different, and we will briefly review the mechanism of each. Other technical considerations include probe types and number, device settings, patient positioning (patients must tolerate being in the prone position), and the use of local or general anesthesia.

Treatment Types

Radiofrequency Ablation (RFA)

RF energy is part of the electromagnetic (EM) spectrum, specifically, the frequencies between 450 Hz and 1200 kHz. Molecules become heated due to the rapidly alternating current being applied by the electrode, through a process called dielectric hysteresis, causing intense vibration and heat. The RFA electrode itself is not the source of heat. It is the molecules adjacent to the electrode that become heated and transmit heat farther through conductivity [17]. The further the molecules are from the probe, the vibration (energy) and temperature drop exponentially.

When performing RFA, the goal is the slowly heat the entire target area to 50–100 °C (ideally 70–100 °C) for 5–8 minutes in order to cause cell death without charring or vaporization. Charring or vaporization have an insulating effect, thereby limiting energy transmission to tissue and decreasing ablation size. As use of RFA has expanded, improvements to the technology have also occurred. This includes probes that are able to limit tissue charring, and probes that have expandable, multitined/clustered ("Christmas tree vs. umbrella") electrodes that result increased electrode surface area and ability to treat more complex tumors [16].

Advantages of using RFA are that the technology is widely available, RFA typically only requires one probe and one procedure for treatment, the probe is relatively small (14–17 gauge), the technology is cheaper compared to other types of ablative therapies, it has a hemostatic effect on tissue to minimize bleeding and an acceptable safety profile [16, 18]. Disadvantages to using RFA are the susceptibility to "heat sinks", size limitation (efficacy of ablation decreases over 4 cm), it requires image guidance and patients can receive skin burns if the grounding pads are not positioned correctly (monopolar systems) [16, 18].

Microwave Ablation

The use of microwave ablation (MWA) to ablate tumors in humans was first described in Japan during the late 1990s [19, 20]. Microwave ablation (MWA) induces heat-based cellular death through a mechanism similar to RFA. It uses EM radiation within the microwave spectrum (3 MHz–3GHz). MWA can heat tissues more rapidly and at higher temperatures than RFA. This has the potential to ablate larger tumors within a shorter treatment time [21]. However, MWA differs from RFA in that the probe (antenna) emits microwave energy that radiates into the tissue surrounding the antenna, causing direct heating [22]. This allows microwaves to be propagated through many types of tissue, even charred or desiccated tissue. Furthermore, multiple microwave probes can be placed in close proximity to each other, allowing for thermal synergy, or they can be widely spaced apart to treat several tumors at once [23]. MWA also offers other advantages over RFA in that no grounding pads are required, thereby eliminating the risk of skin burns and MWA is less susceptible to "heat sinks" than RFA [24].

While MWA has many advantages over RFA, it does have limitations. Microwave energy is more difficult to generate and deliver efficiently and safely to tissue compared to RFA, as the energy must be carried in coaxial cables. Coaxial cables are larger in diameter and more prone to heating than wires used for RFA. This cable and shaft heating can be an obstacle to delivering energy to tissue [25]. Furthermore, this heating effect of the probe can result in proximal tissue thermal damage, creating an unwanted "tail" of ablation and damage to the body wall or other more proximal structures [22]. Many companies have attempted to overcome this limitation by having shaft cooling systems [26]. Furthermore, currently available microwave systems and probes are heterogeneous in their power, frequency, wavelength and probe design. This results in differences in ablation zone characteristics that can make predictability of treatment zones difficult. Finally, many have reported a steeper learning curve with MWA compared to other technologies [21]. This could result in high complication rates and poorer oncologic outcomes for clinicians adopting this technology.

Thermal Ablative Technique that Utilize Cooling

Cryoablation

The origins of cryotherapy began in the 1800s when James Arnott used salt and crushed ice to improve pain and bleeding in tumors [27]. Cryoablation (CRA) of tumors utilizes freezing and thawing cycles, both of which result in cell death through different mechanisms. Cryoablation efficacy can be influenced by cooling rate, treatment time, target temperature, and thawing rate. The temperature will be lowest closest to the cryoprobe and highest at the periphery of the ice ball. Clinicians therefore must ensure that peripheral portion of the ice ball is within the lethal treatment temperature zone to ensure complete cell death [28].

The basic technique for cryoablation utilizes freeze thaw cycles. Tissue cooling should be as rapid as possible and thawing slow and complete. Then this cycle repeated. Most clinician will treat with an initial freeze cycle of 8–10 min, followed by a second cycle of 6–8 min [29]. Different cryoprobes can produce different sizes and/or shapes of ice balls, depending on the treatment area required. Furthermore, multiple probes can be used if needed. A major advantage of cryoablation is the ability to monitor the ablation zone in real time [30]. Cryoablation tends to be less painful than heat-based ablative techniques due to anesthetic effect of cooling [30]. Each cryoprobe acts independently of each other, allowing for multiple probes to be used simultaneously, allowing for ablation zones that conform to the individual tumor shape. Furthermore, CRA invokes an inflammatory response which produces antibodies to the tumor antigen which may result in death of tumor cells outside the treatment zone [31]. Unfortunately, this inflammatory response can also rarely trigger, a systemic inflammatory response, known as cryoshock, resulting in shock, multiorgan failure and disseminated intravascular coagulation [32]. Bleeding complications tend to be more common with cryoablation as the cautery and coagulative effects of heat do not occur. Care must be taken to avoid excessive torque or force on the cryoprobe, as the ice ball may fracture, resulting in bleeding [33]. Finally, as cryoablation systems use argon and helium gas to result in rapid cooling, the cost is higher than other ablative therapies [34].

Non Thermal Ablative Therapies

Irreversible Electroporation

Initially an unwanted byproduct of reversible electroporation, irreversible electroporation (IRE) was eventually investigated as means of tumor treatment in the mid-2000s [35]. IRE is a non-thermal ablative technique that passes an electric current between multiple probes across the ablative zone. This current increases the permeability of the cell membrane, by creating nanopores, resulting in cell death [35, 36]. Connective tissue (blood vessels, collecting system, biliary system) surrounding cells is spared. Since IRE is non-thermal, it has the potential utility of being able to treat central tumors, tumors within close proximity to other structures (ureter, bowel) and tumors near larger vessels (as IRE is not effected by "heat sinks") [36]. Furthermore, IRE induces cell death through apoptosis without areas of necrosis while preserving extracellular structures allowing for faster tissue regeneration.

While IRE shows promise with its ability to ablate tumors, limitations exist. First, IRE requires ECG synchronization (to avoid arrhythmias), full muscle paralysis (electrical current causes muscle contractions) and the use of multiple probes for successful treatment [37]. Finally, as IRE is the newest technology to be approved, its cost are the highest of all ablative therapies and it lacks longer term efficacy data [38]. Furthermore, for effective treatment, device settings needs to be optimized [39].

Outcomes

Oncological Outcomes

Ablative therapy outcomes are comparable to surgical treatment, however, currently there are no randomized controlled studies comparing the two directly. Long-term oncological outcomes have now been published for CRA and RFA, while long-term data is still lacking for MWA and IRE. As ablative therapies have traditionally treated patients who are older, are medically unfit for surgery or have limited survival, overall survival has been lower [40, 41]. Five to ten year cancer specific survival (CSS) for both CRA and RFA are reported in the literature to be 95–100%, which is similar to

PN [41]. Furthermore, there appears to be no significant difference in metastasis-free survival (MFS) between thermal ablation and PN, however, local recurrence free survival (LRFS) is lower for thermal ablation (98.9% for PN and 93.0% for thermal ablation) [41]. A recent systematic review and meta-analysis by Uhlig et al. compared CRA, RFA and MWA to PN. Select results of the their meta-analysis are summarized in Table 2 [42]. As IRE is the newest treatment modality, oncologic data are still maturing. However, preliminary data appear acceptable [43].

Renal Function and Complication Rates

While PN has been reported to have improved preservation of renal function compared to radical nephrectomy, meta-analyses have reported that ablative therapies have similar, if not improved preservation of renal function compared to PN (Table 2) [41, 42, 44]. Due to the less invasive, non-surgical nature of percutaneous ablative therapies, complication rates tend to be significantly lower than PN (Table 2) [41, 42].

Nuances

Treatment Planning

When considering a patient for ablative treatment, tumor size, imaging characteristics, location and patient factors need to be considered. The acronym, ABLATE, was developed by Schmit et al. to aid in ablation planning [45]. ABLATE stands for:

Table 2 Network Meta-Analysis Outcomes for Ablative Treatments compared to Partial Nephrectomy. (Adapted from Uhlig et al. 2019)

Treatment	All Cause Mortality (IRR)	Cancer Specific Mortality (IRR)	Local Recurrence (IRR)	Preservation of Renal Function (MD)	Complications (OR)
CRA	2.58 (1.92–3.46), p < 0.001	2.27 (0.79–6-49), p = 0.13	4.13 (2.28–7.47), p < 0.001	0.66 (−3.2–4.5), p = 0.74	0.67 (0.48–0.92), p = 0.013
RFA	2.58 (1.9–3.51), p < 0.001	2.03 (0.81–5.08), p = 0.13	1.79 (1.16–2.76), p = 0.009	6.49 (2.87–10.1), p < 0.001	0.89 (0.59–1.33), p = 0.56
MWA	3.8 (0.15–93.2), p = 0.4	1.27 (0.03–63.8), p = 0.9	2.52 (1.09–5.83), p = 0.03	−4.4 (−14.08–5.28), p = 0.37	0.26 (0.11–0.6), p < 0.001

CRA cryoablation, *RFA* radiofrequency ablation, *MWA* microwave ablation, *IRE* irreversible electrophoresis, *IRR* Incidence rate ratio, *MD* Mean difference, *OR* Odds ratio

Axial tumor diameter, bowel proximity, location within kidney, adjacency to the collecting system, touching renal sinus fat, endo- or exophytic [45]. If the tumor is located too close to the body wall, bowel or liver, hydrodissection with 5% dextrose can be used prior to treatment [46]. Furthermore, if the ureter is in close proximity to the treatment zone, some clinicians have found heat injury to be minimized by placing a stent and irrigating the collecting system with cold saline to prevent thermal injury [18, 24].

New Technology

As the minimally invasive treatment approach for small renal masses has gained popularity, other treatments have emerged. Newer treatment technologies include high intensity focal ultrasonography (HIFU) and stereotactic ablative body radiation (SABR). As clinical data is still in its infancy, it remains to be seen whether these treatments will continue to be used.

Conclusion

As long-term oncological data have matured for thermal ablative therapies, it has been shown to be a viable option for the treatment of small renal masses. While local recurrence rates may be higher than surgical treatment, the lower cost, lower complication rate, comparable cancer free survival rate and ability to retreat make ablative therapies a viable treatment option that clinicians should discuss with patients. RFA and CRA have the most data as they are the oldest of the ablative treatments, however, early MWA data has been comparable. IRE is still in the early stages and long term outcomes are lacking. Given the new data available, clinicians should discuss percutaneous ablation as a first line option in the treatment of T1a renal masses with patients.

Key Points

1. Percutaneous ablation of renal masses offers a less invasive treatment option than conventional surgery and can be performed as an outpatient procedure with either local or general anesthetic.
2. The ablation technologies currently available are cryoablation (CRA), radiofrequency ablation (RFA), microwave ablation (MWA) and irreversible electroporation (IRE).
3. For RFA, radiofrequency energy causes molecules to become heated due to the rapidly alternating current being applied by the electrode, through a process called dielectric hysteresis, causing intense vibration and heat.

4. Disadvantages of RFA are the susceptibility to "heat sinks", size limitation, image guidance is required and patients can receive skin burns.
5. MWA causes cell death using microwave energy in a manner similar to RFA but it is faster and can treat larger areas. MWA differs from RFA in that the probe (antenna) emits microwave energy that radiates into the tissue surrounding the antenna, causing direct heating. This allows microwaves to be propagated through many types of tissue, even charred or desiccated tissue.
6. Disadvantages to MWA are that it requires more energy than RFA, the heating effect of the probe can cause thermal damage to proximal tissue and probes are heterogeneous in their ablation zone characteristics, making treatment zone predictability difficult.
7. Cryoablation (CRA) utilizes freezing and thawing cycles, both of which result in cell death through different mechanisms. Different cryoprobes can produce different sizes and/or shapes of ice balls, depending on the treatment area required.
8. Disadvantages of CRA are that bleeding complications tend to be more common and the cost is higher.
9. Irreversible electroporation is a non-thermal ablative technique that uses electric currents to create nanopores, resulting in cell death. Connective tissue (blood vessels, collecting system, biliary system) surrounding cells is spared, allowing for treatment of tumors in close proximity to vital structures.
10. While currently there are no randomized controlled trials comparing partial nephrectomy (PN) to ablative therapies, cancer specific survival for RFA and CRA are reported in the literature to be 95–100%, roughly similar to PN. Overall survival is lower, however, that may be due to selection bias. Local recurrence rates are higher than surgery. Long term data for MWA and IRE have not yet matured.

References

1. SEER NCI. Stat fact sheets: kidney and renal pelvis cancer. Cancer Statistics 2019.
2. Mazziotti S, Cicero G, D'Angelo T, et al. Imaging and Management of Incidental Renal Lesions. Biomed Res Int. 2017;2017:1854027. https://doi.org/10.1155/2017/1854027.
3. Patel HD, Gupta M, Joice GA, et al. Clinical stage migration and survival for renal cell carcinoma in the United States. Eur Urol Oncol. 2018;2(4):343–8. https://doi.org/10.1016/j.euo.2018.08.023.
4. Johnson DC, Vukina J, Smith AB, et al. Preoperatively misclassified, surgically removed benign renal masses: a systematic review of surgical series and United States population level burden estimate. J Urol. 2015;193(1):30–5. https://doi.org/10.1016/j.juro.2014.07.102.
5. Cadeddu JA, Chang A, Clark PE, et al. American urological association (AUA) renal mass and localized renal cancer : AUA guideline American urological association (AUA) renal mass and localized renal cancer. Am Urol Assoc. 2017;1-49. http://auanet.org/guidelines/renal-mass-and-localized-renal-cancer-new-(2017)
6. Daugherty M, Sedaghatpour D, Shapiro O, Vourganti S, Kutikov A, Bratslavsky G. The metastatic potential of renal tumors: influence of histologic subtypes on definition of small renal masses, risk stratification, and future active surveillance protocols. Urol Oncol Semin Orig Investig. 2017; https://doi.org/10.1016/j.urolonc.2016.11.009.

7. Ljungberg B, Albiges L, Bensalah K, et al. Renal Cell Carcinoma EAU Guidelines. 2018; http://uroweb.org/wp-content/uploads/EAU-RCC-Guidelines-2018-large-text.pdf
8. Atwell TD, Schmit GD, Boorjian SA, et al. Percutaneous ablation of renal masses measuring 3.0 cm and smaller: comparative local control and complications after radiofrequency ablation and cryoablation. Am J Roentgenol. 2013;200(2):461–6. https://doi.org/10.2214/AJR.12.8618.
9. Finelli A, Ismaila N, Bro B, et al. Management of small renal masses: American society of clinical oncology clinical practice guideline. J Clin Oncol. 2017;35(6):668–80. https://doi.org/10.1200/JCO.2016.69.9645.
10. Jonasch E, Agarwal N, Alva A, et al. NCCN Guidelines Version 2.2020 Kidney Cancer. 2019.
11. Bhindi B, Mason RJ, Haddad MM, et al. Outcomes after Cryoablation versus partial nephrectomy for sporadic renal tumors in a solitary kidney: a propensity score analysis. Eur Urol. 2018;73(2):254–9. https://doi.org/10.1016/j.eururo.2017.09.009.
12. Caputo PA, Zargar H, Ramirez D, et al. Cryoablation versus partial nephrectomy for clinical T1b renal tumors: a matched group comparative analysis. Eur Urol. 2017;71(1):111–7. https://doi.org/10.1016/j.eururo.2016.08.039.
13. Atwell TD, Carter RE, Schmit GD, et al. Complications following 573 percutaneous renal radiofrequency and cryoablation procedures. J Vasc Interv Radiol. 2012;23(1):48–54. https://doi.org/10.1016/j.jvir.2011.09.008.
14. Uppot RN, Silverman SG, Zagoria RJ, Tuncali K, Childs DD, Gervais DA. Imaging-guided percutaneous ablation of renal cell carcinoma: a primer of how we do it. Am J Roentgenol. 2009;192(6):1558–70. https://doi.org/10.2214/AJR.09.2582.
15. Van Poppel H, Becker F, Cadeddu JA, et al. Treatment of localised renal cell carcinoma. Eur Urol. 2011;60(4):662–72. https://doi.org/10.1016/j.eururo.2011.06.040.
16. Higgins LJ, Hong K. Renal ablation techniques: state of the art. Am J Roentgenol. 2015; https://doi.org/10.2214/AJR.15.14752.
17. Organ LW. Electrophysioloic principles of radiofrequency lesion making. 39th ed. Appl Neurophysiol. 1977;39(2):69–76.
18. Hong K, Georgiades C. Radiofrequency ablation: mechanism of action and devices. J Vasc Interv Radiol. 2010;21(SUPPL. 8):S179. https://doi.org/10.1016/j.jvir.2010.04.008.
19. Sato M, Watanabe Y, Ueda S, et al. Microwave coagulation therapy for hepatocellular carcinoma. Gastroenterology. 1996;110(5):1507–14. https://doi.org/10.1053/gast.1996.v110.pm8613057.
20. Ohmoto K, Miyake I, Tsuduki M, et al. Percutaneous microwave coagulation therapy for unresectable hepatocellular carcinoma. Hepato-Gastroenterology. 1999;46(29):2894–900. http://www.ncbi.nlm.nih.gov/pubmed/10576369. Accessed August 13, 2019
21. Thompson SM, Schmitz JJ, Houston Thompson R, et al. Introduction of microwave ablation into a renal ablation practice: valuable lessons learned. Am J Roentgenol. 2018;211(6):1381–9. https://doi.org/10.2214/AJR.18.19775.
22. Lubner MG, Brace CL, Hinshaw JL, Lee FT. Microwave tumor ablation: mechanism of action, clinical results, and devices. J Vasc Interv Radiol. 2010;21(SUPPL. 8):S192. https://doi.org/10.1016/j.jvir.2010.04.007.
23. Brace CL, Laeseke PF, Sampson LA, Frey TM, van der Weide DW, Lee FT. Microwave ablation with multiple simultaneously powered small-gauge triaxial antennas: results from an in vivo swine liver model. Radiology. 2007;244(1):151–6. https://doi.org/10.1148/radiol.2441052054.
24. Brace CL. Microwave ablation technology: what every user should know. Curr Probl Diagn Radiol. 2009;38(2):61–7. https://doi.org/10.1067/j.cpradiol.2007.08.011.
25. Floridi C, De Bernardi I, Fontana F, et al. Microwave ablation of renal tumors: state of the art and development trends. Radiol Med. 2014;119(7):533–40. https://doi.org/10.1007/s11547-014-0426-8.
26. Liang P, Wang Y, Yu X, Dong B. Malignant liver tumors: treatment with percutaneous microwave ablation–complications among cohort of 1136 patients. Radiology. 2009;251(3):933–40. https://doi.org/10.1148/radiol.2513081740.
27. Cooper SM, Dawber RP. The history of cryosurgery. J R Soc Med. 2001;94(4):196–201. https://doi.org/10.1177/014107680109400416.
28. Baust JG, Gage AA, Robilottto AT, Baust JM. The pathophysiology of thermoablation: optimizing cryoablation. Curr Opin Urol. 2009;19(2):127–32. https://doi.org/10.1097/MOU.0b013e328323f654.

29. Kim EH, Tanagho YS, Bhayani SB, Saad NE, Benway BM, Figenshau RS. Percutaneous cryoablation of renal masses: Washington university experience of treating 129 tumours. BJU Int. 2013;111(6):872–9. https://doi.org/10.1111/j.1464-410X.2012.11432.x.
30. Erinjeri JP, Clark TWI. Cryoablation: mechanism of action and devices. J Vasc Interv Radiol. 2010;21(SUPPL. 8):S187. https://doi.org/10.1016/j.jvir.2009.12.403.
31. Sabel MS. Cryo-immunology: a review of the literature and proposed mechanisms for stimulatory versus suppressive immune responses. Cryobiology. 2009;58(1):1–11. https://doi.org/10.1016/j.cryobiol.2008.10.126.
32. Washington K, Debelak JP, Gobbell C, et al. Hepatic cryoablation-induced acute lung injury: histopathologic findings. In: Journal of surgical research, vol. 95. Elsevier; 2001. p. 1–7. https://doi.org/10.1006/jsre.2000.5976.
33. Hruby G, Edelstein A, Karpf J, et al. Risk factors associated with renal parenchymal fracture during laparoscopic cryoablation. BJU Int. 2008;102(6):723–6. https://doi.org/10.1111/j.1464-410X.2008.07735.x.
34. Hunter TD, Palli SR, Rizzo JA. Cost comparison of radiofrequency catheter ablation versus cryoablation for atrial fibrillation in hospitals using both technologies. J Med Econ. 2016;19(10):959–64. https://doi.org/10.1080/13696998.2016.1187153.
35. Miller L, Leor J, Rubinsky B. Cancer cells ablation with irreversible electroporation. Technol Cancer Res Treat. 2005;4(6):699–705. https://doi.org/10.1177/153303460500400615.
36. Jourabchi N, Beroukhim K, Tafti BA, Kee ST, Lee EW. Irreversible electroporation (NanoKnife) in cancer treatment. Gastrointest Interv. 2014;3(1):8–18. https://doi.org/10.1016/j.gii.2014.02.002.
37. Ball C, Thomson KR, Kavnoudias H. Irreversible electroporation: a new challenge in "out of operating theater" anesthesia. Anesth Analg. 2010;110(5):1305–9. https://doi.org/10.1213/ANE.0b013e3181d27b30.
38. Astani S, Brown ML, Getzen TM, Steusloff K. Comparison of procedure cost of various percutaneous tumor ablation modalities: microwave ablation, radiofrequency ablation, cryoablation, and irreversible electroporation. J Vasc Interv Radiol. 2014;25(3):S187. https://doi.org/10.1016/j.jvir.2013.12.505.
39. Silk M, Tahour D, Srimathveeravalli G, Solomon SB, Thornton RH. The state of irreversible electroporation in interventional oncology. Semin Intervent Radiol. 2014;31(2):111–7. https://doi.org/10.1055/s-0034-1373785.
40. Hu X, Shao YX, Wang Y, Yang ZQ, Yang WX, Li X. Partial nephrectomy versus ablative therapies for cT1a renal masses: a systematic review and meta-analysis. Eur J Surg Oncol. 2019;45(9):1527–35. https://doi.org/10.1016/j.ejso.2019.05.010.
41. Pierorazio PM, Johnson MH, Patel HD, et al. Management of Renal Masses and Localized Renal Cancer: systematic review and meta-analysis. J Urol. 2016;196(4):989–99. https://doi.org/10.1016/j.juro.2016.04.081.
42. Uhlig J, Strauss A, Rücker G, et al. Partial nephrectomy versus ablative techniques for small renal masses: a systematic review and network meta-analysis. Eur Radiol. 2019;29(3):1293–307. https://doi.org/10.1007/s00330-018-5660-3.
43. Canvasser NE, Sorokin I, Lay AH, et al. Irreversible electroporation of small renal masses: suboptimal oncologic efficacy in an early series. World J Urol. 2017;35(10):1549–55. https://doi.org/10.1007/s00345-017-2025-5.
44. Patel HD, Pierorazio PM, Johnson MH, et al. Renal functional outcomes after surgery, ablation, and active surveillance of localized renal tumors: a systematic review and meta-analysis. Clin J Am Soc Nephrol. 2017;12(7):1057–69. https://doi.org/10.2215/CJN.11941116.
45. Schmit GD, Kurup AN, Weisbrod AJ, et al. ABLATE: a renal ablation planning algorithm. Am J Roentgenol. 2014;202(4):894–903. https://doi.org/10.2214/AJR.13.11110.
46. Farrell MA, Charboneau JW, Callstrom MR, Reading CC, Engen DE, Blute ML. Paranephric water instillation: a technique to prevent bowel injury during percutaneous renal radiofrequency ablation. Am J Roentgenol. 2003;181(5):1315–7. https://doi.org/10.2214/ajr.181.5.1811315.

Open Radical Nephrectomy

P. Brousil, D. Manson-Bahr, L. Stroman, and T. O'Brien

Introduction

The first elective nephrectomy was performed in 1869 by German surgeon Gustav Simon after many failed surgical attempts to treat multiple ureteric fistulae. It was performed through a dorsal lumbotomy incision; it took an impressive 40 minutes with just 50 ml blood loss. There have been vast advances in surgical care in the last 150 years, yet there remain compelling reasons to continue with open nephrectomy. The BAUS nephrectomy audit of National UK practice in 2017 showed 19% of radical nephrectomy continues to be performed with the open approach [1].

Indications

With the introduction of minimally invasive technology, the default approach to radical nephrectomy is currently laparoscopic (with or without robotic assistance). Open surgery is reserved for when there is concern about compromise in patient

P. Brousil (✉)
Department of Urology, Epsom and St Helier University Hospitals NHS Trust, Epsom, UK
e-mail: philip.brousil@nhs.net

D. Manson-Bahr
Department of Urology, Norfolk and Norwich University hospitals, Norwich, UK

L. Stroman
Department of Urology, St. Georges University Hospital, London, UK

T. O'Brien
Department of Urology, Guys and St. Thomas' NHS Foundation Trust, London, UK

C. Anderson, M. Afshar (eds.), *Renal Cancer*,
https://doi.org/10.1007/978-3-030-84756-2_10

safety or achieving clear oncological margins of resection with minimally invasive strategies. The goals of radical nephrectomy are:

1. Extraction of the tumour with clear margins
2. Preservation of surrounding organs
3. Reasonable operative time and blood loss

If these objectives cannot be achieved laparoscopically, then open surgery is indicated. Sometimes, an initial laparoscopic approach with an expectation of conversion in a predicted difficult case may be reasonable, but bear in mind the open incision to convert may not provide as good access as an open incision of original intent.

Laparoscopy is most often anticipated to be unrealistic in the context of advanced tumours either by virtue of size, local (T4) or venous (T3b, T3c) extension up the IVC or incidental abdominal pathology that would make surgery challenging, especially previous surgery. Lymphadenopathy around the renal hilum is another factor which can severely impede access to the renal vasculature.

CT can be helpful in anticipating intraoperative problems and steering the surgeon towards choosing the correct approach for resection. Consider the size of the tumour: large tumours (>13 cm) can distort anatomy, with compression and effacement of the great vessels; in particular, left sided large tumours can be difficult to manipulate for safe mobilisation and dissection of hilar structures. Larger tumours are also more likely to invade the renal vein, and secrete vasoactive proteins, recruiting extra blood supply, and leading to poor views from bleeding as one tries to dissect. With exceptionally large tumours, at some stage the incision to retrieve the specimen becomes so large that the benefits to the patient of minimally invasive surgery can become diminished. Assessment of the peri-nephric fat on pre-operative imaging can also predict a difficult dissection laparoscopically; this is seen especially surrounding tumours with poorly demarcated edges where T3 disease is suspected. One must be suspicious of difficult dissection in seemingly straightforward primary tumours in the context of metastatic disease; at cytoreductive nephrectomy, one can often encounter ‘sticky’ or highly vascularised perinephric fat, or occult renal vein invasion, as these tumours are more likely to be ‘vasoactive’.

Surgery for tumours extending into the IVC deserve special mention. It can present some of the most challenging surgery in abdomen. Open surgery for such cases is still the mainstay of practice because of the degree of vascular control required to extract the tumour without catastrophic bleeding. Robotic assisted laparoscopic has recently sought to challenge this well established paradigm. However the literature remains Spartan; several centres have began publishing small series on successful extractions, initially with Level 1–2 thrombi by Neves-Zincke classification [2] in 2011 [3], then some centres trialling the robotic approach with level 3 [4] and even level 4 tumour thrombi with operative times up to 11 hours [5]. The authors all raise the issue of exceptional challenge in performing such surgery, and whether such techniques can be generalised to the wider surgical community is unclear. Robotic surgery for IVC tumours is like climbing Everest without oxygen: it can be done, but only with extensive prior experience and the conditions have to be just right.

Broadly speaking, indications for open radical nephrectomy are cases complicated by:

1. Involvement of contiguous organs
2. IVC tumour thrombus
3. Previous abdominal surgery
4. Extensive lymphadenopathy
5. Very large tumours

Pre-Operative Embolisation of the Kidney

Once a well-debated topic, pre-operative embolisation is rarely used in modern practice. 75% of patients are thought to get post-embolisation syndrome [6], not to mention pain, and therefore its only practical setting is within 24 hours of surgery. Further concern of causing ischaemia to the tumour and subsequent tumour embolisation into the chest have been reported [7, 8] and overall, many authors question its value [8, 9]. It can be of value however. Whereas early ligation of the right renal artery is achievable intraoperatively (described later), the left can be more difficult, and in the context of huge tumours and peri-hilar lymphadenopathy, a pre-operative embolisation can be considered.

The Incision

There are many ways to approach the kidney; the choice should be made in consideration of patient and tumour factors.

The Flank Approach

A flank incision has been the mainstay for many surgeons over the years, with the advantage of leaving the peritoneum and its contents intact. Particularly with large left sided tumours where the spleen is at risk, dissection and possible removal of the 11th or 12th rib with this approach is more straightforward. In patients with multiple previous intra-peritoneal surgery or a large pannus from obesity, this approach is relatively advantageous. The incision can be made subcostal or supra-costal. Subcostal incisions give poor access to the upper pole of the kidney and are generally reserved for open pyeloplasty and perhaps lower pole partial nephrectomy. To optimise exposure of the upper pole of the kidney, a supra-costal approach serves best. An incision is made along the line of the 11th or 12th rib, and extended anteriorly. Once dissection through the muscle layers to the rib is complete, the pleura is carefully dissected off the superior border of the rib. It is fragile fascia, and can be easily opened inadvertently. Preservation of the neurovascular bundle should be attempted. Once fully dissected free, the rib can be dislocated or dismembered if required. The kidney is mobilised and lifted to reveal the hilum posteriorly for control. There are some downsides to this approach. The patient is managed in the lateral decubitus position with the operating table in a flexed position to approximately 30–70°; for some patients with cardio-pulmonary disease this may not be appropriate. Access to the great vessels is limited until the kidney is mobilised. When the tumour has incited intense venous collateralisation, the blood loss incurred from dissection before eventual vascular control of the kidney may be considerable; extending the incision gives limited extra exposure to the hilum. Further, some feel that patients can experience considerable pain from excision or fracture of the rib exposed and retracted in dissection. Several focussed studies have not found significant differences in pain scores by surgical approach, however pain score studies are notoriously difficult to reproduce [10–12]. One of the long standing issues with this approach is the risk of flank bulge or hernia, which may be as high as half the patients, although most series report rates of 8–23% for retroperitoneal open access [13–15]. To add to this concern, the repairs are traditionally considered fairly futile. Bulge and hernia are different. Whereas a hernia is a gap in a myofascial layer, bulge is an eventration of all 3 muscles layers leading to the visual defect. It is likely that 'bulge' has a worse outcome than true hernia when repaired, since the cause is denervated muscle which remains intact. Some authors recommend excision to prevent recurrence [16]. In experienced hands of surgeons that have developed a specific interest, good outcomes are achievable however [16]. Diblasio et al. have reported a modification of this incision which minimises the risk of hernia/bulge to 3% [17].

Thoraco-Abdominal Approach

This incision is effectively a much higher version of the flank supra-costal approach. It gives excellent access to the upper abdomen and chest. It is particularly useful for difficult upper pole tumours. It's contemporary use has waned however. It is a very large morbid incision; chest drains can be uncomfortable post-operatively, and the lung is usually collapsed intra-operatively for access, increases the chances of cardio-pulmonary complications. The costo-chrondral border of the rib cage which is divided, never fully heals.

The patient is managed in the lateral decubitus position once again with table broken. It is most commonly used in right sided approached with excellent access to the IVC posteriorly, even above the hepatic veins. The incision is made over the eighth, ninth or tenth rib space and the chest cavity is entered. Removing a segment of rib to aid retraction can be done without long-term impunity; if the rib is left fractured or dislocated, this tends to leave the patient with more post-operative pain. The incision is extended anteriorly across the costal cartilage and then angled down towards the umbilicus. The peritoneum is entered beneath the inferior border of the ribcage. Returning to the chest cavity, the lung is collapsed and gently retracted superiorly by pads or swabs and the diaphragm is opened on the superior surface close to the chest wall to avoid injury to the phrenic nerve. Through this incision, the spleen or liver can be retracted superiorly, and dissection of the kidney and its tumour from its superior relations can be achieved before completion nephrectomy in the abdomen. Closure of pleura and diaphragm and costal cartilage is required (if divided) and placement of a post-operative chest drain.

Anterior Subcostal Approach

Possibly the most commonly used approach in open surgery, yielding access to the hilum and great vessels, and laterally for renal mobilisation. It can be extended superiorly to the xiphoid process for improved IVC access (as a Mercedes-benz shaped incision), and across the midline for access to the contralateral great vessel. Unlike flank and thoraco-abdominal approaches, it is usually easier to approach the hilum before mobilisation of the kidney. The patient is managed prone for this incision, and a kidney rest may be placed under the patient to elevate the resection target. The incision is typically made 2 finger breaths beneath the costal margin of the rib cage and not higher, to ensure adequate sheath for a comprehensive closure following resection.

Lexus or L-Shaped Incision

This incision begins in the midline at the xiphoid process and extends inferiorly towards the umbilicus before turning 90 degrees left or right towards the nephrectomy site. The flap is sutured to the abdominal wall supero-laterally to hold it away for the duration of surgery. It affords excellent access to the entire upper abdomen and is most commonly used in nephrectomy with IVC thrombectomy. The inferior border of the ribs can be lifted with a Thompson or Omnitract retractor to afford excellent views under the diaphragm where an upper pole tumour has made dissection difficult. The intention of this incision is to give access laterally for safe dissection off the abdominal wall and bowel, and medially for IVC and aortic access and tumour dissection.

Radical Nephrectomy

Irrespective of the incision chosen the principles of dissection remain the same: maintenance of patient safety with avoidance of severe bleeding and injury to abdominal organs, and good oncological resection with clear margins.

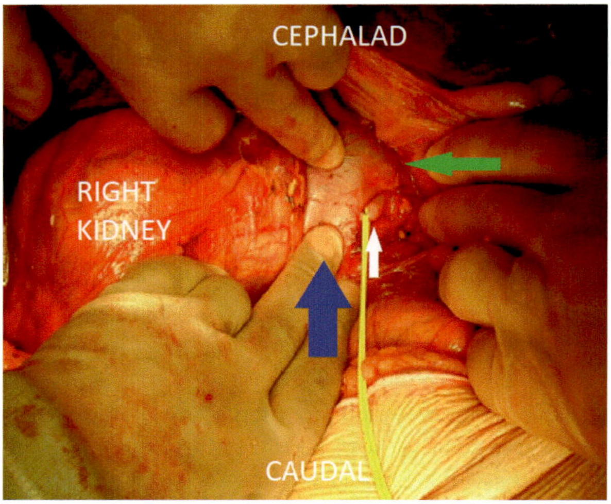

Fig. 1 Refection of the IVC (blue arrow) and Left renal vein (green arrow) to identify and ligate the right renal artery (white arrow). Photograph courtesy of Tim O'Brien

In order to limit bleeding, one can consider early ligation of the renal artery as the first step in the nephrectomy. For both left and right sided tumours, dissection of the lateral border of the distal duodenum with medial reflection to the right gives exposure to the aorta upon opening the mesentery of the descending colon up to the course of the inferior mesenteric vein. The left renal vein is a key landmark which usually runs over both the right and left renal artery on their respective sides of the aorta (see Fig. 1).

Large tumours and lymphadenopathy distort anatomy and can efface the great vessels; fastidious dissection until anatomical surety must be achieved as ligation of the SMA or incorrect renal artery is a disaster. This approach to the renal vasculature is very similar to the technique in exploration of severe renal trauma.

Many of the tumours selected for open renal surgery are advanced, and paraneoplastic angiogenesis leave them with a complex array of diaphanous vessels under high pressure surrounding the kidney within gerotas fascia. Studies have shown angiogenesis forms 25% of tumour volume and the endothelium of tumour vasculature is phenotypically different: higher permeability, abnormal sprouts, deranged vessel hierarchy and genetic alterations making them 'leaky' and very easy to tear [18] (see Fig. 2).

Consequently, assiduous control of these vessels does not always prevent bleeding during mobilisation of the kidney until the artery is controlled. It is often the case that one might merely tie off the artery early and proceed with renal mobilisation as it may be too onerous at that stage to achieve adequate exposure to formally divide it.

An anterior approach nephrectomy on either side requires mobilisation of the colon off the kidney by incising the white line of Toldt and developing the plane between the colon mesentery and Gerota's fascia. It is here that the great vessels, hilum and ureter can be identified. The gonadal vein is closely associated with the ureter; it is a potential source of heavy bleeding, especially if the renal vein/IVC is

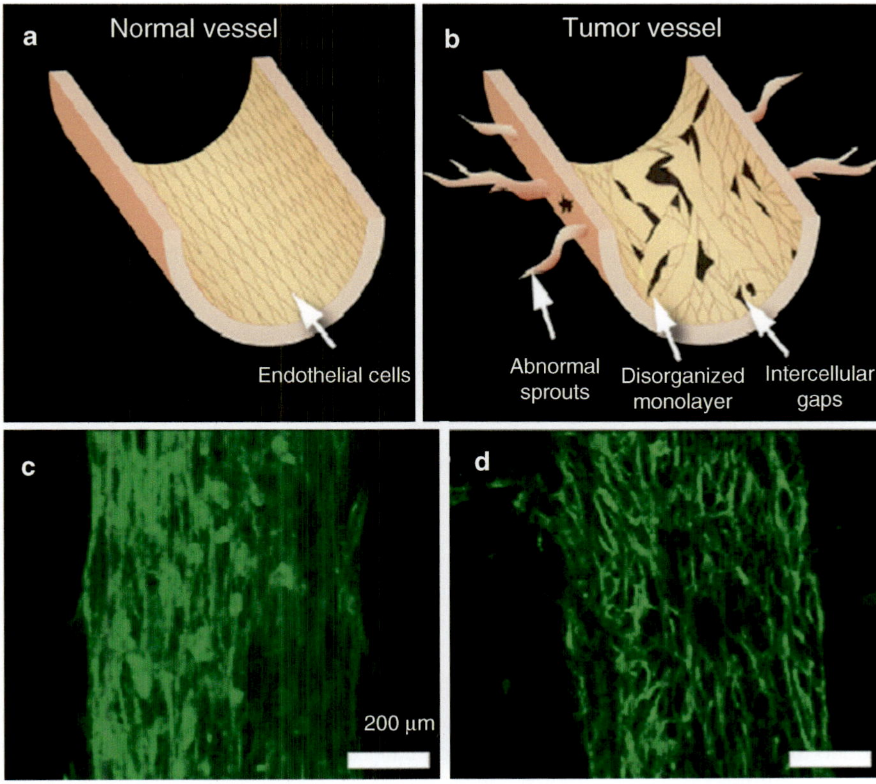

Fig. 2 Electron microscope comparison of normal vs tumour vessels, taken from Jimenez et al. [18]

involved with tumour thrombus and can be divided with impunity. This is not a mandatory manoeuvre, however on the left, where it drains into the renal vein, it may impede dissection. Early mobilisation of the spleen or liver off the kidney is important, as it is possible to tear these organs easily with minimal retraction of the kidney; sometimes splenic tears cannot be resolved without splenectomy. Further mobilisation of the diaphragmatic attachments of the spleen or liver can be further performed to gain greater access in the context of difficult upper pole renal tumours. The pancreas can be adherent to the medial border of the left kidney when tumour present, and if dissection is impossible without injury, the tail can be taken with the specimen with the free end oversewn or closed with vascular stapler. A drain should be left in these circumstances.

Mobilisation of the kidney is typically undertaken layer by layer and in 'high risk' areas, with the aid of a right angled Mixter-*O'Shaughnessy* or Lahey vascular clamp to discover vasculature and ligating as one dissects. These areas are namely along the border of the great vessels, and around the splenic hilum and adrenal gland. Inadvertent vascular injury in these areas can be difficult control, and in some cases, not possible until the kidney is removed.

One consideration to bear before the hilar dissection is completed is whether one should take the adrenal gland with the specimen. Clearly nodular disease on pre-op imaging in the context of advanced tumours would indicate a ipsilateral adrenalectomy, but what about micro-metastasis? O'Malley and colleagues conclude in a systematic review [19] that risk factors for involvement were:

1. renal vein tumour thrombus to the level of the adrenal vein
2. upper pole tumours ≥7 cm
3. radiographic abnormalities on pre-operative imaging (non-visualisation, nodular, enlargement or irregular borders).

One must take great care, especially on the right when mobilising the adrenal gland; with the short adrenal vein draining straight into the IVC, avulsion is easy, and repair of the IVC can be difficult to control if the kidney and caudate lobe of the liver have not been mobilised.

Control of the renal vasculature can be performed with a variety of methods. Whereas power devices such as the Harmonic™ (Ethicon), LigaSure™ (Medtronic) or Thunderbeat™ (Olympus) scalpel are extremely effective for almost bloodless fascial dissection, with good control of minor vessels, sutures and clips remain the mainstay of major vessel ligation. Surgeons may elect to apply a transfixation suture with 4–0 prolene to the lumbar vein if exposure has been difficult and there is concern of retraction and bleeding.

Closure of anterior wounds are typically performed en-mass with a heavy PDS suture. For flank incision, there is some data to suggest a multi-layered closure may reduce the incidence of flank bulge (which can be up to 50%) with vicryl for the internal oblique fascia and PDS for the anterior sheath (reference single vs multi layer closure trial).

Surgery for Kidney Tumours with IVC Thrombus

Before undertaking surgery for tumours extending into the IVC, good quality images of the venous invasion are required. There are several pertinent characteristics: cephalad extension, distal bland thrombus, signs of complete or partial IVC obstruction and expansion of the IVC. The Mayo Classification of IVC thrombus [20, 21] (See Fig. 3) offers a very practical assessment of RCC venous extension in terms of operative consideration:

Mayo Classification of IVC [21] Tumour Thrombus

1. Thrombus limited to renal vein
2. Thrombus extending ≤2 cm above the renal vein
3. Thrombus extending >2 cm above the renal vein but below the hepatic veins
4. Thrombus at or above the hepatic veins but below the diaphragm
5. Thrombus extending above the diaphragm

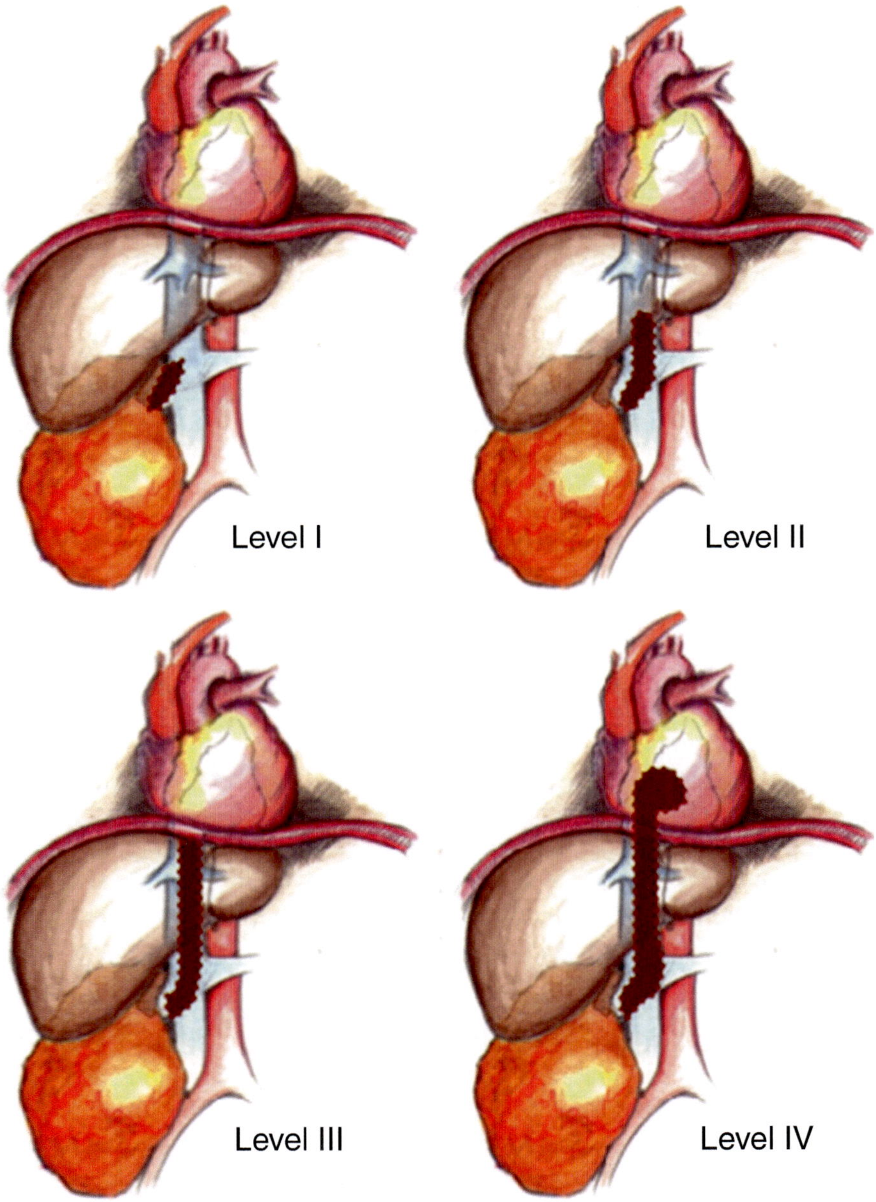

Fig. 3 Diagramatic representation of the Mayo classification of IVC thrombus, taken from Gonsalez et al. [20]

The classification is pertinent and superior to the TNM staging system as it provided more description to the exact degree of IVC extension. Whereas TNM classification can predict prognosis, the Mayo classification will accurately portend to the degree of dissection required and therefore complexity of the procedure. The technique of dissection will be discussed based on the Mayo classification of the tumour.

Pre-Operative Imaging

RCC tumours with IVC extension tend to progress quickly. Patients can develop metastasis, including tumour emboli in the pulmonary arteries or extension within weeks of previous imaging. Many surgeons insist on restaging the week before surgery.

With respect to surgical planning, 2 aspects of venous tumour thrombus need to be known:

1. The extent of cephalad extension
2. The possibly of IVC wall infiltration
3. Presence and extent of bland thrombus

Where the CT may be equivocal or unclear, MR venogram is helpful. Flow void on T2 weighted signal strongly correlates with flow through the IVC. Lack of flow void not only helps highlight the cephalad extend of a thrombus, but also partial vs complete obstruction of the IVC. Bland thrombus can be differentiated from tumour thrombus also using MRI: diffusion weighted imaging provides differentiation between the two. Bland thrombus is important to consider: it can obstruct the lumbar collaterals, promoting high pressure collateralisation of the peri-nephric space with diaphanous veins and contributing to significant operative blood loss, and the risk of pulmonary embolus once the tumour has been removed. In general, bland thrombus should be removed at the time of cavotomy, unless it is solid and fixed to the IVC wall. High volume centres such as the Mayo Clinic, have explored whether to leave an IVC filter in situ post cavotomy and thrombectomy where the patient is left with mobile bland thrombus [22], however this is not routine practice in the UK. Pre-operative placement of IVC filter is considered hazardous, as the tumour can grow into it, increasing the likelihood of IVC resection [23].

Bland thrombus can indicate of complete obstruction on MRI, and expansion of the IVC raises the possibility of IVC infiltration of tumour and the need for IVC excision; one study found the need to staple or resect the IVC in 22% of patients with bland thrombus [22]. A further study demonstrated the need to ligate or resect the IVC is increased from 12% to 53% of patients in the presence of bland thrombus [24]. Further work from the Mayo clinic concluded that there are three major risk factors predicting not only need for IVC interruption, but invasion of tumour into the IVC intima on pathologic analysis: right renal tumour (the vein is shorter), expansion of the IVC and radiographic evidence of complete occlusion [25]. Presence of all three factors increases the likelihood of IVC resection from 2% to 66% for level II to IV thrombi tumours.

The discussion of whether the IVC can be excised and merely tied off without reconstruction remains debated. In the context of IVC obstruction from RCC,

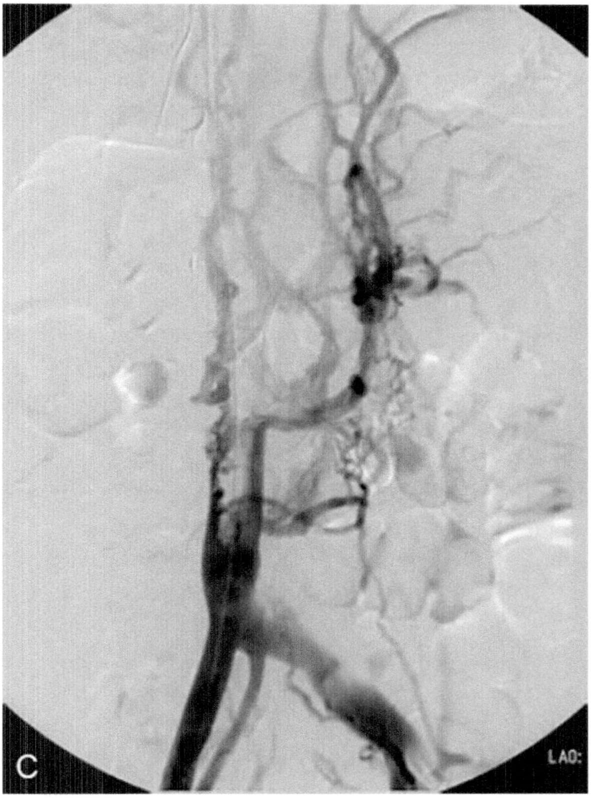

Fig. 4 Venous angiogram of IVC shows extensive azygous collateralisation. Taken from Campbell-Walsh Urology [6]

shunting tends to occur via 3 systems: the lumbar venous plexus, hemi-azygous system via the left renal vein (see Fig. 4) and via the haemorrhoidal plexus (into the inferior mesenteric vein and portal system) [26]. The left renal vein can develop further collateral drainage via peri-nephric veins communicating with the splenic vein or inferior phrenic vein, however the right kidney is more vulnerable to supra-renal IVC obstruction and does not have the ability to collateralise in the same way. These are important considerations when the decision to interrupt the IVC has been made; the right renal vein would require reconstruction, whilst the left does not.

Further Pre-Operative Considerations

Pulmonary Emboli

Approximately 3–4% of RCC patients with IVC thrombus have PE at presentation; the higher the thrombus, the greater the risk of emboli [24, 27]. It cannot be known if this is tumour or vascular emboli. It would be natural to be reluctant to offer these patients surgery, however retrospective data does not demonstrates worse outcomes in these patients [27]; conversely one may be encouraged to perform surgery to reduce the risk of further life-threatening emboli (vascular or tumour) being thrown off. Tumours with IVC thrombus can cause significant disruption to the venous return of many organs, and surgical resection remains a strong argument to prevent renal, hepatic and cardiac failure: surgery for 'local' symptoms, not purely oncology.

Budd-Chiari Syndrome

Budd-Chiari syndrome describes the consequent hepatic congestion from obstruction of the hepatic veins that drain into the IVC. Level III tumour thrombi can obstruct these veins and cause significant physiological abnormalities pertinent to delivering safe surgery. Hyper- and hypocoagulopathy can be seen in these cases, and although surgical resection remains the only way to correct these abnormalities definitively, coagulopathy increases post-operative mortality significantly; one should consider surgery for patients with a pre-operative INR > 1.5 with great caution [28]. Such patients are typically experiencing extreme variations in fluid balance and post-operative invasive haemodynamic monitoring on ITU should be utilised, particularly when venous obstruction has been rapidly corrected with surgical removal of tumour and bland thrombus.

Anaemia

Anaemia is very commonly seen at presentation in advanced renal cell carcinoma. The patient is usually in an iron deficient state. IVC surgery has the potential for significant blood loss; mean blood loss in a series of IVC thrombectomy patients with budd-chiari was 4.2 litres [29], and therefore one should consider IV iron replacement several weeks before surgery to optimise the patient.

Resection

For tumours extending into the IVC, an anterior approach is typical, usually with an L-shaped incision for right sided tumours, and a Mercedes incision for left sided tumours when hepatic mobilisation is required. The Chevron incision is also commonly used, given access to the pelvis is not required. Some authors advocate a right thoraco-abdominal approach, irrespective of tumour laterality, to spare the patient needing cardio-pulmonary bypass in cases of level IV thrombi [30], although this is not standard practice within our region.

As mentioned previously, early ligation of the renal artery is a key step to minimising blood loss during surgery. In most cases, intense collateralisation of fragile vessels under high pressure makes dissection and manipulation of the specimen difficult without significant blood loss. Ligation of the artery takes the pressure out of this abnormal venous system, facilitating progress [9]. For right sided tumours, ligation within the aorto-caval space avoids tumour manipulation; for left sided tumours, pre-operative embolization may be considered as discussed previously.

Mobilisation of the kidney is performed as described before, leaving the renal vein intact. The adrenal gland should routinely be taken with the specimen because of the expectation of involvement. Further dissection is based on the level of tumour extension into the renal vein/IVC; the Mayo classification is helpful here to detail the variation in technique.

Mayo Level 0

Here the IVC is not involved, with the tumour sitting within the renal vein only. Usually the tumour can be milked back into the renal vein to leave an adequate length for ligation, however one may still require control of the IVC: on the right, the renal vein is short and ligation at the renal ostium may be required; on the left, high pressure collateral can make dissection difficult as the gonadal, inferior adrenal and lumbar veins that drain into the left renal vein can be obstructed. Early ligation of the renal artery here can avoid significant blood loss; an audit at Guy's and St Thomas' Hospital, UK, demonstrated a mean reduction in blood loss of 1 litre when his is achieved. In the case of a retro-aortic vein, the aorta may need to be mobilised, augmenting the dissection, and extraction of the tumour with a negative margin can be very challenging. Suture closure over a clamp of the renal ostium is typically achieved with a fine non-absorbable suture such as 4–0 prolene.

Mayo Level 1

It is rare for these tumours to completely obstruct the IVC but they may be associated with bland thrombus. Manipulation of the tumour within the IVC risks fracture and embolism with potentially disastrous consequences; one must therefore take great care when establishing extent of the thrombus intra-operatively. Milking the tumour back should only be done when the surgeon is ready to clamp the IVC. Dissection and control of the contralateral renal vein, distal and proximal IVC should have been performed. The L1 lumbar vein can drain into the IVC posteriorly near the level of the renal ostium and is usually under increased pressure with IVC thrombi; injury and bleeding to this vein can be notoriously difficult to control because of difficulty achieving exposure. Classically, no lumbar veins are known to drain into the IVC superior to the renal vein insertion. Lumbar veins however are prone to considerable variation [31], and whereas dissection at the front of the IVC is generally safe and free of tributaries, posteriorly it requires exhaustive vigilance.

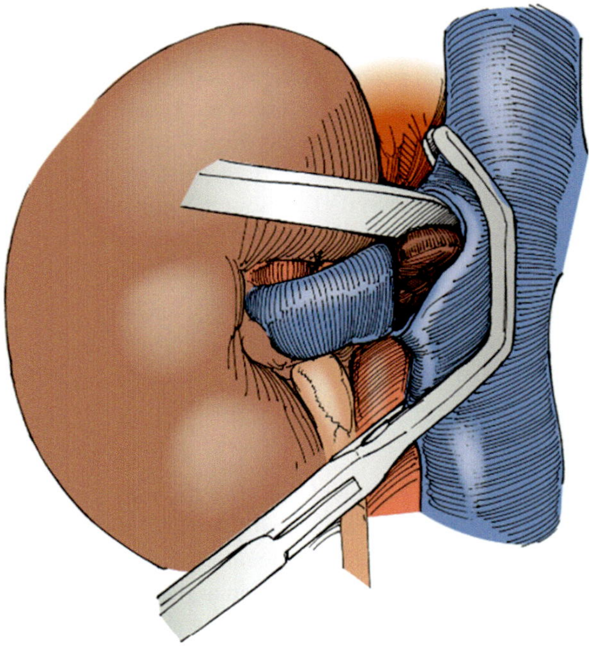

Fig. 5 Satinsky clamp across renal vein ostium for a right sided tumour. Taken from 'Hinman Atlas of Urologic Surgery' [32]

Many tumours can be milked back into the renal vein and a clamp across the ostium provides ligation for resection. Where this cannot be achieved, a Satinsky clamp can be applied in parallel to the IVC, taking a bite out of the IVC which contains the tumour (see Fig. 5). Closure of the IVC with running 3 or 4–0 prolene suture can then be performed without interrupting venous return to the heart. Reducing the calibre of the IVC by 50% with this closure can lead to morbidity, and a patch may be required in those cases. Making the incision over the renal ostium, parallel to the IVC and extending longitudinally generally avoids this issue.

Mayo Level 2

It is less likely the tumour can be milked back into the renal vein here and complete control of the IVC is required. Various methods can be used to interrupt the veins: we typically use fabric Rummel tourniquets and a combination of atraumatic Dardik and Satinsky clamps (see Fig. 6).

If more clearance is required caudally on the IVC to get above the thrombus, the caudate lobe is mobilised by dividing the short hepatic veins which drain directly into the IVC. This can provide an additional 4–5 cm of IVC exposure (see Fig. 7).

These short veins can be clipped or ligated with 3/0 ligatures. Bleeding from the liver from these ostia should be controlled with 5–0 prolene suture. One might consider a test run of IVC control before cavotomy to check for haemodynamic collapse although this is rarely seen if the portal and lumbar collateral circulation has been maintained. Upon cavotomy as previously described, the tumour is removed in continuity with the kidney. Meticulous inspection of the cava is then required to ensure no residual tumour.

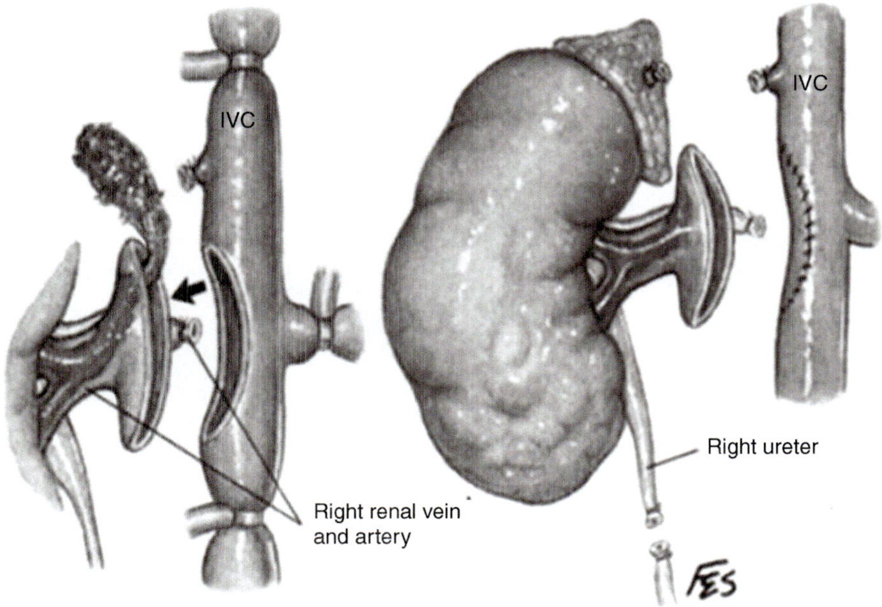

Fig. 6 Resection of the right renal vein ostium with level II IVC tumour after application of Rummel tourniquets to proximal and distal IVC and left renal vein. Taken from 'Renal Cancer' [33]

Fig. 7 Mobilisation of the caudate lobe (blue arrow) with division of the short hepatic veins draining into the IVC. This yield a further IVC exposure anteriorly. Photograph courtesy of Tim O'Brien

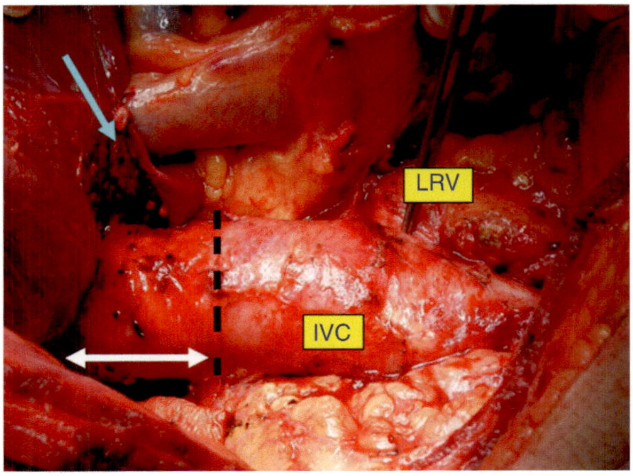

Mayo Level 3

A level 3 thrombus is potentially a game changer: advanced liver transplant techniques are required to mobilise the liver for access to the supra-hepatic IVC and a cardiac surgeon may be required to provide bypass to facilitate safe cavotomy. At level 3 the tumour extends at or above the hepatic veins but below diaphragm. The key technical step for level 3 extension is full mobilisation of the right lobe of the

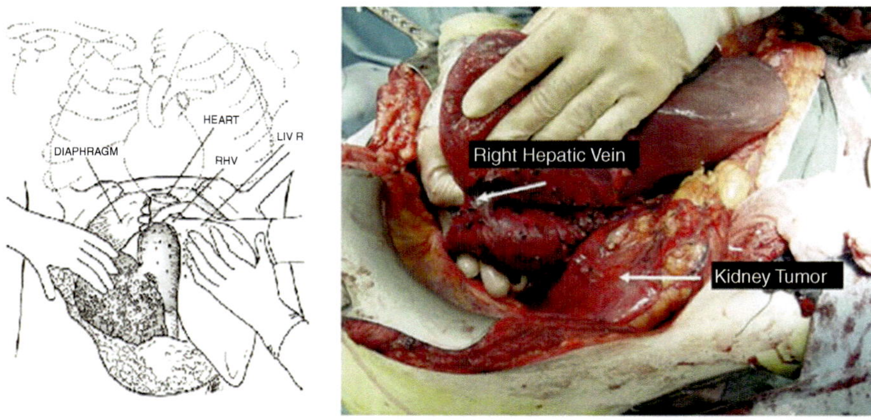

Fig. 8 Piggybacking of the liver for posterior supra and infra IVC exposure. Surgeon has his hand around the suprahepatic IVC and will try to milk the tumour down below the hepatic veins before applying the clamp. Picture from Ciancio et al. [34]

liver to allow access to the retrohepatic IVC with folding of the right liver over the left, known as piggybacking [34]. This is demonstrated in Fig. 8.

Once the short hepatics are freed, the diaphragmatic ligaments of the liver (round and cardinal) are dissected and the larger right lobe of the liver can be rotated anteriorly to sit on top of the left liver. The surgeon is then left with excellent access to the IVC above and below the hepatic veins to either milk back the tumour below then clamp or clamp above the hepatic veins having applied temporary ligation to the portal system (Pringle manoeuvre) followed by cavotomy.

Mayo Level 4

Tumours extending above the diaphragm are the most complex. Within the abdomen, they are more likely to invade the IVC and require interruption with resection or graft. To resect the majority of these tumours, cardiopulmonary bypass, without or without deep hypothermic circulatory arrest, is required. Some authors advocate tackling these scenarios without bypass [35, 36], however the mainstay remains with bypass and these teams concede the need for cardiovascular surgeons to be involved. Recent multicentre studies show no difference in post-operative outcomes using cardio-pulmonary bypass [37]. In our institution, a median sternotomy provides peerless exposure to the supradiaphragmatic IVC and right atrium. The incision is extended into the abdomen in a hockey stick incision. The kidney is mobilised first before proceeding to the proximal end of the tumour resection. Hypothermia to 22 °C, if used, is limited to 30 minutes to prevent post-operative neurological complication. Long term neurological deficit is remarkably rare since improvements in technique since its first attempt in the 1950s. 30 day mortality from these advanced tumours is 7–10% [37, 38].

IVC Ligation and Grafting

For the most part, IVC thrombi float freely endo-luminally, merely tethered distally, however a small proportion of tumours are inseparably adherent or invading the IVC wall. Complete clearance may only be achievable with partial excision of the caval wall. Primary closure is likely to yield complications if the IVC is left with less than 50% of its original calibre. A patch repair to widen or repair an excised segment can be undertaken. Bovine pericardium or autologous vein grafts give excellent handling and repair is relatively straightforward. An interposition graft is more complex; use of xenograft with bovine pericardium or synthetic grafts with PTFE or Dacron are widely reported, but only in small series, given the rarity of the circumstance. For a completely obstructed IVC, it may be resected and ligated without impunity, if the contralateral kidney and distal IVC have had the opportunity to collateralise already. As discussed previously, it is reasonable to consider this following right sided nephrectomy, but not with tumours of the left. Ultimately, if a large distal bland thrombus cannot be removed as adherent, the safest precaution against pulmonary embolus is to leave the IVC ligated proximally.

IVC grafts are at risk of two main complications: infection and thrombosis/occlusion. Whereas infection is rare unless there has been a concurrent bowel resection [39], occlusion can occur with ensuing morbidity. The rate of reported graft occlusion is variable owing to a paucity of data: small series as one might expect as the need to graft is uncommon. The occlusion rate is variable in the literature, from 0–35% [40–42]. Figure 9 shows PTFE and Bovine graft interposition of the IVC.

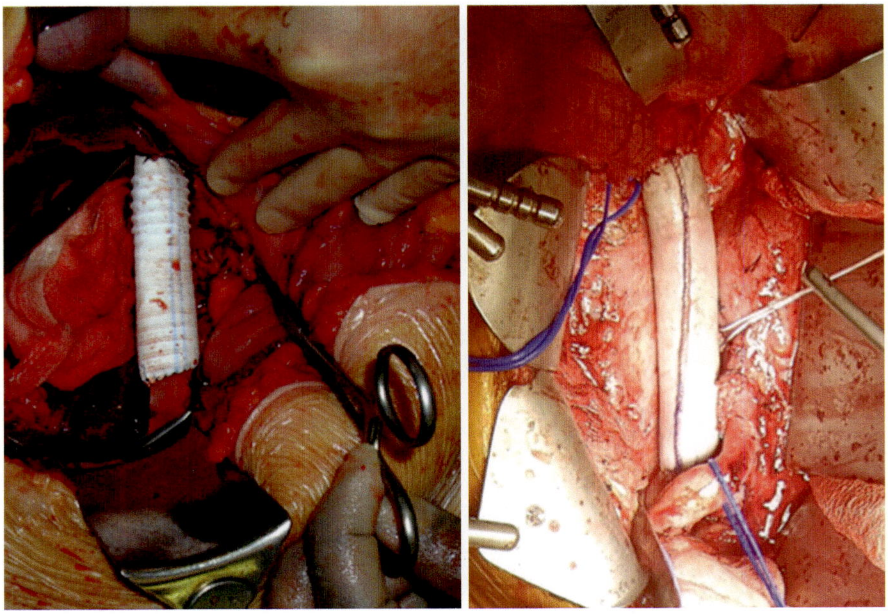

Fig. 9 IVC veins grafts, synthetic (left) and Bovine (right) following right nephrectomy. Note left renal vein reconstruction was not required. Photographs courtesy of Tim O'Brien

Most patients are managed with extended courses of prophylactic LMWH following graft surgery, but acute thrombosis of an interposition graft or even patch grafts can occur regardless. To this end, it is important that the collateral venous circulation of the IVC, in particular the lumbar veins, are not ligated during dissection. Distal lumbar veins should be preserved if practical, however proximal ones usually need control in order to mobilise the IVC adequately for dissection and ligation.

Key Points

- The BAUS nephrectomy audit of National UK practice in 2017 showed 19% of radical nephrectomy continues to be performed with the open approach
- The goals of radical nephrectomy are:
  - Extraction of the tumour with clear margins
  - Preservation of surrounding organs
  - Reasonable operative time and blood loss

  If these objectives cannot be achieved laparoscopically, then open surgery is indicated
- Surgery for tumours extending into the IVC presents some of the most challenging surgery in the abdomen. Open surgery for such cases is still the mainstay of practice because of the degree of vascular control required to extract the tumour without catastrophic bleeding.
- The Mayo Classification of IVC thrombus offers a very practical assessment of RCC venous extension in terms of operative consideration
- Mayo classification of IVC [21] tumour thrombus
  - Thrombus limited to renal vein
  - Thrombus extending ≤2 cm above the renal vein
  - Thrombus extending >2 cm above the renal vein, below hepatic veins
  - Thrombus at or above the hepatic veins but below the diaphragm

For tumours extending into the IVC, an anterior approach is typical, usually with an L-shaped incision for right sided tumours, and a Mercedes incision for left sided tumours when hepatic mobilisation is required. The Chevron incision is also commonly used, given access to the pelvis is not required.

References

1. Devlin CM, Fowler S, Biyani CS, Forster JA. Changes in UK renal oncological surgical practice from 2008 to 2017: implications for cancer service provision and surgical training. BJU Int. n/a:n/a.
2. Neves RJ, Zincke H. Surgical treatment of renal cancer with vena cava extension. Br J Urol. 1987;59(5):390–5.

3. Abaza R. Initial series of robotic radical nephrectomy with vena caval tumor thrombectomy. Eur Urol. 2011;59(4):652–6.
4. Meng M. Urologic oncologic survey robotic level III inferior vena cava tumor thrombectomy: initial series. Gill IS, Metcalfe C, Abreu A, Duddalwar V, Chopra S, Cunningham M, Thangathurai D, Ukimura O, Satkunasivam R, Hung A, Papalia R, Aron M, Desai M, Gallucci M. J Urol. 2015 Oct;194(4):929-938. [Epub 2015 Apr 6]. Urol Oncol. 2017;35(5):311. https://doi.org/10.1016/j.juro.2015.03.119.
5. Wang B, Huang Q, Liu K, Fan Y, Peng C, Gu L, et al. Robot-assisted level III-IV inferior vena cava Thrombectomy: initial series with step-by-step procedures and 1-yr outcomes. Eur Urol. 2020;78(1):77–86.
6. Wein AJ, Kavoussi LR, Partin AW, Peters CA. Campbell-Walsh urology. 11th ed. Elsevier; 2016.
7. Jennings SB, Austenfeld MS, Basham K. Fatal pulmonary embolus from ischemic necrosis of Intracaval tumor thrombus: a case report. J Urol. 1993;150(5 Part 1):1492–5.
8. Subramanian VS, Stephenson AJ, Goldfarb DA, Fergany AF, Novick AC, Krishnamurthi V. Utility of preoperative renal artery embolization for management of renal tumors with inferior vena caval thrombi. Urology. 2009;74(1):154–9.
9. Ciancio G, Vaidya A, Soloway M. Early ligation of the renal artery using the posterior approach: a basic surgical concept reinforced during resection of large hypervascular renal cell carcinoma with or without inferior vena cava thrombus. BJU Int. 2003;92(4):488–9.
10. Chiavegato L, Medina-Pestana J, Tedesco-Silva H, Paisani D, Fiore J Jr, Faresin S. Surgical approach does not affect perioperative respiratory morbidity in living donor nephrectomy: comparison between anterior subcostal incision and flank incision. Transplant Proc. 2010;42(5):1472–5.
11. Hager B, Herzog SA, Sandner-Kiesling A, Zigeuner R, Pummer K. Comparison of early postoperative pain after partial tumour nephrectomy by flank, transabdominal or laparoscopic access. Br J Pain. 2019;13(3):177–84.
12. Kumar S, Duque JL, Guimaraes KC, Dicanzio J, Loughlin KR, Richie JP. Short and long-term morbidity of thoracoabdominal incision for nephrectomy: a comparison with the flank approach. J Urol. 1999;162(6):1927–9.
13. Honig MP, Mason RA, Giron F. Wound complications of the retroperitoneal approach to the aorta and iliac vessels. J Vasc Surg. 1992;15(1):28–33. Discussion -4
14. Ballard JL, Abou-Zamzam AM, Teruya TH, Harward TR, Flanigan DP. Retroperitoneal aortic aneurysm repair: long-term follow-up regarding wound complications and erectile dysfunction. Ann Vasc Surg. 2006;20(2):195–9.
15. Gardner GP, Josephs LG, Rosca M, Rich J, Woodson J, Menzoian JO. The retroperitoneal incision. An evaluation of postoperative flank 'bulge'. Arch Surg. 1994;129(7):753–6.
16. Purnell CA, Park E, Turin SY, Dumanian GA. Postoperative flank defects, hernias, and bulges: a reliable method for repair. Plast Reconstr Surg. 2016;137(3):994–1001.
17. Diblasio CJ, Snyder ME, Russo P. Mini-flank supra-11th rib incision for open partial or radical nephrectomy. BJU Int. 2006;97(1):149–56.
18. Jimenez-Torres JA, Virumbrales-Munoz M, Sung KE, Lee MH, Abel EJ, Beebe DJ. Patient-specific organotypic blood vessels as an in vitro model for anti-angiogenic drug response testing in renal cell carcinoma. EBioMedicine. 2019;42:408–19.
19. O'Malley RL, Godoy G, Kanofsky JA, Taneja SS. The necessity of adrenalectomy at the time of radical nephrectomy: a systematic review. J Urol. 2009;181(5):2009–17.
20. González J, Ciancio G. Surgery of the inferior vena cava. Cham: Springer; 2017.
21. Blute ML, Leibovich BC, Lohse CM, Cheville JC, Zincke H. The Mayo Clinic experience with surgical management, complications and outcome for patients with renal cell carcinoma and venous tumour thrombus. BJU Int. 2004;94(1):33–41.
22. Blute ML, Boorjian SA, Leibovich BC, Lohse CM, Frank I, Karnes RJ. Results of inferior vena caval interruption by greenfield filter, ligation or resection during radical nephrectomy and tumor thrombectomy. J Urol. 2007;178(2):440–5. Discussion 4
23. Gershman B, Leibovich BC. Assessing the evidence for the surgical Management of Renal Cell Carcinoma with venous tumor thrombus: room to grow. Eur Urol. 2016;70(2):281–2.

24. Ayyathurai R, Garcia-Roig M, Gorin M, González J, Manoharan M, Kava B, et al. Bland thrombus association with tumour thrombus in renal cell carcinoma: analysis of surgical significance and role of inferior vena caval interruption. BJU Int. 2012;110
25. Psutka SP, Boorjian SA, Thompson RH, Schmit GD, Schmitz JJ, Bower TC, et al. Clinical and radiographic predictors of the need for inferior vena cava resection during nephrectomy for patients with renal cell carcinoma and caval tumour thrombus. BJU Int. 2015;116(3):388–96.
26. Dahan H, Arrivé L, Monnier-Cholley L, Le Hir P, Zins M, Tubiana JM. Cavoportal collateral pathways in vena cava obstruction: imaging features. AJR Am J Roentgenol. 1998;171(5):1405–11.
27. Abel EJ, Wood CG, Eickstaedt N, Fang JE, Kenney P, Bagrodia A, et al. Preoperative pulmonary embolism does not predict poor postoperative outcomes in patients with renal cell carcinoma and venous thrombus. J Urol. 2013;190(2):452–7.
28. O'Brien T, Fernando A, Thomas K, Van Hemelrijck M, Bailey C, Austin C. Raised preoperative international normalised ratio (INR) identifies patients at high risk of perioperative death after simultaneous renal and cardiac surgery for tumours involving the peri-diaphragmatic inferior vena cava and right atrium. BJU Int. 2017;119(3):424–9.
29. Shirodkar SP, Soloway MS, Ciancio G. Budd-Chiari syndrome in urology: impact on nephrectomy for advanced renal cell carcinoma. Indian J Urol. 2011;27(3):351–6.
30. Patil MB, Montez J, Loh-Doyle J, Cai J, Skinner EC, Schuckman A, et al. Level III-IV inferior vena caval thrombectomy without cardiopulmonary bypass: long-term experience with intrapericardial control. J Urol. 2014;192(3):682–8.
31. Baniel J, Foster RS, Donohue JP. Surgical anatomy of the lumbar vessels: implications for retroperitoneal surgery. J Urol. 1995;153(5):1422–5.
32. Smith JAJMD, Howards SSMD, Preminger GMMD, Dmochowski RRMDF. Copyright. In: Smith JAJMD, Howards SSMD, Preminger GMMD, RRMDF D, editors. Hinman's atlas of urologic surgery; 2019. p. iv.
33. Libertino JA. Renal cancer: contemporary management. New York: Springer; 2013.
34. Ciancio G, Soloway MS. Renal cell carcinoma with tumor thrombus extending above diaphragm: avoiding cardiopulmonary bypass. Urology. 2005;66(2):266–70.
35. Ciancio G, Shirodkar SP, Soloway MS, Livingstone AS, Barron M, Salerno TA. Renal carcinoma with supradiaphragmatic tumor thrombus: avoiding sternotomy and cardiopulmonary bypass. Ann Thorac Surg. 2010;89(2):505–10.
36. Kaag MG, Toyen C, Russo P, Cronin A, Thompson RH, Schiff J, et al. Radical nephrectomy with vena caval thrombectomy: a contemporary experience. BJU Int. 2011;107(9):1386–93.
37. Nguyen HG, Tilki D, Dall'Era MA, Durbin-Johnson B, Carballido JA, Chandrasekar T, et al. Cardiopulmonary bypass has no significant impact on survival in patients undergoing nephrectomy and level III-IV inferior vena cava Thrombectomy: multi-institutional analysis. J Urol. 2015;194(2):304–8.
38. Abel EJ, Thompson RH, Margulis V, Heckman JE, Merril MM, Darwish OM, et al. Perioperative outcomes following surgical resection of renal cell carcinoma with inferior vena cava thrombus extending above the hepatic veins: a contemporary multicenter experience. Eur Urol. 2014;66(3):584–92.
39. Bower TC, Nagorney DM, Cherry KJ Jr, Toomey BJ, Hallett JW, Panneton JM, et al. Replacement of the inferior vena cava for malignancy: an update. J Vasc Surg. 2000;31(2):270–81.
40. Caldarelli G, Minervini A, Guerra M, Bonari G, Caldarelli C, Minervini R. Prosthetic replacement of the inferior vena cava and the iliofemoral vein for urologically related malignancies. BJU Int. 2002;90(4):368–74.
41. Morris PD, Furtado R, Pulitano C, Crawford M, Yeo D, Vasilaras A, et al. Inferior vena cava resection and reconstruction with bovine pericardium for renal cell carcinoma: complications and outcomes. Urology. 2019;134:143–7.
42. Tomimaru Y, Eguchi H, Wada H, Doki Y, Mori M, Nagano H. Surgical outcomes of liver resection combined with inferior vena cava resection and reconstruction with artificial vascular graft. Dig Surg. 2019;36(6):502–8.

Radical Nephrectomy for Renal Cell Carcinoma: Non-robotic Minimally Invasive Approaches

Ryan L. Steinberg, Brett A. Johnson, Jeffrey A. Cadeddu, and Abhay Rane

Introduction

Since the original report 150 years ago by Gustav Simon [1], the nephrectomy has undergone multiple landmark changes including the adoption of the retroperitoneal flank approach in the early twentieth century to reduce the incidence of intraabdominal complications, as well as a more radical, Halsted-esque, resection to remove the peri-renal fat and Gerota's fascia [2]. More recently, the use of laparoscopy has shown improved recovery after surgery [3, 4] and patient-reported quality of life [5]. Since the initial report of laparoscopic nephrectomy, minimally invasive surgery for renal cell carcinoma has rapidly evolved. We now aim to review the multiple, non-robotic based approaches that have been reported.

Contraindications

Few absolute contraindications to minimally invasive surgery for radical nephrectomy exist. Uncorrected coagulopathy increases the risk of peri-operative bleeding and should be corrected. Though, for patients on anti-coagulation for cardiac or vascular reasons, individual risk/benefit assessment should be undertaken as to whether these medications can safely be held. There have been reports that laparoscopic renal procedures can be safely performed during anti-platelet therapy [6]. In addition, the inability to tolerate general anesthesia [7] or pneumoperitoneum [8, 9],

R. L. Steinberg · B. A. Johnson · J. A. Cadeddu
University of Texas Southwestern Department of Urology, Dallas, TX, USA

A. Rane (✉)
Surrey and Sussex Healthcare NHS Trust, East Surrey Hospital, Surrey, UK

C. Anderson, M. Afshar (eds.), *Renal Cancer*,
https://doi.org/10.1007/978-3-030-84756-2_11

particularly in patients with advanced cardiopulmonary disease, would negate the ability to perform laparoscopy. Various adjustments to minimize the effects of insufflation, including working at lower pressures, use of helium instead of carbon dioxide [10], and use of specialized instruments [11] have been reported.

A thorough history and physical examination can identify potential difficulties during surgery and can help determine which approach would be best for the patient (laparoscopic vs open, transperitoneal vs. retroperitoneal). Prior transperitoneal or retroperitoneal surgery and obesity can increase surgical difficultly but do not preclude the ability to safely complete procedures. Ultimately, careful patient selection can optimize outcomes and minimize surgical risk.

Approaches

Transperitoneal

The transperitoneal approach is the traditional and most widely utilized minimally invasive method for performing a nephrectomy since the initial report by Clayman et al. [12] in 1991. It provides the largest working space of all approaches and is often the most familiar approach to urologists. Though, entry into the peritoneal cavity risks potential bowel or other intraperitoneal injury during insufflation or port placement.

After induction of anesthesia and appropriate tube placement (intravenous line, orogastric tube, urethral catheter), the patient is positioned in a modified (30–45°) flank position with the contralateral arm placed on an arm board and the ipsilateral arm secured in one of a number of positions (at patient's side, on a folded pillow across the chest or on a Kraus armboard). The patient is appropriately padded and secured to the table, allowing for table tiliting. Significant bed flexion and the use of the kidney rest is not required as with open surgery. Figure 1 demonstrates the above positioning with the arm secured at the patient's side. Pneumoperitoneum is obtained and ports are placed allowing for triangulation toward the 11th rib. Multiple trocar configurations have been reported [13]. The most common configuration utilizes ports located in the anterior axillary line at the level of the umbilicus and just off the costal margin approximately 1/3 of the way from the xiphoid to the umbilicus for instrumentation, as well as peri-umbilically for the camera. In the case of obese patients, trocar placement further lateral is required.

Retroperitoneal

The retroperitoneal approach was first described by Kerbl et al. in 1993 [14]. This technique more closely mimics an open flank approach given the avoidance of the bowel and the use of psoas muscle as a surgical landmark. Though, as noted in the

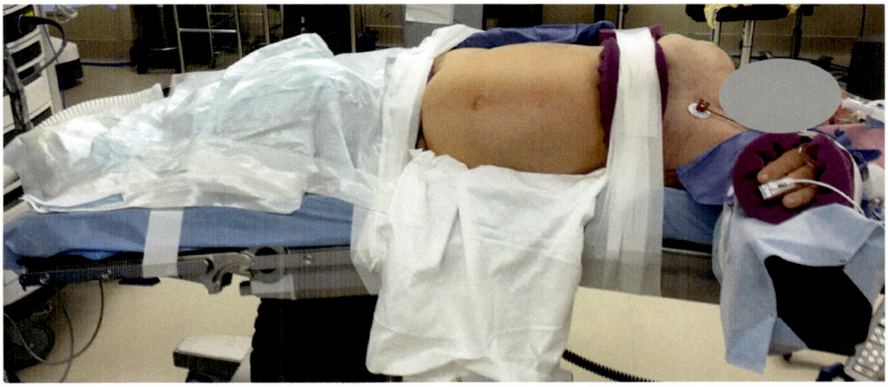

Fig. 1 Patient positioning for a right transperitoneal laparoscopic nephrectomy. A modified flank position is used with left (contralateral) arm on an arm board and right (ipsilateral) arm secured at patient's side

original report, the working space is substantially smaller than traditional laparoscopy, thereby reducing triangulation of the instruments and leading to increased instrument clashing.

The primary theoretical advantage of this approach is in avoiding the peritoneal cavity, thereby leading to earlier recovery of bowel function. This also negates the need for lysis of adhesions in patients with multiple prior intra-abdominal procedures. Though, a randomized prospective trail comparing traditional and retroperitoneal laparoscopic nephrectomy found only operative time to be different between the 2 approaches, but not blood loss, analgesic use, hospitalization time, or complication rate [15]. Disadvantages of this approach include the aforementioned smaller working envelope, as well as the subtlety of the anatomic landmarks. Considering the latter, entry too anterior can violate the peritoneum and risks colonic injury while too posterior risks bleeding from the psoas muscle or quadratus lumborum.

In this approach, patients are placed in a full flank position with an axillary roll to prevent a brachial plexus injury, as well as moderate bed flexion in order to open the retroperitoneal space between the 12th rib and iliac crest. An incision is made in the soft spot midway between the 12th rib and iliac crest which typically corresponds with the posterior axillary line. Dissection proceeds down to the lumbodorsal fascia which his opened and the retroperitoneum entered. Development of a potential space can then be performed bluntly with a finger, a balloon dilator, or with a laparoscope to create a working space along the psoas fascia. Typically, one of the instrument ports can then be placed posterior and cephalad to the camera port, just lateral to erector spinae muscles. Through this port, a blunt instrument can be used to dissect the peritoneum off the anterior abdominal wall medially, creating space for the other instrument port, often located just off the tip of the 12th rib. Figure 2 demonstrates port placement.

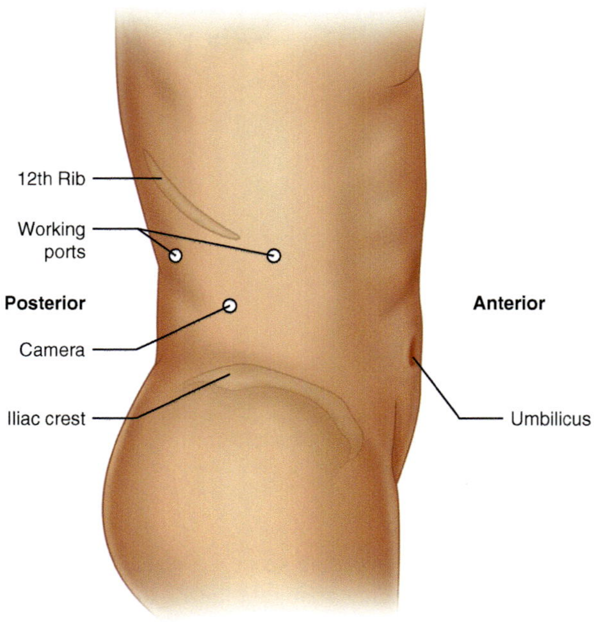

Fig. 2 Retroperitoneal laparoscopic nephrectomy port configuration. The camera port should be placed midway between the 12th rib and iliac crest and the working instrument ports placed cephalad. Care should be taken with placement of the posterior port to avoid the erector spinae muscles and the anterior port to avoid the peritoneal cavity

Hand-Assisted

The hand-assisted laparoscopic nephrectomy (HALN) was initially described by Nakada et al. in 1997 [16]. This technique combines the tactile feedback of open surgery with the minimal invasiveness of laparoscopy. Pneumoperitoneum is maintained by utilizing one of several commercial devices (e.g. *GelPort*, Applied Medical (Rancho Santa Margarita, CA, USA), *HandPort*, Smith and Nephew (Andover, MA, USA)) that allows a gloved hand to be inserted into the abdomen in an airtight manner (Fig. 3). Typically, the surgeon's non-dominant hand is placed intra-abdominally for retraction, palpation, and blunt dissection while the dominant hand manipulates a laparoscopic instrument via a traditional port. Figure 4 demonstrates the port placement for a right-handed surgeon performing a (a) right and (b) left hand-assisted nephrectomy.

The primary benefit of HALN is that it allows the technical challenges of laparoscopy to be easier for a more novice surgeon. Further, it allows for directly tissue palpation, making hilar anatomy more easily identifiable and allows for the treatment of masses with renal vein involvement [17]. Also, in the case of large tumors, hand-assisted retraction may be stronger and provide better exposure than laparoscopic instruments. In the event of a hilar injury, the presence of a hand in the abdomen can allow for better vascular control [18]. Traditional laparoscopic technique can be converted to hand-assisted by extending the non-dominant hand trocar incision and placing a hand-assist device.

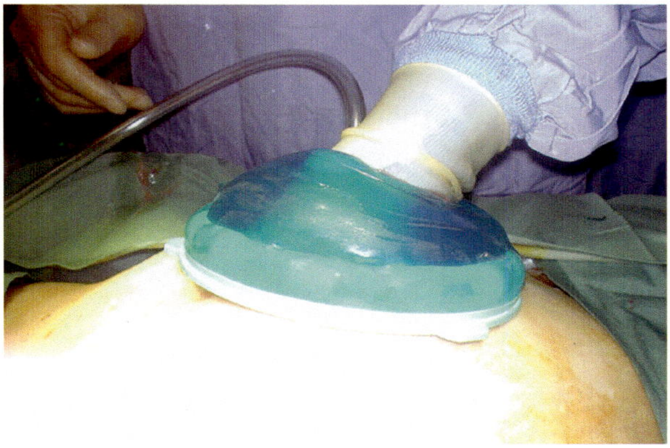

Fig. 3 Image of a commercial hand-assist device to maintain pneuoperitoneum with placement of a hand within the peritoneal cavity

Retrospective analysis of HALN compared to traditional laparoscopy is difficult as surgeons tend to elect for HALN for more challenging cases (large tumors or significant scaring). However, HALN has been showed to reduce operative time by 90 min [19]. A prospective randomized comparison demonstrated no difference in post-operative pain, hospitalization time, and complications [20]. Drawbacks of HALN include increased cost of the hand-assistance device, poorer cosmesis of the larger incision. There also the possibility of more pain and longer convalescence with the large incision, however, several studies have demonstrated these to be similar [18]. Ultimately, the HALN can be a valuable tool for challenging cases or as an intermediate means to manage intra-operative complications without conversion to open surgery [21].

Single-Site

Laparoendoscopic Single-Site (LESS) surgery refers to a laparoscopic technique that consolidates all ports within a single skin incision (typically peri-umbilically) [22]. The conceptual drive of LESS is minimization of skin incisions, and therefore, reduced port-related complications/pain and improved cosmesis. Non-randomized studies have demonstrated LESS is non-inferior to traditional laparoscopy with regards to peri-operative outcomes and minor improvements in post-operative pain and cosmesis [23]. A randomized trial demonstrated reduced recovery time and positive subjective cosmesis [24]. This technique has also be applied in robotic surgery [25].

LESS is a technical challenge and makes ergonomics unfavorable. Given the instruments are entering the abdominal cavity in close proximity, they often collide. Also, in some cases, the instruments must be crossed, leading to simple tasks becoming very technically demanding. Often, specialized equipment (curved, cross armed instruments) are required. Significant experience with laparoscopy is needed prior embarking on LESS.

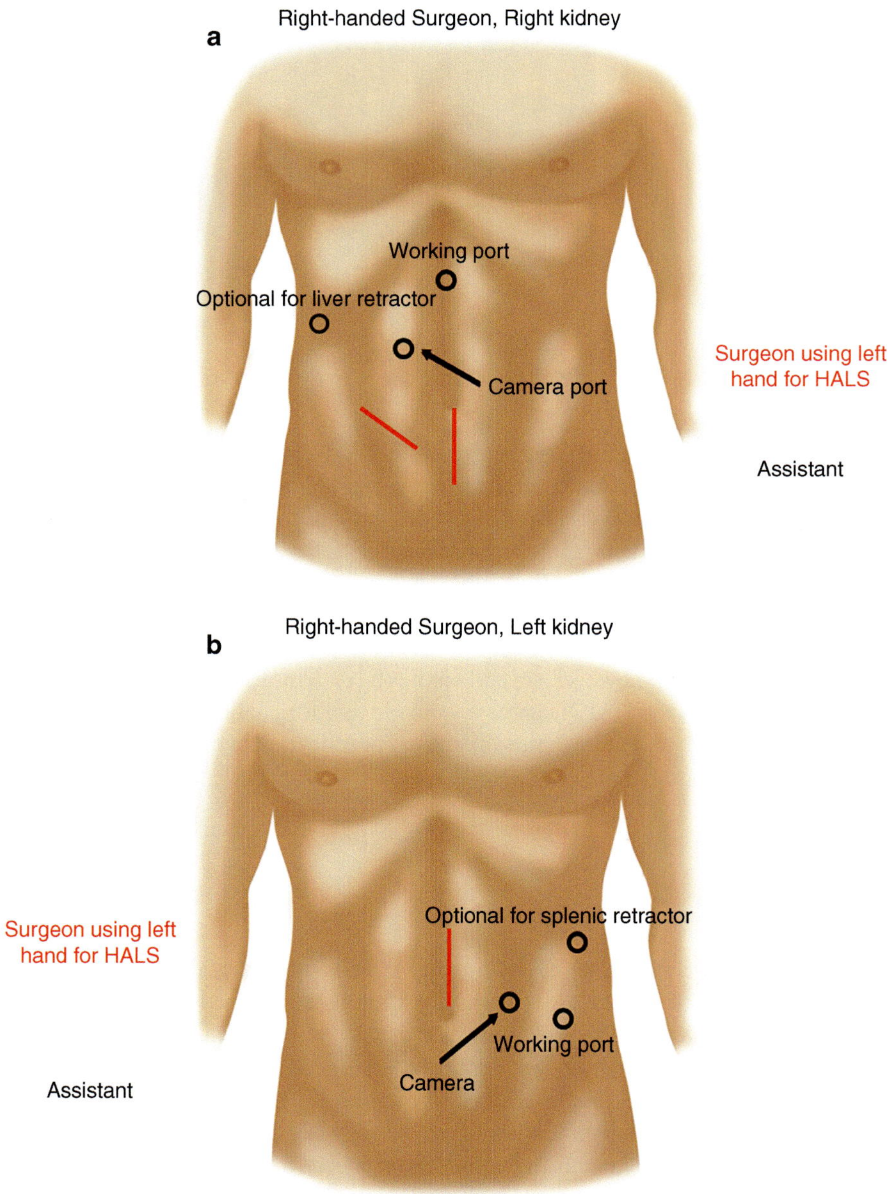

Fig. 4 Port configuration and surgeon/assistant positioning for a right-handed surgeon performing a (**a**) right and (**b**) left hand-assisted laparoscopic nephrectomy. Note, the red lines represent the location of the hand-assist device while circles represent the placement of traditional laparoscopic ports

LESS has been utilized extensively for laparoscopic donor nephrectomies as these tend to be healthy patients with favorable renal anatomy. A recent Cochrane review compared LESS donor nephrectomy to traditional laparoscopy and found no difference with regard to operative time, blood loss, complication rate, ischemia time, or graft loss. LESS demonstrated improved pain scores [26]. Ultimately, LESS technique offers a means to reduce the number of ports and improve cosmesis, but this trade-off must be balanced with the increase in the technical challenge.

Natural Orifice Transluminal Endoscopic Surgery (NOTES)

The Natural Orifice Transluminal Endoscopic Surgery (NOTES) approach, as its name implies, utilizes natural orifices (e.g., the mouth, vagina, rectum) for placement of ports or multi-channel access devices through which the surgery is performed and specimens extracted. The appeal of this technique is to access the peritoneal cavity but avoid the need for abdominal incisions. Theoretical advantages of NOTES include reduced post-operative pain, reduced incision-related complications, and improved cosmesis. Though, as with single port surgery, this approach is very technically demanding given the loss of triangulation and the inadequate instrumentation for the approach [27]. Further, the unfamiliar camera angle when approaching the kidney given the orifice access can be disorienting.

Proof of concept for NOTES nephrectomy was first reported using vaginal access in a porcine model by Gettman et al. in 2001 [28]. More recently, transvesical peritoneal access was explored, again in an animal model [29]. The first human case was reported by Kaouk et al. in 2010 [30]. In this case, dense pelvic adhesions from a prior hysterectomy required intraperitoneal port placement for introduction of the vaginal port and colonic retraction. All subsequent reports, comprising multiple single patient reports and small series) have utilized a combination of NOTES and traditional laparoscopy [31–34]. To our knowledge, there are no comparative studies assessing the NOTES approach. As such, this approach should be undertaken only by those with significant laparoscopic experience and without known comparative efficacy to other techniques.

Current Nuances

The laparoscopic nephrectomy gained widespread popularity in the 1990's and has since been modified in a number of ways as discussed above. The most significant current consideration is the debated whether radical nephrectomy should utilize a robotic surgical system. While traditional laparoscopy is more technically challenging than robotic surgery, it is also possibly less resource-intensive. However, this comparison is very complex depending on the clinical environment and outside the scope of this chapter.

There continue to be technological advances in the field of laparoscopy. The FlexDex platform (FlexDex Surgical, Brighton, MI) is a mechanical laparoscopic instrument that translates the surgeon's hand, wrist and arm movements into corresponding movements inside the patient. This device confers the benefits of wrist movements and multiple degrees of freedom without the cost and complexity of a surgical robot [35]. Advances in endoscopic camera systems including stereoscopic three-dimensional imaging, 4 K-high definition, and near-infrared imaging, as well as flexible tip endoscopes continue to improve visualization. The advent of newer electrosurgical technology including ultrasonic shears, electrothermical bipolar vessel sealing, and thermal tissue fusion have improved hemostasis and dissection. Laparoscopic suturing devices (e.g. *Endo Stitch*™, Medtronic Minimally Invasive Therapies, *Suture Assistant*, Ethicon, and *OverStitch*®,Apollo Endosurgery Inc) have also reduced the technical challenge of suturing laparoscopically [36].

All of these technological advances continue to make non-robotic laparoscopy safer and less technically challenging. Laparoscopic skills remain a critical component in the modern urologist's armamentarium.

Key Points

Technique	Basics	Advantages	Disadvantages
Transperitoneal laparoscopy	• Most widely utilized • Trans-abdominal access and pneumoperitoneum is established • 3–5 ports are placed	• Common operation most urologists are comfortable with • Minimal additional costs and required equipment	• Still technically challenging
Retroperitoneal laparoscopy	• Completely extra-peritoneal • Retroperitoneum is dissected and insufflated	• Avoids abdominal cavity (and any adhesions that may be present)	• Less familiar approach for many • Less working space • Subtle anatomical landmarks • Difficult to maintain insufflation
Hand-assisted laparoscopy	• Utilizes device to place the non- dominant hand intra-abdominal while maintaining pneumoperitoneum • Combines benefits of open surgery (tactile feedback, manual dissection) with laparoscopy	• Technically easier • Allows less experience surgeon to deal with larger tumors or greater case complexity • Allows easier control of a hilar injury	• Larger incision • Worse cosmesis • Specialized equipment needed
Laparoendo-scopic single-site surgery (LESS)	• All laparoscopic ports enter through one incision • Incision is typically peri-umbilical	• Excellent cosmesis	• More technically challenging • Specialized equipment required • Loss of triangulation

Technique	Basics	Advantages	Disadvantages
Natural orifice transluminal endoscopic surgery (NOTES)	• Abdominal access obtained via natural orifice (typically trans-vaginally)	• No scars or abdominal port sites	• Disorientating anatomy • Minimal working space • Loss of triangulation

References

1. Herr HW. Surgical management of renal tumors: a historical perspective. Urol Clin N Am. 2008;35(4):543–9.
2. Robson CJ. Radical nephrectomy for renal cell carcinoma. J Urol. 1963;89:37–42.
3. Perry KT, Freedland SJ, Hu JC, Phelan MW, Kristo B, Gritsch AH, et al. Quality of life, pain and return to normal activities following laparoscopic donor nephrectomy versus open mini-incision donor nephrectomy. J Urol. 2003;169(6):2018–21.
4. Rassweiler J, Frede T, Henkel TO, Stock C, Alken P. Nephrectomy: a comparative study between the transperitoneal and retroperitoneal laparoscopic versus the open approach. Eur Urol. 1998;33(5):489–96.
5. Pace KT, Dyer SJ, Stewart RJ, Honey RJ, Poulin EC, Schlachta CM, et al. Health-related quality of life after laparoscopic and open nephrectomy. Surg Endosc. 2003;17(1):143–52.
6. Kefer JC, Desai MM, Fergany A, Novick AC, Gill IS. Outcomes of partial nephrectomy in patients on chronic oral anticoagulant therapy. J Urol. 2008;180(6):2370–4. discussion 734
7. Monk TG, Weldon BC. Anesthetic considerations for laparoscopic surgery. J Endourol. 1992;6(2):89–94.
8. Nunn JF. Applied respiratory physiology. Oxford: Butterworth-Heinemann; 2013.
9. Lew J, Gin T, Oh T. Anaesthetic problems during laparoscopic cholecystectomy. Anaesth Intensive Care. 1992;20(1):91–2.
10. Wolf JS, Clayman VR, McDougall EM, Shepherd DL, Folger WH, Monk TG. Carbon dioxide and helium insufflation during laparoscopic radical nephrectomy in a patient with severe pulmonary disease. J Urol. 1996;155(6):2021.
11. Herati AS, Andonian S, Rais-Bahrami S, Atalla MA, Srinivasan AK, Richstone L, et al. Use of the valveless trocar system reduces carbon dioxide absorption during laparoscopy when compared with standard trocars. Urology. 2011;77(5):1126–32.
12. Clayman RV, Kavoussi LR, Soper NJ, Dierks SM, Meretyk S, Darcy MD, et al. Laparoscopic nephrectomy: initial case report. J Urol. 1991;146(2):278–82.
13. Harper JD, Leppert JT, Breda A, Schulam PG. Standardized linear port configuration to improve operative ergonomics in laparoscopic renal and adrenal surgery: experience with 1264 cases. J Endourol. 2011;25(11):1769–73.
14. Kerbl K, Figenshau RS, Clayman RV, Chandhoke PS, Kavoussi LR, Albala DM, et al. Retroperitoneal laparoscopic nephrectomy: laboratory and clinical experience. J Endourol. 1993;7(1):23–6.
15. Desai MM, Strzempkowski B, Matin SF, Steinberg AP, Ng C, Meraney AM, et al. Prospective randomized comparison of transperitoneal versus retroperitoneal laparoscopic radical nephrectomy. J Urol. 2005;173(1):38–41.
16. Nakada SY, Moon TD, Gist M, Mahvi D. Use of Pnumo sleeve as an adjunct in laparoscopic nephrectomy. J Urol. 1997;49:612–3.
17. Henderson A, Murphy D, Jaganathan K, Roberts WW, Wolf JS Jr, Rané A. Hand-assisted laparoscopic nephrectomy for renal cell cancer with renal vein tumor thrombus. Urology. 2008;72(2):268–72.

18. Wolf JS. Hand-assisted laparoscopy: pro. J Urol. 2001;58:310–2.
19. Wolf JS, Moon TD, Nakada SY. Hand assisted laparoscopic nephrectomy: comparison to standard laparoscopic nephrectomy. J Urol. 1998;160(1):22–7.
20. Venkatesh R, Belani JS, Chen C, Sundaram CP, Bhayani SB, Figenshau RS, et al. Prospective randomized comparison of laparoscopic and hand-assisted laparoscopic radical nephrectomy. Urology. 2007;70(5):873–7.
21. Gettman MT, Box G, Averch T, Cadeddu JA, Cherullo E, Clayman RV, et al. Consensus statement on natural orifice transluminal endoscopic surgery and single-incision laparoscopic surgery: heralding a new era in urology? Eur Urol. 2008;53(6):1117–20.
22. Box G, Averch T, Cadeddu J, Cherullo E, Clayman R, Desai M, et al. Nomenclature of natural orifice translumenal endoscopic surgery (NOTES) and laparoendoscopic single-site surgery (LESS) procedures in urology. J Endourol. 2008;22(11):2575–81.
23. Autorino R, Cadeddu JA, Desai MM, Gettman M, Gill IS, Kavoussi LR, et al. Laparoendoscopic single-site and natural orifice transluminal endoscopic surgery in urology: a critical analysis of the literature. Eur Urol. 2011;59(1):26–45.
24. Tugcu V, Ilbey Y, Mutlu B, Tasci A. Laparoendoscopic single-site surgery versus standard laparoscopic simple nephrectomy: a prospective randomized study. J Endourol. 2010;24(8):1315–20.
25. Kaouk JH, Autorino R, Kim FJ, Han DH, Lee SW, Yinghao S, et al. Laparoendoscopic single-site surgery in urology: worldwide multi-institutional analysis of 1076 cases. Eur Urol. 2011;60(5):998–1005.
26. Gupta A, Ahmed K, Kynaston HG, Dasgupta P, Chlosta PL, Aboumarzouk OM. Laparoendoscopic single-site donor nephrectomy (LESS-DN) versus standard laparoscopic donor nephrectomy. Cochrane Database Syst Rev. 2016;2016(5):CD010850.
27. Autorino R, Haber GP, White MA, Khanna R, Altunrende F, Yang B, et al. Pure and hybrid natural orifice transluminal endoscopic surgery (NOTES): current clinical experience in urology. BJU Int. 2010;106(6b):919–22.
28. Gettman MT, Lotan Y, Napper CA, Cadeddu JA. Transvaginal laparoscopic nephrectomy: development and feasibility in the porcine model. Urology. 2002;59(3):446–50.
29. Metzelder M, Vieten G, Gosemann J, Ure B, Kuebler J. Endoloop© closure of the urinary bladder is safe and efficient in female piglets undergoing transurethral NOTES nephrectomy. Eur J Pediatr Surg. 2009;19(06):362–5.
30. Kaouk JH, White WM, Goel RK, Brethauer S, Crouzet S, Rackley RR, et al. NOTES transvaginal nephrectomy: first human experience. Urology. 2009;74(1):5–8.
31. Branco AW, Branco Filho AJ, Kondo W, Noda RW, Kawahara N, Camargo AA, et al. Hybrid transvaginal nephrectomy. Eur Urol. 2008;53(6):1290–4.
32. Alcaraz A, Musquera M, Peri L, Izquierdo L, García-Cruz E, Huguet J, et al. Feasibility of transvaginal natural orifice transluminal endoscopic surgery–assisted living donor nephrectomy: is kidney vaginal delivery the approach of the future? Eur Urol. 2011;59(6):1019–25.
33. Porpiglia F, Fiori C, Morra I, Scarpa RM. Transvaginal natural orifice transluminal endoscopic surgery–assisted minilaparoscopic nephrectomy: a step towards scarless surgery. Eur Urol. 2011;60(4):862–6.
34. Paparel P, Golfier F. Vaginal extraction after laparoscopic nephrectomy. BJU Int. 2011;108(11):1934–7.
35. Criss C, Ralls M, Johnson K, Awtar S, MD J, Geiger J. A novel intuitively controlled articulating instrument for Reoperative foregut surgery: a case report. J Laparoendosc Adv Surg Tech. 2017;9:983–6.
36. Rassweiler JJ, Teber D. Advances in laparoscopic surgery in urology. Nat Rev Urol. 2016;13(7):387–99.

Radical Nephrectomy: Role of Robotic Assisted Approach

A. L. Walsh and B. J. Challacombe

Introduction

While slow to be adopted, robot-assisted laparoscopic nephrectomy (RALN) is gaining momentum for the treatment of large and complex renal tumours. Robotic surgery has a very well established role in urologic surgery with robot-assisted radical prostatectomy and robot-assisted partial nephrectomy (PN) now accounting for 90% and 67% respectively of all prostatectomies and PN's in the UK BAUS audit 2018. The role of robotics in radical nephrectomy is less well defined and consequently we have been slower to adopt the robotic approach regarding radical nephrectomy for large renal tumours. Many would advocate open surgery for large complex tumours with caval involvement and the laparoscopic approach for those with smaller tumours not amenable to or suitable for PN.

Arguments against RALN include the perceived increased cost, more limited access to robotic theatre time, loss of haptic feedback and some report longer operating time of robotic surgery. Arguments for RALN however are numerous and include shorter hospital stay, decreased morbidity and pain, better visualisation of key structures and increased dexterity. RALN can also act as a key training modality for robotic surgeons to allow them to acquire the skills required for more complex renal surgery such as pyeloplasty and robot assisted partial nephrectomy.

Open radical nephrectomy confers significant morbidity on the patient with a large painful incision, either flank/subcostal or midline. This results in increased analgesia requirements, longer length of hospital stay and a higher incidence of wound herniation and chronic wound pain. RALN offers a minimally invasive approach to complex renal tumours. The degree of movement and anatomical control offered by the robot allows for retroperitoneal lymph node dissection and caval

A. L. Walsh (✉) · B. J. Challacombe
Department of Urology, St Georges Hospital, London, UK
e-mail: anna.walsh@stgeorges.nhs.uk; ben.challacombe@gstt.nhs.uk

C. Anderson, M. Afshar (eds.), *Renal Cancer*,
https://doi.org/10.1007/978-3-030-84756-2_12

thrombectomy in the right hands. Both of which are extremely challenging laparoscopic undertakings.

Indications for Radical Nephrectomy

Radical nephrectomy is the gold standard of care for larger renal tumours which are not suitable for nephron-sparing surgery (NSS). This includes where there would be an insufficient volume of parenchyma remaining to maintain the functionality of the kidney or if there is evidence of renal vein thrombosis. EAU guidelines recommend NSS for all T1 renal tumours. There are no reported differences in oncological outcomes between laparoscopic or open radical nephrectomy, however there are no randomised control trials assessing this. Open is traditionally preferred for very large tumours (>T2b), those invading the inferior vena cava or with visible nodal disease. NCCN guidelines state radical nephrectomy can be performed via an open, laparoscopic or robotic approach [1].

Training

RALN provides a training platform for surgeons and fellows to develop their robotic skills prior to performing complex PN resections, nephroureterectomies or tackling larger, more complex tumours. RALN encompasses five of the key eight steps involved in PN, most crucially the dissection of the hilum. It provides an excellent training platform and is not encompassed into the BAUS robotic training curriculum for robotic surgery [2]. RALN enables not only the surgeon but the whole theatre team to increase their familiarity with robotic upper tract surgery prior to embarking on the stressful 'on clamp' dissection at PN.

With the increased availability of the robot and more surgical and fellowship training programmes we see a fall-off in laparoscopic training and skill development. The skill set required to perform complex laparoscopic procedures will not be there and potentially laparoscopic surgery may become a thing of the past.

Large Renal Masses

Minimally invasive radical nephrectomy reduces morbidity and hospital stay when compared to open surgery with equivalent oncological outcomes [3]. The therapeutic indications for minimally invasive surgery continue to expand with surgical experience and technological advances. There are many case series reporting outcomes of laparoscopic nephrectomy for large renal masses which would traditionally have been managed with open surgery [4, 5].

Steinberg et al. examined outcomes in laparoscopic nephrectomy for tumours >7 cm, but all tumours >14 cm were excluded from analysis. Larger tumours did have more blood loss (200 ml v 100 ml in the <7 cm group) but similar operating times, complications rates and length of stay [5]. They reported no open conversions in their series of 65 patients [5]. Pierorazio's series of 64 patients with median tumour size of 12.9 cm reported an average 400 ml blood loss with a 13.8% conversion rate. Abaza et al.'s [6], albeit small, robotic series comprised 15 patients all with tumours >15 cm with no open conversions and a median estimated blood loss of 159 ml, this is compared to 500 ml reported for open nephrectomy in Steinberg's group which had a median tumour size of 9.9 cm. The average reported conversion rate across laparoscopic series is approximately 5% with reasons for conversion being failure to progress, uncontrolled massive bleeding and unknown IVC tumour thrombus.

Reported operative times in laparoscopic series for large tumours range around 192–240 min compared to robotic 234 min robotically for tumours over 15 cm. Laparoscopic resection of these large tumours is extremely challenging and high volume experience is required. A multi-centre study found that of 26 sites included in the trial only 10 centres performed laparoscopic nephrectomy for tumours >7 cm [4]. Robotics allows for easier dissection of the hilum, more dexterity and ability to reach around tight spaces where they may encounter bulky lymph node disease and ease of retraction with the robotic fourth arm. Extreme challenges such as IVC thrombus, lymph node dissection and solid organ invasion can all be managed robotically with only case reports of these challenges reported laparoscopically. These challenges are discussed in later sections.

Lymph Node Dissection

The role of lymph node dissection (LND) for localised RCC is debated with the only randomised control trial to date showing no benefit [7]. Over 70% of the cases in this trial however were T1/T2 tumours and unlikely to have lymph node metastasis and therefore benefit from LND. There was also no data on the number of nodes resected during the trial. With us performing surgery for larger, more advanced tumours, there is a definite need for LND in certain cases to improve chances of disease free survival.

Several large retrospective cohort studies have suggested that in patients with large tumours, visible lymph node disease and even metastatic disease there is a survival benefit with adequate LND [8]. While technically feasible, laparoscopic retroperitoneal lymph node dissection is a challenging undertaking requiring a skilled surgeon and high volume unit. The precision and ergonomics of robotics allows excellent control of tension and planes to facilitate RPLND in this setting. The ability to salvage bleeding from major structures is also far easier to control robotically than laparoscopically.

Evidence suggest that the benefit from LND is proportional to lymph node yield [9] with >12 nodes resulting in almost a 50% increase in the likelihood of detecting a positive node. A more extensive laparoscopic dissection or template is difficult to achieve. To date there are only a few retrospective studies in the literature championing laparoscopic lymph node dissection [10]. This could in part be due to lower stage tumours undergoing laparoscopic nephrectomy and those requiring LND having open nephrectomy as described by Terrone et al.

In those laparoscopic series that do look at LND the yield ranged from 2.7 to 7.8 (Chapman series), with a demonstrable improvement in yield with experience. In comparison to this, Abaza et al. [11] in a smaller series had an average lymph node yield of 13.9 with minimal morbidity equivocal to that with open surgical series highlighting the easier learning curve of this minimally invasive technique.

Caval Thrombectomy

4–10% of locally advanced cases of RCC are found to have IVC thrombosis. This cohort has traditionally been managed with open surgery given the complexity and potential hazards of opening the IVC laparoscopically and performing an adequate lymphadenectomy. Laparoscopically this is a significant undertaking and there are only a small number of studies in the literature reporting laparoscopic IVC thrombectomy and its outcomes. While it is possible, it is extremely challenging and requires immense skill and support.

Robotic-assisted thrombectomy maybe a more appropriate approach to minimally invasive IVC surgery and thrombectomy. The improved ergonomics allow for easier slinging of the cava while the fourth arm allows for easy retraction of the kidney freeing the assistant (see Fig. 1). The quicker suturing time reduces cross clamping time and blood loss is significantly less via the robotic approach. In cases of extensive thrombosis where cross-clamping is required the robot allows for swifter and more dynamic application of a tourniquet.

The largest laparoscopic series from China contains 11 patients, some with level IV IVC thrombus and joint thoracic resections [12]. In total under there are under 100 reported cases of laparoscopic IVC thrombectomy with robot-assisted thrombectomy rapidly taking over and likely halting the progression of the laparoscopic technique. Recently focus has shifted to more challenging robotic cases with IVC patch cavoplasty for caval wall invasion and fogarty balloon occlusion for intra- and retro-hepatic IVC control [13]. Current series are reporting outcomes of level II and III IVC thrombectomy with comparable morbidity to open surgery [14].

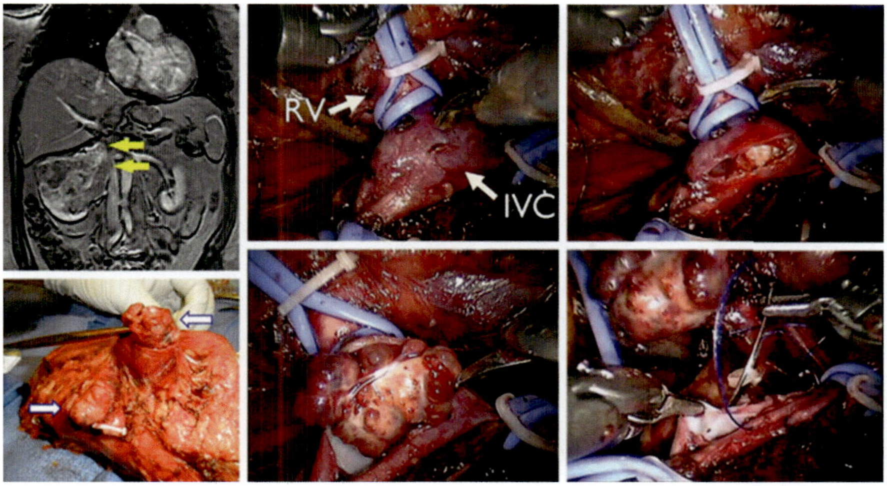

Fig. 1 Patient with two renal veins each with caval tumor thrombus, as seen on magnetic resonance imaging (upper left), after extraction (lower left) and intraoperatively with modified Rommel tourniquets for cross-clamping of the inferior vena cava (IVC) and lightly applied to prevent back bleeding from the right renal vein (RV) to open and deliver lower thrombus in a bloodless filed (right)

Other Challenges: Pushing the Boundaries of Robotic Nephrectomy

RALN enables a minimally invasive surgical approach for large, and even massive renal tumours. With this comes the challenge of caval thrombectomy and lymphadenectomy as described but also solid organ invasion where resection of other organs may also be required. RALN with partial hepatectomy, partial duodenectomy, cholecystectomy and distal pancreatectomy have all been described [15]. While such procedures are not commonplace with increasing robotic experience and skill we can expect more reports.

Recent interest has moved to robotic laparoendoscopic single site surgery (R-LESS). The proposed benefits would be almost no scarring and potentially reduced pain scores and incidence of incisional hernias. The robotic platform may help reduce the main issues of LESS with regards to intra-corporeal triangulation of instruments, external instrument clashes and enhanced ergonomics with reduced working space (see Fig. 2). To date there are several small case series and case reports looking at R-LESS in radical nephrectomy but the jury is out as to its role.

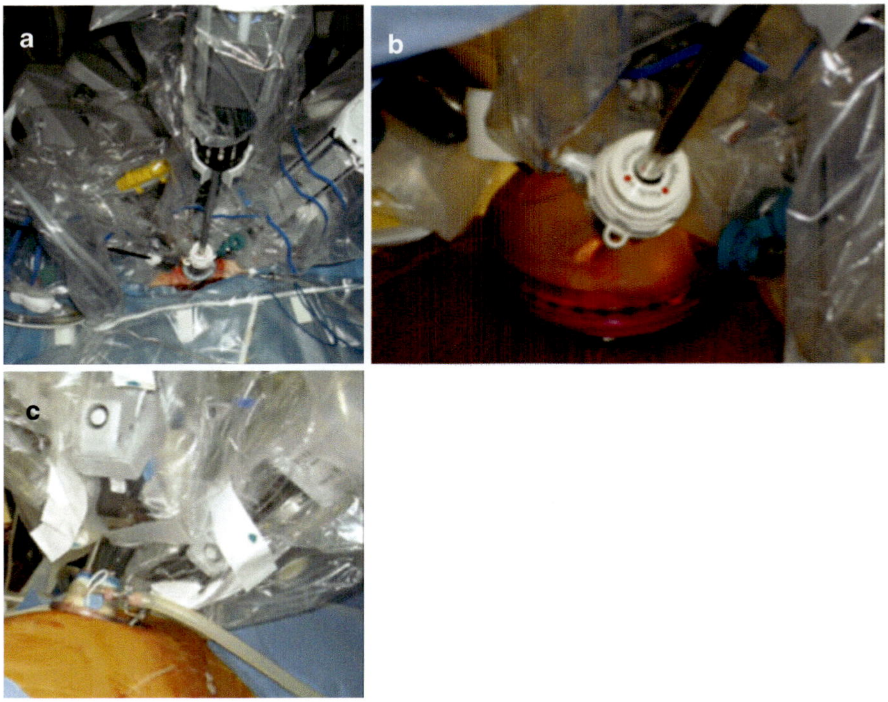

Fig. 2 Access devices to perform robotic laparoendoscopic single-site surgery: (**a**) SILS Port (Covidien), (**b**) Gelpoint (Applied), and (**c**) TriPort (Olympus). Courtesy of Jihad Koauk, Cleveland Clinic, Cleveland, OH, USA

Controversies in RALN

Data from the U.S.A. shows a dramatic increase in the use of RALN since the turn of the century with 1.5% of radical nephrectomies performed robotically in 2003 and 27% in 2015 [16]. While suggested that RALN was associated with a higher operating time and cost than laparoscopic surgery this point has subsequently been disputed. If the robot is already available in the department operating costs do not exceed that of laparoscopy and robotic surgery may actually be more cost effective [17]. Robotic surgery decreases requirements for disposables such as harmonic scalpels as only diathermy is required, ports are re-usable and instruments can be kept to a minimum.

Several analyses to date have proposed that RALN is associated with an increased operating time compared to laparoscopic or open surgery. It is also not however the experience of these authors in our centre. Operating time reflects surgical experience and case complexity and substantial variation has been seen in all three techniques. Often operating time reflects the case load volume of a centre, experience of the surgeon and depends on whether the procedure is performed in a training centre.

Loss of haptic feedback is a concern in robotic surgery across the board. This is not unique to RALN. Undoubtedly caution is required especially at dissection of the hilum to ensure excessive force is not applied to vessels or the tumour. This is a skill that is required of all robotic surgeons and takes time to develop. Similarly off screen injury with instruments in the fourth arm can be a perceived issue in robotic surgery that requires caution to avoid.

Conclusion

RALN it allows for a minimally invasive approach to complex and large renal tumours. It also provides an ideal training platform in the more 'routine' cases prior to surgeons embarking on more complex upper tract cases such as robotic partial nephrectomy or robotic pyeloplasty's. Laparoscopy has limitations even in the most skilled hands when faced with nodal disease, vascular invasion and invasion into other solid organs. To date there is no studies to support the superiority of RALN over LN, likewise many argue that it does not extend indications for minimally invasive surgery. However absence of evidence doesn't equal evidence of absence. Currently we have no level 1 evidence to support RARP or robotic pyeloplasty but both are superseding their open and laparoscopic counterparts.

If we do not try we do not progress.

Robotic surgery is constantly evolving with new robotic systems continuously being developed. The potential is there for quicker, slicker and safer surgery with an increased ability to perform complex cases.

Key Points

1. Robotic radical nephrectomy is feasible and safe.
2. Standard indications include T1a-T2 tumours where partial nephrectomy isn't possible.
3. Robotic radical nephrectomy may act as a training platform for more complex robotic renal procedures.
4. With increasing robotic availability the extra costs associated with robotic nephrectomy are reduced.
5. Robotic nephrectomy may allow for quicker and smoother surgery permitting rapid recovery and minimising hospital stay.
6. Intra-operative complications are more easily correctable with robotics compared to standard laparoscopic surgery.
7. The robotic approach is being extended to include renal tumours with vascular invasion including caval thrombus in experienced centres.

8. Robotic para-caval and para-aortic lymphadenectomy is feasible in selected cases and may be safer than the laparoscopic approach.
9. The intraoperative pneumoperitoneum minimises blood loss from collaterals in larger tumours. This may reduce the overall operative blood loss compared to the open approach.
10. Robotic nephrectomy is a common and important part of the portfolio of the modern upper tract minimally invasive surgeon.

References

1. Motzer RJ, Agarwal N, et al. *NCCN clinical practice guidelines in oncology.* Kidney Cancer Version 2.2019, NCCN Clinical Practice Guidelines in Oncology 2019 [cited 2020 02–01-20]; Available from: www.nccn.org/professionals.
2. Challacombe C, A.K.e.a. *BRITISH ASSOCIATION OF UROLOGICAL SURGEONS (BAUS) ROBOTIC SURGERY CURRICULUM - GUIDELINES FOR TRAINING.* [cited 2020 15-01-2020]; Guideline]. Available from: http://www.baus.org.uk/_userfiles/pages/files/Publications/RoboticSurgeryCurriculum.pdf.
3. Dunn MD, et al. Laparoscopic versus open radical nephrectomy: a 9-year experience. J Urol. 2000;164(4):1153–9.
4. Jeon SH, et al. Comparison of laparoscopic versus open radical nephrectomy for large renal tumors: a retrospective analysis of multi-center results. BJU Int. 2011;107(5):817–21.
5. Steinberg AP, et al. Laparoscopic radical nephrectomy for large (greater than 7 cm, T2) renal tumors. J Urol. 2004;172(6 Pt 1):2172–6.
6. Abaza R, Gerhard RS, Martinez O. Robotic radical nephrectomy for massive renal tumors. J Laparoendosc Adv Surg Tech A. 2020;30(2):196–200.
7. Blom JH, et al. Radical nephrectomy with and without lymph node dissection: preliminary results of the EORTC randomized phase III protocol 30881. EORTC genitourinary group. Eur Urol. 1999;36(6):570–5.
8. Whitson JM, et al. Lymphadenectomy improves survival of patients with renal cell carcinoma and nodal metastases. J Urol. 2011;185(5):1615–20.
9. Terrone C, et al. The number of lymph nodes examined and staging accuracy in renal cell carcinoma. BJU Int. 2003;91(1):37–40.
10. Chapman TN, et al. Laparoscopic lymph node dissection in clinically node-negative patients undergoing laparoscopic nephrectomy for renal carcinoma. Urology. 2008;71(2):287–91.
11. Abaza R, Lowe G. Feasibility and adequacy of robot-assisted lymphadenectomy for renal-cell carcinoma. J Endourol. 2011;25(7):1155–9.
12. Shao P, et al. Laparoscopic radical nephrectomy and inferior vena cava Thrombectomy in the treatment of renal cell carcinoma. Eur Urol. 2015;68(1):115–22.
13. Kundavaram C, et al. Advances in robotic vena cava tumor Thrombectomy: Intracaval balloon occlusion, patch grafting, and vena Cavoscopy. Eur Urol. 2016;70(5):884–90.
14. Chopra S, et al. Robot-assisted level II-III inferior vena cava tumor Thrombectomy: step-by-step technique and 1-year outcomes. Eur Urol. 2017;72(2):267–74.
15. Petros FG, Angell JE, Abaza R. Outcomes of robotic nephrectomy including highest-complexity cases: largest series to date and literature review. Urology. 2015;85(6):1352–8.
16. Jeong IG, et al. Association of Robotic-Assisted vs laparoscopic radical nephrectomy with perioperative outcomes and health care costs, 2003 to 2015. JAMA. 2017;318(16):1561–8.
17. Abaza R, Gonsenhauser I, Box G, Sharp D, Sabsigh A. Robotic nephrectomy is not costlier than standard laparoscopy when a robot is available. J Urol. 2015;193(4S):e388.

Contemporary Role of Open Nephron Sparing Surgery

Eduard Roussel, Mattias Willem van Hattem, Maarten Albersen, Steven Joniau, and Hendrik Van Poppel

Introduction

The incidence of renal cell carcinoma (RCC) has steadily increased over the past two decades and represents a considerable part of global cancer burden [1, 2]. However, localized disease can in many cases be curatively treated by surgery. Over a century after the first partial nephrectomy (PN) was accidentally performed in 1884 in an attempt to excise a perirenal fibroadenoma, this procedure has become the gold standard of care for the surgical extirpation of renal masses as stated by most guideline panels [3–6]. Historically, most patients presented with large symptomatic tumours whereas this day incidental diagnosis of asymptomatic small renal masses is much more common due to the increased and routine use of abdominal imaging modalities such as ultrasound, computed tomography and magnetic resonance imaging [1, 2]. Nephron sparing surgery (NSS) was initially reserved for imperative indications such as tumours in solitary kidneys or hereditary cancer syndromes but became more widely practiced as the technique of open partial nephrectomy (OPN) was refined throughout the twentieth century [3, 4]. It has become clear that the maximal preservation of functional renal parenchyma is paramount for functional outcome whilst a substantial body of evidence supporting oncological equivalence of PN and radical nephrectomy (RN) has been established [7–14]. However, the role of OPN has been challenged since the introduction of minimally invasive surgery (MIS) such as laparoscopic partial nephrectomy (LPN) and, more recently, robot assisted partial nephrectomy (RAPN). Although complex renal tumours are increasingly being treated with MIS modalities, OPN remains extremely valuable in the treatment of clinically challenging cases and certainly holds a firm place in the urologist's treatment armamentarium of kidney tumours.

E. Roussel · M. W. van Hattem · M. Albersen · S. Joniau · H. Van Poppel (✉)
Department of Urology, University Hospitals Leuven, Leuven, Belgium
e-mail: Hendrik.vanpoppel@uzleuven.be

C. Anderson, M. Afshar (eds.), *Renal Cancer*,
https://doi.org/10.1007/978-3-030-84756-2_13

Indications for NSS

Numerous studies have compared functional and oncological outcomes of PN compared to RN in favour of PN due to accumulating evidence on morbidity and mortality associated with decreased renal function while oncological equivalence has been established [7–9]. A recent Cochrane systematic review comparing RN and PN for clinically localised RCC found that PN was associated with a lower all-cause mortality, whereas cancer specific survival, serious adverse events and recurrence free survival were comparable to RN [9]. This is attributed to the preservation of functional renal parenchyma and the concomitant avoidance of iatrogenic chronic kidney disease (CKD) or need for renal replacement therapy [7]. Moreover, PN is associated with improved overall survival (OS) compared to RN in patients with unanticipated benign tumours, where the confounding effect of cancer is absent [10]. Contrarily, following a re-analysis of the prospective randomized controlled trial by the European Organisation for Research and Treatment of Cancer (EORTC), the beneficial effect of PN compared to RN on estimated glomerular filtration rate (eGFR) did not result in an improved OS [11]. It is thought that moderate renal dysfunction arising from surgery may not have the same negative implications as when arising from medical causes [12]. Patients with preoperative CKD, as well as those who have significant comorbidities are most likely to benefit from NSS [13, 14]. Therefore, RN could be better suited for patients for whom NSS is not imperative and have complex renal tumours for which the technical and oncological safety of NSS is not guaranteed [15, 16].

The feasibility of PN compared to RN is mainly determined by the amount of preservable renal parenchyma rather than tumour size [17–20]. Furthermore, since increasing tumour size is associated with metastatic potential, patients at higher risk for metastatic disease may be exactly those who benefit most from preserved renal function to allow for potential additional therapies [18].

Different clinical scenarios, such as initial, repeat or salvage PN entail different surgical approaches and OPN could be preferred in technically challenging tumours. Contrarily, the choice between RN and PN for the appropriate indication should never be dictated by the surgical access approach.

Surgical techniques in NSS

Different surgical approaches for NSS have been adopted by urologists in an attempt to minimize morbidity without compromising oncological or functional outcomes. During OPN a retroperitoneal approach via lumbotomy for mobilisation and vascular control is often used, leaving the peritoneum intact. The incision is preferentially made on the 12th rib, although larger, upper pole tumours may require more cranial lumbotomies. However, very large or bilateral tumours may require a transperitoneal approach via chevron incision. Both RAPN and LPN can equally be carried out via retroperitoneal or transperitoneal approach based on the surgeon's preference and experience [21].

Subsequently, the kidney is mobilized within the perinephric fat to allow for vascular control at the renal hilum. Mobilization of the kidney can be of particular difficulty due to the presence of so-called toxic fat. The Mayo adhesive probability (MAP) score is a helpful tool to preoperatively assess the presence of adherent perinephric fat on cross-sectional imaging [22]. It is often advocated to preserve the perinephric fat overlying the tumoral surface during excision since possible occult perinephric fat invasion can be present [23].

Renal ischaemia has been extensively studied since minimizing ischaemia related injury is of importance secondary to the maximal preservation of healthy, functional renal parenchyma. Although zero ischaemia (off-clamp) techniques have been described, clamping of the renal vasculature (either the main renal artery or segmental arteries) provides a bloodless field for tumour resection and reconstruction of the renal parenchyma and avoids excessive blood loss as well [21, 24]. Additionally, the reduction in surrounding renal tissue turgor eases tumour excision as well as external renorraphy. The higher venous backflow in OPN often requires clamping of the renal vein as well, due to the absence of a pneumoperitoneum providing intra-abdominal pressure.

A large multi-institutional study, including patients with solitary kidneys, concluded that warm ischaemia time (WIT) should be limited to less than 20 min and cold ischaemia time (CIT) to less than 35 min in order to avoid an increased risk of chronic or acute kidney injury [25]. However, these values are fairly arbitrary, and it is advocated to keep ischaemia time to a minimum in order to maximise the preservation of functional renal tissue [26]. A recent meta-analysis of 156 studies however, found that the net effect of ischemia techniques on surgical, functional or oncological outcome is debatable due to the plethora of confounding factors such as patient selection criteria, surgical technique and the amount of preserved functional renal parenchyma [27].

Since laparoscopic and robotic systems have become more widely accessible, experience with MIS has increased and WIT during MIS has drastically decreased, reaching comparable results to OPN [27]. Although cold ischaemia in MIS has been described and technically feasible, renal hypothermia is considered a main advantage of OPN [28]. Surface hypothermia is achieved after hilar clamping using ice slush for 10–20 min prior to resection of the tumour in order to reduce kidney metabolism. This is especially of concern in complex tumours where technically challenging dissection or reconstruction is needed, and prolonged ischaemia time is expected. Nephrometry scores such as the established RENAL and PADUA score can be of aid to objectively classify the complexity of renal tumours in preoperative planning [29–31].

Extirpation of the tumour can be performed by enucleation, where the natural plane between the tumoral pseudocapsule and the healthy renal parenchyma is followed, or enucleoresection where a rim of renal parenchyma is excised with the tumour (see Fig. 1a–f). Enucleation has been found to be oncologically equivalent to enucleoresection or wedge resection [32]. Completely endophytic tumours may

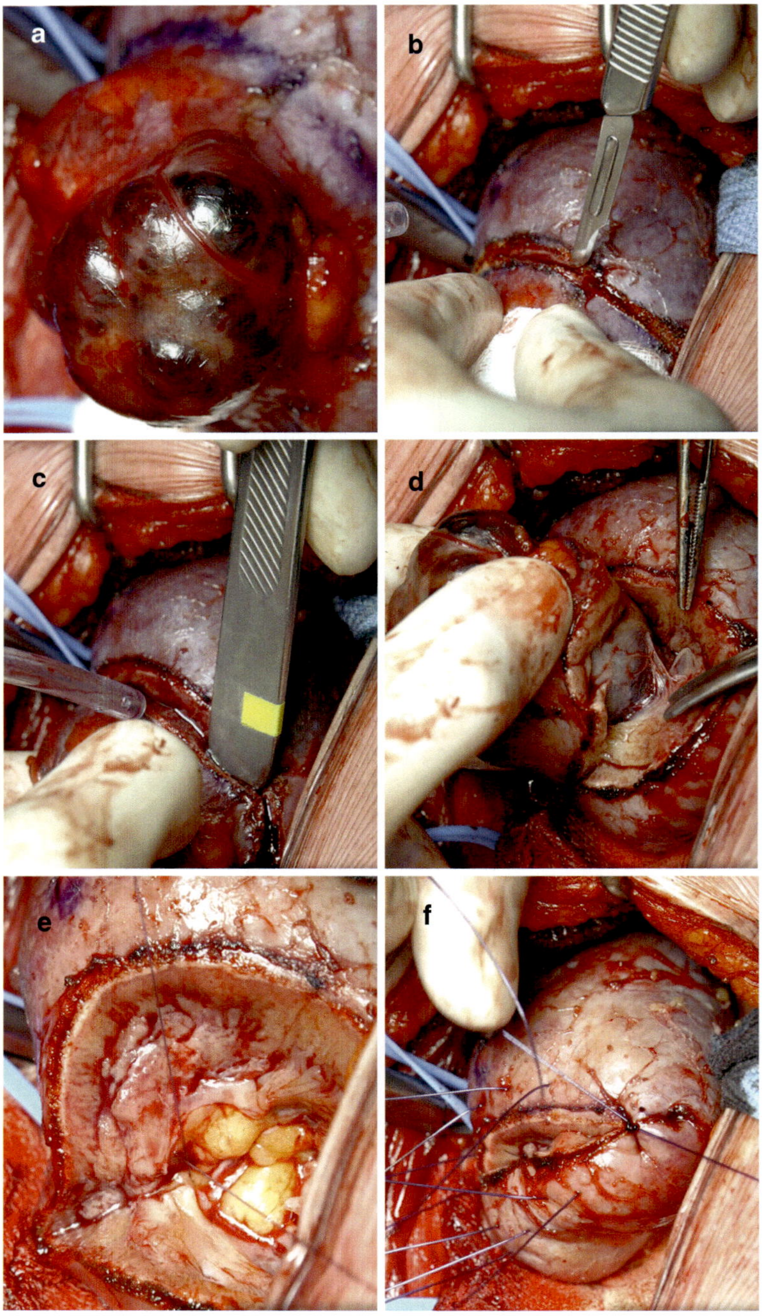

Fig. 1 (**a**) Exophytic part of renal tumour. (**b**) Circumcision of the renal tumour. (**c**) Development of the enucleoresection plane. (**d**) Enucleoresection of the renal tumour. Both the enucleation and the enucleoresection plane are visible. (**e**) Closure of the renal sinus. Protruding renal sinus fat is visible. (**f**) External renorraphy with full thickness stitches using a double flat knot. Link to video of the full OPN procedure: https://youtu.be/_zktrg8y0Cc

require a wedge resection of the healthy parenchyma covering the underlying tumour, which can be subsequently enucleated.

Visible open vessels on the cut renal surface can be controlled with fine absorbable figure-of-eight sutures. If the urinary collecting system is breached during tumour extirpation, it is reconstructed with fine absorbable sutures. When large parenchymal defects are present a bolster composed of absorbable haemostatic agents can be utilised to replace the excised volume. The renal vasculature can be unclamped prior to the renorraphy, which reapproximates the renal cortex tension-free (early unclamping) to reduce ischaemia time. Alternatively, the renal vasculature stays clamped until after the renorraphy. However, clamping a second time should be avoided due to repeated unclamping-reperfusion injury.

Morbidity

Most frequent intra-operative complications associated with OPN include haemorrhage, pleural damage and damage to adjacent organs. Early postoperative complications include haematoma formation, pneumonia or atelectasis, acute kidney injury, ileus, urinary leak and infection whereas late postoperative complications include urinary fistula formation, arteriovenous fistula formation, arteriocaliceal fistula formation, incisional hernias and chronic pain [24].

The morbidity associated with NSS is slightly higher compared to RN. A large, prospective randomized controlled trial by the EORTC, comparing NSS and RN for the management of small, low stage, solitary renal tumours found that severe haemorrhage as well as re-intervention rates were higher in the NSS compared to the RN group (3.2% vs 1.2% and 4.4% vs 2.4%, respectively) [33]. Patard et al. reported on a large multicentre series and found that morbidity increases when expanding the tumour size indication for NSS with a higher mean operative time, increased blood loss and higher transfusion rates [34].

A recent systematic review and meta-analysis by Tsai et al. compared OPN and RAPN and included 34 studies and over 60,000 patients. They reported less blood loss, lower transfusion rates, longer operative times, lower overall postoperative complications, lower readmission rates, shorter hospital stay and less postoperative eGFR decline for RAPN vs OPN, concluding that RAPN was associated with lower morbidity and better renal function preservation when compared to OPN [35]. Retroperitoneal vs transperitoneal approach in RAPN does not seem to result in any significant difference in complications [36].

Although any survival benefit of lymphadenectomy in RCC remains controversial, even in the case of clinically node positive disease, it is certainly of prognostic significance as it provides important additional staging information [37, 38]. Additionally, tumours at high risk of pathological node positive disease are good candidates to undergo lymphadenectomy [39]. Arguably, the extent of lymphadenectomy could be greater in OPN compared to minimally invasive procedures. However, studies have demonstrated the feasibility and favourable early oncological outcomes of minimally invasive extensive retroperitoneal lymphadenectomy, despite the current lack of tactile feedback with these techniques [40, 41].

Outcome

Oncological outcomes of OPN, LPN and RAPN seem to be equivalent, although it has to be noted that OPN still has the longest oncological follow-up data [42–45]. Large collaborative efforts are needed and currently ongoing to compare long term oncologic outcomes of PN via different surgical access approaches. Due to oncological equivalence and reduced morbidity, indications for MIS are thus rapidly expanding. Although minimally invasive NSS techniques are reported in increasingly complex cases, the possibility of MIS should never be prioritized over the maximum preservation of healthy renal parenchyma in those patients who deserve it [41].

It is likely that the use of OPN will further decline in the future. Nonetheless, it holds an extremely valuable place for certain clinical scenarios. Complex, large, endophytic, tumours, redo PN, horseshoe kidneys or unique kidneys might be better suited for OPN as compared to MIS. Additionally, hereditary kidney cancer patients often present with multiple and bilateral tumours and represent technically challenging cases who are at high risk of local tumour recurrence. In these patients an open approach could be preferred over MIS.

Furthermore, it is evident that not all centres are equipped with the currently available MIS technology and that not all urologists have the required expertise to carry out these procedures.

Several studies have evaluated the cost of different surgical access approaches as this is an increasingly important healthcare concern. It is clear that the purchase and maintenance of laparoscopic and robotic equipment is associated with a higher cost, but it is believed that this cost can be compensated by decreased morbidity and shorter length of hospital stay. Laydner et al. found no significant difference in the cost of NSS comparing all surgical access approaches for renal tumours of low and intermediate complexity [46–48].

Conclusions

Nephron sparing surgery is the preferred treatment for all renal tumours when oncologically and technically safe, regardless of surgical approach. Indications for MIS are rapidly expanding, and increasingly complex tumours can be treated with LPN or RAPN. However, oncological, functional or perioperative outcomes should not be compromised by the choice of surgical approach. OPN holds a firm place among the increasingly available robotic and laparoscopic systems and stays essential in the treatment of localized RCC. Open approaches could be considered superior to

MIS in clinically challenging cases, making OPN all but obsolete in an era of technological advances.

Key Points

- Nephron sparing surgery is the gold standard treatment for clinically localised RCC whenever technically feasible and oncologically safe, irrespective of the surgical approach.
- Technological innovations and their expanding utilization have resulted in comparable outcomes for MIS and open approaches, making MIS preferable for standard cases if the technology, experience and skill set is available.
- Open partial nephrectomy holds an extremely valuable place in the treatment of complex tumours (large, endophytic, multiple or bilateral) in complex patients (hereditary renal cancer syndromes or solitary kidneys) to preserve as much nephrons as possible when longer ischemic times and challenging reconstructions are expected.

References

1. Hsieh JJ, Purdue MP, Signoretti S, Swanton C, Albiges L, Schmidinger M, et al. Renal cell carcinoma. Nat Rev Dis Prim. 2017;3(1):17009.
2. Ljungberg B, Campbell SC, Cho HY, Jacqmin D, Lee JE, Weikert S, et al. The epidemiology of renal cell carcinoma. Eur Urol. 2011;60(4):615–21.
3. W. HH. A history of partial nephrectomy for renal tumors. J Urol. 2005;173(3):705–8.
4. Herr HW. Surgical management of renal tumors: a historical perspective. Urol Clin North Am. 2008;35(4):543–9.
5. Ljungberg B, Albiges L, Abu-Ghanem Y, Bensalah K, Dabestani S, Fernández-Pello S, et al. European association of urology guidelines on renal cell carcinoma: the 2019 update. Eur Urol. 2019;75(5):799–810.
6. Campbell S, Uzzo RG, Allaf ME, Bass EB, Cadeddu JA, Chang A, et al. Renal mass and localized renal cancer: AUA guideline. J Urol. 2017;198(3):520–9.
7. Go AS, Chertow GM, Fan D, McCulloch CE, Hsu C. Chronic kidney disease and the risks of death, cardiovascular events, and hospitalization. N Engl J Med. 2004;351(13):1296–305.
8. Van Poppel H, Da Pozzo L, Albrecht W, Matveev V, Bono A, Borkowski A, et al. A prospective, randomised EORTC intergroup phase 3 study comparing the oncologic outcome of elective nephron-sparing surgery and radical nephrectomy for low-stage renal cell carcinoma. Eur Urol. 2011;59(4):543–52.
9. Kunath F, Schmidt S, Krabbe LM, Miernik A, Dahm P, Cleves A, et al. Partial nephrectomy versus radical nephrectomy for clinical localised renal masses. Cochrane Database Syst Rev. 2017;5(5):CD012045.
10. Weight CJ, Lieser G, Larson BT, Gao T, Lane BR, Campbell SC, et al. Partial nephrectomy is associated with improved overall survival compared to radical nephrectomy in patients with unanticipated benign renal tumours. Eur Urol. 2010;58(2):293–8.
11. Scosyrev E, Messing EM, Sylvester R, Campbell S, Van Poppel H. Renal Function After Nephron-sparing Surgery Versus Radical Nephrectomy: Results from EORTC Randomized Trial 30904. Eur Urol. 2014;65(2):372–7.

12. Lane BR, Campbell SC, Demirjian S, Fergany AF. Surgically induced chronic kidney disease may be associated with a lower risk of progression and mortality than medical chronic kidney disease. J Urol. 2013;189(5):1649–55.
13. Woldu SL, Weinberg AC, Korets R, Ghandour R, Danzig MR, RoyChoudhury A, et al. Who really benefits from nephron-sparing surgery? Urology. 2014;84(4):860–8.
14. Larcher A, Capitanio U, Terrone C, Volpe A, De Angelis P, Dehó F, et al. Elective nephron sparing surgery decreases other cause mortality relative to radical nephrectomy only in specific subgroups of patients with renal cell carcinoma. J Urol. 2016;196(4):1008–13.
15. Van Poppel H, Joniau S, Albersen M. Nephron sparing for renal cell carcinoma: whenever possible? Eur Urol Focus. 2016;2(6):656–9.
16. Van Poppel H, Sylvester R. Is overall survival not influenced by partial vs radical nephrectomy? BJU Int. 2018;121(3):319.
17. Lane BR, Fergany AF, Weight CJ, Campbell SC. Renal functional outcomes after partial nephrectomy with extended ischemic intervals are better than after radical nephrectomy. J Urol. 2010;184(4):1286–90.
18. Bratslavsky G. Argument in favor of performing partial nephrectomy for tumors greater than 7 cm: The metastatic prescription has already been written. Urol Oncol Semin Orig Investig. 2011;29(6):829–32.
19. Mir MC, Derweesh I, Porpiglia F, Zargar H, Mottrie A, Autorino R. Partial nephrectomy versus radical nephrectomy for clinical T1b and T2 renal tumors: a systematic review and meta-analysis of comparative studies. Eur Urol. 2017;71(4):606–17.
20. Veys R, Abdollah F, Briganti A, Albersen M, Van PH, Joniau S. Oncological and functional efficacy of nephron-sparing surgery versus radical nephrectomy in renal cell carcinoma stages ≥cT1b: a single institution, matched analysis. Cent Eur J Urol. 2018;71(1):48–57.
21. Kenney PA, Wotkowicz C, Libertino JA. Contemporary open surgery of the kidney. Campbell-Walsh Urol. 2012;2:1567–8.
22. Martin L, Rouviere O, Bezza R, Bailleux J, Abbas F, Schott-Pethelaz A-M, et al. Mayo adhesive probability score is an independent computed tomography scan predictor of adherent perinephric fat in open partial nephrectomy. Urology. 2017;103:124–8.
23. Casilla-Lennon MM, Kenney PA, Wszolek M, Libertino JA. Open partial nephrectomy. In: Renal cancer. Berlin: Springer; 2020. p. 221–42.
24. Anastasiadis E, O'Brien T, Fernando A. Open partial nephrectomy in renal cell cancer – Essential or obsolete? Int J Surg. 2016;36:541–7.
25. Becker F, Van Poppel H, Hakenberg OW, Stief C, Gill I, Guazzoni G, et al. Assessing the impact of ischaemia time during partial nephrectomy. Eur Urol. 2009;56(4):625–35.
26. Thompson RH, Lane BR, Lohse CM, Leibovich BC, Fergany A, Frank I, et al. Every minute counts when the renal hilum is clamped during partial nephrectomy. Eur Urol. 2010;58(3):340–5.
27. Greco F, Autorino R, Altieri V, Campbell S, Ficarra V, Gill I, et al. Ischemia techniques in nephron-sparing surgery: a systematic review and meta-analysis of surgical, oncological, and functional outcomes. Eur Urol. 2019;75(3):477–91.
28. Rogers CG, Ghani KR, Kumar RK, Jeong W, Menon M. Robotic partial nephrectomy with cold ischemia and on-clamp tumor extraction: recapitulating the open approach. Eur Urol. 2013;63(3):573–8.
29. Kutikov A, Uzzo RG. The RENAL nephrometry score: a comprehensive standardized system for quantitating renal tumor size, location and depth. J Urol. 2009;182(3):844–53.
30. Ficarra V, Novara G, Secco S, Macchi V, Porzionato A, De Caro R, et al. Preoperative aspects and dimensions used for an anatomical (PADUA) classification of renal tumours in patients who are candidates for nephron-sparing surgery. Eur Urol. 2009;56(5):786–93.
31. Canter D, Kutikov A, Manley B, Egleston B, Simhan J, Smaldone M, et al. Utility of the R.E.N.A.L. nephrometry scoring system in objectifying treatment decision-making of the enhancing renal mass. Urology. 2011;78(5):1089–94.

32. Andrea M, Vincenzo F, Francesco R, Alessandro A, Roberto B, Giorgio C, et al. Simple enucleation is equivalent to traditional partial nephrectomy for renal cell carcinoma: results of a nonrandomized, retrospective. Comparative Study. J Urol. 2011;185(5):1604–10.
33. Van Poppel H, Da Pozzo L, Albrecht W, Matveev V, Bono A, Borkowski A, et al. A prospective randomized EORTC intergroup phase 3 study comparing the complications of elective nephron-sparing surgery and radical nephrectomy for low-stage renal cell carcinoma. Eur Urol. 2007;51(6):1606–15.
34. Patard J-J, Pantuck AJ, Crepel M, Lam JS, Bellec L, Albouy B, et al. Morbidity and clinical outcome of nephron-sparing surgery in relation to tumour size and indication. Eur Urol. 2007;52(1):148–54.
35. Tsai S-H, Tseng P-T, Sherer BA, Lai Y-C, Lin P-Y, Wu C-K, et al. Open versus robotic partial nephrectomy: Systematic review and meta-analysis of contemporary studies. Int J Med Robot Comput Assist Surg. 2019;15(1):e1963.
36. Mittakanti HR, Heulitt G, Li H-F, Porter JR. Transperitoneal vs. retroperitoneal robotic partial nephrectomy: a matched-paired analysis. World J Urol. 2020;38(5):1093–9.
37. Bhindi B, Wallis CJD, Boorjian SA, Thompson RH, Farrell A, Kim SP, et al. The role of lymph node dissection in the management of renal cell carcinoma: a systematic review and meta-analysis. BJU Int. 2018;121(5):684–98.
38. van Hattem MW, Roussel E, Van Poppel H, Albersen M. Role of Lymphadenectomy in renal cell cancer. In: Renal cancer. Berlin: Springer; 2020. p. 281–94.
39. Van Poppel H. Lymph node dissection is not obsolete in clinically node-negative renal cell carcinoma patients. Eur Urol. 2011;59(1):24–5.
40. Prasad SM, Shalhav AL. Comparative effectiveness of minimally invasive versus open lymphadenectomy in urological cancers. Curr Opin Urol. 2013;23(1):57–64.
41. Petros FG, Angell JE, Abaza R. Outcomes of robotic nephrectomy including highest-complexity cases: largest series to date and literature review. Urology. 2015;85(6):1352–9.
42. Xia L, Wang X, Xu T, Guzzo TJ. Systematic review and meta-analysis of comparative studies reporting perioperative outcomes of robot-assisted partial nephrectomy versus open partial nephrectomy. J Endourol. 2017;31(9):893–909.
43. Wu Z, Li M, Liu B, Cai C, Ye H, Lv C, et al. Robotic versus open partial nephrectomy: a systematic review and meta-analysis. PLoS One. 2014;9(4):e94878.
44. Luciani LG, Porpiglia F, Cai T, D'Elia C, Vattovani V, Giusti G, et al. Operative safety and oncologic outcome of laparoscopic radical nephrectomy for renal cell carcinoma> 7 cm: a multicenter study of 222 patients. Urology. 2013;81(6):1239–45.
45. Vartolomei MD, Foerster B, Kimura S, Autorino R, Shariat SF, Seitz C. Oncologic outcomes after minimally invasive surgery for cT1 renal masses: a comprehensive review. Curr Opin Urol. 2018;28(2):132–8.
46. Castle SM, Gorbatiy V, Avallone MA, Eldefrawy A, Caulton DE, Leveillee RJ. Cost comparison of nephron-sparing treatments for cT1a renal masses. Urol Oncol Semin Orig Investig. 2013;31(7):1327–32.
47. Alemozaffar M, Chang SL, Kacker R, Sun M, DeWolf WC, Wagner AA. Comparing costs of robotic, laparoscopic, and open partial nephrectomy. J Endourol. 2013;27(5):560–5.
48. Laydner H, Isac W, Autorino R, Kassab A, Yakoubi R, Hillyer S, et al. Single institutional cost analysis of 325 robotic, laparoscopic, and open partial nephrectomies. Urology. 2013;81(3):533–9.

Retroperitoneal Robotic Partial Nephrectomy

D. Sri, M. Malki, M. Hussain, and N. Barber

Introduction

Inception

Following Clayman et al.'s first description of transperitoneal (TP) laparoscopic nephrectomy in 1990 [1], the role of minimally invasive surgery in the retroperitoneum (RP) could not be realised till the introduction of the balloon dissector to create the retroperitoneal space. In 1994 the first complete RP laparoscopic lower pole partial nephrectomy was reported, with benefits noted in ambulation, discharge and recovery [2].

The first robot assisted RP partial nephrectomy was described in 2004 by Gettmann et al. in 2004, utilising the DaVinci robotic surgical system (Intuitive). Of 13 patients who underwent robot assisted partial nephrectomy (RAPN), 2 patients with posterior and lateral tumours underwent RP RAPN [3]. **The popularity and uptake of RP minimally invasive surgery has been slow, with a much steeper learning curve compared to TP surgery cited as a major factor**.

Current Myths and Misconceptions

The TP route is considered easier and allows the surgeon to perform in a familiar environment and a wider field (Table 1). The RP route has key advantages (Table 2) over the TP route in upper tract surgery and the aim of this chapter is to focus on the nuances of RP-RAPN and along the way dispel some of the commonly held myths and misconceptions of this approach within mainstream urology.

D. Sri (✉) · M. Malki · M. Hussain · N. Barber
Frimley Renal Cancer Centre, Frimley Park Hospital, Surrey, UK

C. Anderson, M. Afshar (eds.), *Renal Cancer*,
https://doi.org/10.1007/978-3-030-84756-2_14

Table 1 Summary of common advantages and disadvantages of TP-RAPN

Transperitioneal RAPN	
Advantages	Disadvantages
• More anatomic landmarks • Lager working space • Very anterior tumour • Anterior hilar tumour	• Manipulation of posterior tumour • Medial rotation of kidney • Bowel injury • Adhesions because of previous abdominal surgery

Table 2 Summary of common advantages and disadvantages of RP-RAPN

Retroperitoneal RAPN	
Advantages	Disadvantages
• Direct access to hilum • No peritoneal violation • Reduced risk of abdominal bowel injury • Earlier return of bowel habits • Conservation management of post-operative complications (urine leak, haemorrhage)	• Limited working space, reduced triangulation • Less familiar anatomical landmarks • Anterior tumour

Retroperitoneal Robotically Assisted Partial Nephrectomy: Technique and Tips

This section focuses on the technique and nuances in performing a successful RP RAPN. The fundamentals of our approach are as described by the team at the Vattikuti Urology Institute in Detroit, USA [4, 5].

Patient Positioning

The patient is placed in the lateral decubitus (or full flank) position. The hip, spine and shoulders of the patient are horizontally in line and positioned towards the edge of the table. The bottom leg is flexed, and the top leg may require a slight degree of flexion to avoid the risk of common peroneal nerve strain and footdrop. The location and degree of break varies across operating tables. The aim is to achieve a fully flexed table (approximately 230 °) providing maximal space between the 12th rib and the iliac crest. A general rule of thumb is to align the anterior superior iliac spine of the patient over the table break; however, this would require adjustment in patients with high BMI or those with prominent aprons. Patients with a prominent iliac crest also present a challenge, whereby positioning the hip below the level of the break often provides a better working space.

Creating the Retroperitoneal Space

The **surface landmarks required to find and create the retroperitoneal space are the iliac crest, tip of the 12th rib and the axillary lines.** The midaxillary line serves as a good reference point to adjust for patients who may have long/short 12th ribs and for those with absent 12th ribs. The placement of the ports differs subtly to the laparoscopic retroperitoneal approach, as if the camera port is too close to the 12th rib the instruments and camera tend to be too close to the kidney and result in external clashes. A 12–15 mm camera port incision is made approximately 2 cm above the iliac crest in line with the tip of 12th rib. This would broadly be in line with the mid axillary line and lateral to the triangle of petit. In the open approach the aponeurosis of the external oblique and the external oblique muscles are separated using retractors (e.g., a Kocher-Langenbeck), and the thoracolumbar fascia exposed. A curved forceps is used to penetrate this layer and enter the retroperitoneal space. One should be able to feel the 12th rib and posteriorly the belly of quadratus lumborum. The psoas muscle and the kidney may also be palpable. An alternative technique is to use a curved forceps following incision of the skin and subcutaneous tissue to penetrate both the aponeurosis of the external oblique and the thoracolumbar fascia. This provides two distinct 'pops' to suggest one is in the correct plane, and the space developed.

A balloon dilator is then inserted into the created space and, with the port facing the anterior abdomen. The obturator is removed, and the balloon can be expanded under direct vision using a laparoscope. Approximately 40 compressions are required to achieve an adequate space without compromising the peritoneum. This however will vary, with slimmer patients requiring fewer compressions and larger patients perhaps requiring up to 60 compressions. Once the appropriate space has been created the dilator is deflated and an 12 mm robotic camera port is placed.

Port Placement

Figure 1 illustrates optimal port placement for RP-RAPN. The camera port tends to be longer (120–130 mm) with a balloon and seal to secure its position. Pneumoretroperitoneum is established with CO_2 at 12–15 mmHg. The use of valveless pressure barrier insufflators such as Airseal can allow for use of lower pressures. The lateral port is inserted first, and a needle can be used to gauge angle of entry and position. This port is placed approximately 7–8 cm superolateral to the camera port in the superior lumbar triangle. The indentation found at the lateral edge of erector spinae and the inferior border of the 12th rib serve as external landmarks for this port. The medial robotic port is placed 7–8 cm often in line with the camera port. ***A consideration to make if expecting to work predominantly in the lower pole is to place the medial robotic port approximately 1–2 cm lower than the line of the camera port.*** A 12–15 mm assistant port is then placed equidistant to and 1 cm caudal to a line between the camera and the medial robotic port. This translates roughly to the anterior axillary line and should be cephalad to the anterior superior iliac spine. A fourth robotic arm can be utilised in some cases by inserting a port 2 cm inferiorly and 7–8 cm medial to the medial arm. The peritoneum overlying this area may need to be swept away using either laparoscopic instruments or blunt finger dissection. A fourth arm can be particularly useful in patients with

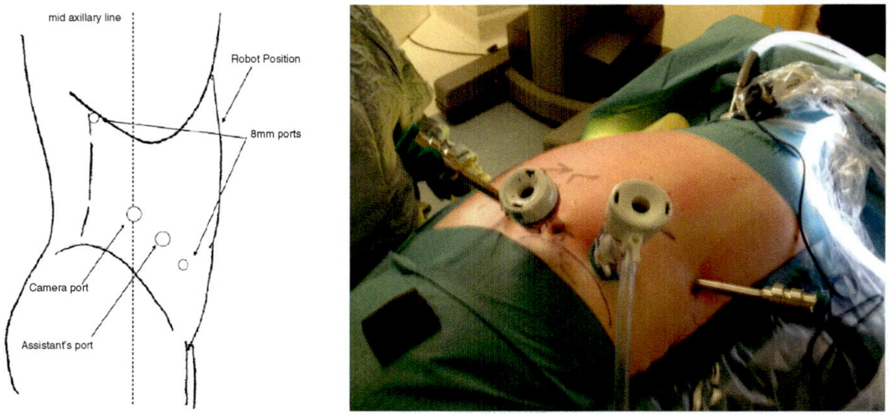

Fig. 1 Optimal port placement for RP-RAPN utilising the Da Vinci Si Surgical System (3 arm technique)

abundant perinephric fat or to allow for retraction during the warm ischaemic time to enable the assistant to concentrate all their efforts on assisting with tumour excision.

Docking

Robotic docking depends on the model that is utilised at a centre. With the Da Vinci Si the room layout should accommodate the entry of the patient side cart from over the patient's head and parallel to the patient's spine. With the Da Vinci Xi the patient side cart can be brought in perpendicular to the bed.

Initial Landmarks

Once instrument control has been gained by the surgeon on the console, orient oneself to the landmarks. **Superiorly the peritoneal fold and the transversus abdominus, inferiorly the psoas tendon and ureter, cranially the diaphragm and caudally the pelvis** (Fig. 2). An assessment of the paranephric fat should be made. **Fat management is an integral component of retroperitoneal surgery.** Where required the paranephric fat is dissected off Gerota's fascia and in some cases overhangs of fat from the peritoneal fold would also require management. When working superiorly it is important to take care so as not to breach the peritoneum.

Next Gerota's fascia is incised and entered parallel to and just above the psoas muscle. This is developed cranio-caudally in line with psoas. Dissection is then carried on cranially and caudally along the muscle to elevate the kidney and perinephric fat. Mobilising the upper and lower pole sufficiently will enable the assistant/the fourth arm to achieve optimal lift during identification of the hilum.

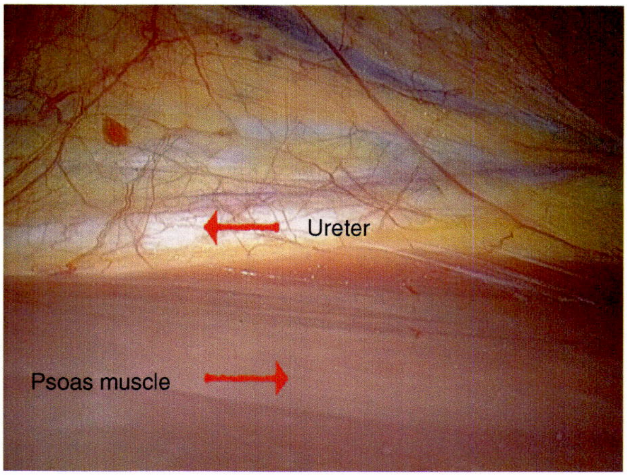

Fig. 2 Initial landmarks encountered during creation of the retroperitoneal space

Hilar Dissection

Adhering to systematic methods and similar principles to laparoscopic retroperitoneal surgery results in safe robotic retroperitoneal renal surgery. During dissection of the hilum the kidney should be placed on stretch to facilitate vessel identification and improve blunt dissection. We would recommend dissection to be parallel, in line with the direction of the vessels going from inferior to superior, to reveal the hilum. This minimises the risk of inadvertent vascular injury or bleeding from smaller vessels and tributaries. Retroperitoneally the renal artery is the first structure encountered and is mobilised to allow application of 2 vascular clamps (Fig. 3). We would recommend isolation of the artery with a vessel loop to facilitate easy location and retraction of the artery. The vein can similarly be identified and isolated, although this is not entirely necessary during retroperitoneal partial nephrectomy. As a result, ligation of the gonadal vein and any bleeding risk incurred from having to dissect or identify the renal vein (as is the case in transperitoneal surgery) is not frequently encountered.

Tumour Identification

Gerota's fascia can now be incised and mobilised off the capsular surface of the kidney to expose the tumour. There remains some debate and controversy as to the location of tumours that are accessible via the retroperitoneal route. In the experience of the authors, at high volume retroperitoneal robotic centres all tumours apart from anterior hilar tumours are accessible and manageable retroperitoneally. A key consideration in ensuring optimal access is managing the para, perinephric fat and peritoneal fold that could potentially obscure one's view. The position at which Gerota's fascia is incised to access the parenchyma is therefore quite important. For

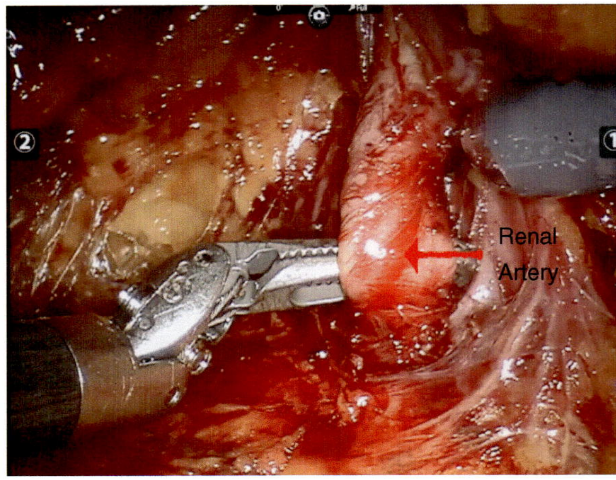

Fig. 3 Intraoperative demonstration of renal artery dissection in RP-RAPN

anterior and lateral tumours dropping the kidney from the peritoneal fold and coming onto the parenchyma at a more anterior location would mean that once the tumour has been identified and mobilised there is less overhanging fat during the warm ischaemia time. For more posterior tumours dropping the kidney this way could be counterproductive as the natural lift provided by the superior attachment to the peritoneal fold will help facilitate excision of the tumour. In these cases, one would tend to incise into Gerota's fascia 1–2 cm below the line of the peritoneal fold. Making these considerations on a case-by-case basis would result in most tumours being accessible retroperitoneally.

Intraoperative robotic ultrasound (US) can and is utilised retroperitoneally to identify the margins of the tumour and aid excision. It is particularly useful in identification of predominantly or completely endophytic tumours. The TilePro™ function displays the live US images on the console screen. Understandably the manipulation and space with which to perform intraoperative US can be restrictive and requires good co-ordination between surgeon and bed side assistant.

Hilar Clamping

All necessary material from sutures to instruments are confirmed to be present prior to hilar clamping. The ports are inspected to ensure they are within the retroperitoneal cavity, so as not to complicate instrument changes during the warm ischaemia time (WIT). The use of the osmotic diuretic Mannitol is controversial. It is thought to both improve renal blood flow and through free radical scavenging properties reduce the ischaemic insult post clamping. A 2018 prospective double-blind trial in patients with normal renal function undergoing RAPN found no statistically significant difference in renal function between mannitol and placebo [6]. Similarly using mannitol had no impact on renal function in patients with solitary kidney undergoing RAPN [7]. In our practice we had discontinued the use of intraoperative mannitol.

Clamping of the renal hilum can be performed with laparoscopically applied bulldog clamps (Fig. 4) or robotically applied bulldog (Klein/Scanlan) clamps. Although ex-vivo studies have claimed robotically applied clamps to provide less clamp force and allow more flow across a clamped segment compared to their laparoscopic counterparts [8], this does not translate into poorer haemostasis in-vivo. Their use has been shown to be safe, feasible and non-inferior to laparoscopic bulldog applicators [9].

The main renal artery is clamped first prior to clamping the renal vein. Not all centres / surgeons preferentially clamp the renal vein. Small exophytic tumours could also be tackled off clamp. Selective arterial clamping (SAC) remains controversial [10, 11]. The rationale is that the limitation of global ischaemia to the kidney reduces the ischaemic damage and improves the long-term functional outlook. SAC is often paired with Indocyanine Green (ICG) instillation and utilisation of Da Vinci's integrated fluorescence capability, FireFly ™, allowing visual assessment of perfusion to the tumour. Paulucci et al. conducted a multi-institution prospective study comparing main arterial clamping (MAC) to SAC in matched patients and found no statistically significant difference between the two [12].

Tumour Excision

Tumour excision is conventionally carried out using sharp dissection with a rim of normal parenchyma to minimise a positive surgical margin. In encapsulated tumours, enucleation can be carried out once onto the right plane, removing the tumour en-bloc with an intact capsule.

Renorrhaphy

Traditionally a 2-layer renorrhaphy is employed for closure. The monopolar scissors and if required the left robotic arm instrument are replaced for robotic needle drivers. Sutures are anchored with a knot and a Hem-O-Lok clip. A continuous

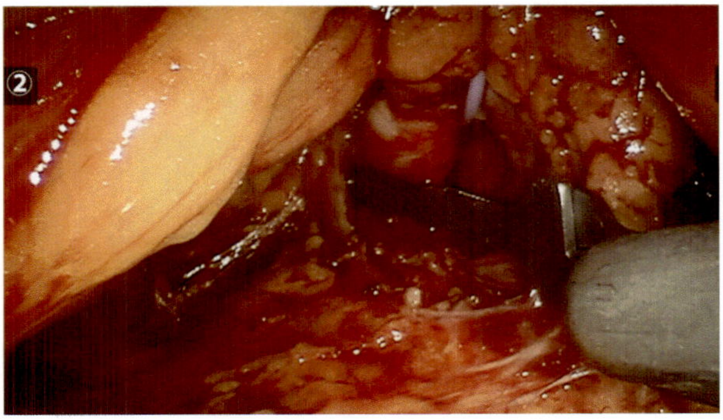

Fig. 4 Intraoperative demonstration of main artery clamping using laparoscopic bulldog applicators in RP-RAPN

inner/deep renorrhaphy is performed using either a braided suture (polyglactin) or a monofilament (poliglecaprone 25) in a continuous fashion. The sutures are secured with a Hem-O-Lok clip using the sliding clip technique [13]. We utilise a 2–0 poliglecaprone 25 in our practice. The advantage of a monofilament suture is the ability to tighten the renorrhaphy retrospectively if required. The outer renorrhaphy is similarly closed using either interrupted or continuous sutures. It is important to ensure the renal capsule is included in this layer to allow adequate tension of the sutures for haemostasis and closure of the defect. We utilise a 1–0 polyglactin suture for the outer layer.

Considerations to be made during retroperitoneal surgery include the direction of travel of the sutures. A general rule of thumb would be to suture from the far end of the defect towards you to prevent instrument clashes and a more awkward angle when progressing with the renorrhaphy. This way the left hand can utilise the previous suture to manipulate the kidney and the defect to an angle that would facilitate easier ergonomics when suturing.

In some centres barbed v-loc sutures have replaced traditional braided and monofilament sutures. The perceived benefit lies in maintaining the applied tension, and has been shown in studies to reduce mean WIT by a statistically significant 6.2 min [14].

Repair of any collecting system entry can be performed either individually or during the inner renorrhaphy. The sliding clip renorrhaphy has seen a steady elimination of the need for collecting system repair (Fig. 5). Omitting collecting system repair and utilising the sliding clip technique reduces the mean WIT with no difference in rate of post-operative complications and urine leak [15]. A contemporary review of factors influencing urine leak in 975 patients who underwent partial nephrectomy found open surgery, high estimated blood loss and not utilising a sliding clip renorrhaphy technique to increase this risk [16].

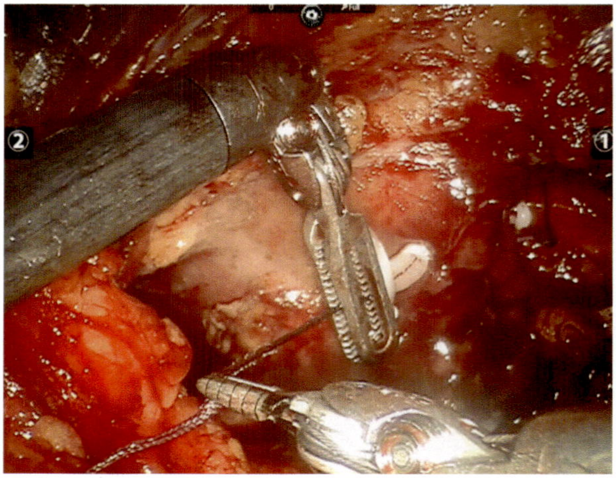

Fig. 5 Intraoperative demonstration of the sliding clip outer renorrhaphy in RP-RAPN

Hilar Unclamping and Tumour Retrieval

After completion of the renorrhaphy the hilar clamps are removed - the renal vein clamp should be removed first in cases where it is applied. Any persistent bleeding can be overcome by cinching the Hem-o-Lok clips to tighten the sutures. Further interrupted sutures can be added if required for haemostasis.

Early unclamping, after successful completion of the inner renorrhaphy, can be utilised to reduce the WIT. This method can also allow for supplementary re-enforcement of the inner layer if required.

The renorrhaphy bed can be further supplemented with haemostatic adjuncts. These are particularly useful in the case of oozing from the parenchymal edge. There are a wide range of absorbable haemostatic agents, haemostatic matrix, fibrin sealants and other adjuncts available for use. In our practice TISSEEL™, FLOSEAL™ (Baxter), VISTASEAL™ and SURGICEL SnOW™ (Ethicon) are the more commonly used agents.

A surgical drain can be left if required. In retroperitoneal surgery we tend not to do so. The tumour is placed in a specimen retrieval bag (Endo Catch™) and retrieved through the 15 mm assistant port. The overlying fascia and skin are closed.

Post-Operative Care

An enhanced recovery pathway (ERP) is utilised post-operatively centring on early mobilisation and return to a normal diet. Discharge criteria include tolerating a normal diet, mobilising and adequate oral analgesia. The median length of stay in our centre for RP-RAPN patients is 1 day.

Is RP-RAPN Safe, Efficacious and Affordable?

The choice of approach when tackling partial nephrectomy tends to be surgeon dependent. Naturally, higher volume centres are more likely to utilise and adopt RP-RAPN [17]. **There are no randomised trials comparing the safety and efficacy of RP and TP RAPN**. Most studies tend to be retrospective in design and are confounded by selection bias. The salient peri-operative, functional and oncological outcomes of the larger volume head-to-head studies are summaries in Table 3.

Perioperative Outcomes

A systematic review and meta-analysis of four eligible studies compared 229 TP-RAPN patients to 220 RP-RAPN patients who shared similar size, location and complexity characteristics. They found **RP-RAPN to be equivalent to TP in terms of complications (both Clavien < 3 and Clavien ≥ 3), conversion rate, warm**

Table 3 Summary of comparative literature of RP-RAPN vs TP-RAPN exploring peri-operative, functional and oncological outcome

Author	RP vs TP	Tumour Size (cm)	Nephrometry Score	Op Time (mins)	WIT (mins)	Complications (%)	Hospital Stay (days)	Positive Margins (%)	Drop in GFR
Hughes- Hallett, 2013 [18]	44 vs 59	2.8 vs 3.1	5.5 vs 5.5	149 vs195	22 vs 19	9 vs 10	2.5 vs 4.6	6.8 vs 5	–
Gin, 2014 [19]	75 vs 116	2.5 vs 3.2	8 vs 7	156 vs 191	24 vs 26	9 vs 17	1.5 vs 2	8 vs 6	2 vs 2 (gain)
Choo, 2014 [20]	43 vs 43	2.8 vs 2.7	6 vs 6.6	120 vs 153	23 vs 26	–	–	0 vs 2	11.4 vs 8.6
Kim, 2015 [21]	116 vs 97	2.5 vs 2.5	8 vs 8	152 vs 149	NR	7 vs 10	1 d 57% vs 10%	–	–
Sharma, 2016 [22]	25 vs 40	–	7 vs 7	224 vs 248	27 vs 30	16 vs 43	2.3 vs 3.0	4 vs 2	–
Maurice, 2017 [23]	74 vs 296	2.4 vs 2.5	8 vs 7	176 vs 176	21 vs 19	12 vs 14	2.2 vs 2.6	1.4 vs 1.7	Statistically insignificant
Stroup, 2017 [24]	141 vs 263	2.9 vs 3.1	7 vs 7	217 vs 232	23 vs 23	11 vs 14	2.2 vs 2.5	2.8 vs 4.2	6.2 vs 6.4
Laviana, 2018 [25]	78 vs 78	–	–	167 vs 191	21 vs 22	24 vs 36	1.8 vs 2.7	3.9 vs 2.6	4 vs 6
Arora, 2018 [26]	99 vs 394	3 vs 3.2	7 vs 7	160 vs 170	17 vs 17	–	1 vs 3	2.1 vs 2	6.8 vs 9.9
Harke, 2019 [27]	203 vs 551	2.6 vs 3.0	9 vs 9	120 vs 143	8 vs 11	14 vs 22	8 vs 9	4 vs 3	6.4 vs 11.5
Paulucci, 2019 [28]	157 vs 157	2.9 vs 3	–	157 vs 185	17 vs 17	12 vs 12	1 vs 2	3.9 vs 2.4	–
Abaza, 2020 [29]	30 vs 107	3.0 vs 3.5	7 vs 7	128 vs 141	11 vs 11	4 (overall)	0.7 vs 0.9	0 vs 0	16.3 vs 13.8
Mittakanti, 2020 [30]	166 vs 166	3.1 vs 3.3	6 vs 6	162 vs 191	18 vs 18	53 vs 47	1.7 vs 1.9	2.8 vs 1.9	4.1 vs 5.9
Frimley Renal Cancer Centre, 2020	**631**	**3.1**	**6.5**	**135**	**21**	**8**	**1**	**4**	**6**

ischaemic time (WIT) and estimated blood loss (EBL). A significant difference in operative time however was noted (p = 0.05), with a mean difference of 28.03 mins in favour of RP-RAPN [31]. Choo et al. demonstrated that this significant difference was present when both techniques were match-paired with nephrometry scores. Although no difference was noted in the WIT (p = 0.139), a **statistically significant (p = 0.028) mean 33 min reduction in operative time in favour of the RP group was noted even when match-paired for tumour complexity** [20]. These findings are corroborated by more contemporary larger volume multicentre series comparing RP and TP RAPN [17, 26, 27]. It has been argued that peri-operative outcome measures can be dependant on the expertise of the surgeon, as has been shown in a systematic review by McLean et al. looking at RP and TP RAPN in posterior tumours (considered a favourable location for RP surgery). They demonstrated no significant difference in the above outcome measures [32].

Where the message is certainly clearer is regarding patient length of stay (LOS) and convalescence. **LOS has been shown to be significantly shorter in RP-RAPN with a 1-day reduction in median LOS (p = <0.0001) in European collaborative data** [17], and **2-day reduction in LOS (p < 0.01) in International collaborations** [26]. This advantage in inpatient stay for RP-RAPN is also reflected in the McLean systematic review [32].

The obese patient presents additional challenges to both operative approaches. The **safety and advantages of RP-RAPN have also been demonstrated in patients with a BMI > 30 kg/m^2**. Median operative time of 130 mins, overall 3% post-operative complication rate, a 1% transfusion rate and a 1 day median length of stay have been established for RP-RAPN in this cohort [33].

Oncological and Functional Outcomes

Oncologically no significant difference in recurrence and disease progression is demonstrated in the literature. Similarly, **no significant difference in drop in eGFR in the immediate or longer term is recognized** (Table 3). Both approaches in the high-volume series display similar positive surgical margin (PSM) rates [18, 20, 26–30]. Low volume single centre experiences tend towards higher PSM rates for RP-RAPN patients and worse oncological outcomes, which highlights the need for centralisation and high volume to achieve equivalent safety and efficacy in an otherwise unfamiliar operative environment [34].

Cost Implications

Using time-driven activity-based costing (TDABC) model for small renal masses, Laviana et al. demonstrated **lower costs for RP-RAPN by $2337.16 per case**. This was predominantly driven by shorter statistically significant mean operative time

(167.0 vs 191.1min, $P = 0.001$) and LOS [1.82 days vs 2.68 days, $P < 0.001$] in the RP-RAPN cohort. The slightly higher disposable instrument costs of RP-RAPN (approximately $207.66 more per case) were offset by the gains in operative time (approximately $37.63/min) and LOS ($1713/day). They deduced equivalent costs in the pre-operative and follow-up stages for both approaches, with **gains in cost variation attributed to intra and post-operative pathway differences** [25].

Challenging the Current Consensus

Based on the advantages and disadvantages of both approaches, as highlighted in Tables 1 and 2, there does seem to be a consensus in the literature about the optimal use of each approach as summarised in Table 4 [35].

Ultimately the **choice of approach should be based on the surgeon's experience and expertise**. Given the wider practice, familiarity and higher volume there is evidence in the literature that TP-RAPN can be utilised safely and effectively to manage patients with posterior and lateral masses and in the 'hostile' abdomen [23, 28, 32, 35]. As our experience and volume with RP-RAPN grows there is **emerging data to suggest similar safety and efficacy to RP-RAPN in cases where traditionally the TP route may have been favoured**. Technical challenges such as a prominent iliac crest can be overcome by utilising a longer assistant port to allow a more optimal fulcrum and less restricted range for the bed side assistant. Technological evolutions and the fourth generation of Intuitive's DaVinci better utilise space and further miniaturise ports allowing for anatomical variations to be less likely to hamper progress during RP surgery. The rotating boom of the Da Vinci Xi allows for much easier docking, resulting in suboptimal approach angles of the patient cart being more forgiving during surgery [30]. Malki et al. have demonstrated the non-inferiority of RP-RAPN in obese patients [33]. Contemporary multicentre studies have demonstrated feasibility and safety of RP-RAPN in anterior, medial and complex tumours, whilst maintaining their advantages of shorter operative times and quicker patient convalescence [17–34].

Table 4 Summary of current consensus when considering the surgical approach to RAPN

RP-RAPN	TP-RAPN
Posterior and lateral renal masses	Anterior and medial masses
Prior abdominal surgery	Highly complex Tumours
Prior intraperitoneal pathology (e.g., Crohn's disease, acute abdomen, ascites, malignancy)	Anatomical kidney variations (horseshoe, pelvic)
	Obese patients
	Prior retroperitoneal/percutaneous renal procedures
	Prominent iliac crest/lumbar spine pathology limiting flexion

Future Trends in RP-RAPN

The authors of this chapter are based at a tertiary upper tract robotic centre in Surrey, UK with a referral radius of over 50 miles spanning Surrey, Hampshire and Sussex. Currently we perform over 300 upper tract procedures per annum, with over 90% of these using the RP route. As technology improves and volume increases, we would expect a natural evolution with RP-RAPN to tackle increasingly complex tumours. **At our centre pT1b and pT2a tumours are managed via the RP route and we would expect this trend to continue to develop**. Meanwhile adapting to and utilising existing technology to hone technique will continue to evolve. Indocyanine Green (ICG) instillation and utilisation of Da Vinci's integrated fluorescence capability, FireFly ™, allows for visual assessment of perfusion to the tumour and aids in selective arterial clamping (SAC). This is already widely used in TP-RAPN [36] and with superior use of limited space offered by the Da Vinci Xi, this can become technically more feasible in RP-RAPN. IRIS™ is an anatomical visualization service using data from diagnostic imaging to construct 3D models of patient anatomy that can be integrated to the surgeon console using TilePro. This should pave the way for better surgical planning and help tackle more complex cases.

Currently various competitor robot assisted surgical (RAS) systems are in production or en-route to the market [37]. Of these CMR Surgical's Versius™ system is already established in clinical practice, whilst Medtronic's HUGO™ RAS is widely considered as the next viable competitor to enter the market. As RAS systems become widely available globally, the boundaries of what is achievable with these newer systems will also continue to be pushed with time, volume, experience and shared evolution between surgeon and surgical system. Although various upper tract procedures have been successfully completed using the Versius™ system, the RAPN procedure eludes this system for the time being. As the system evolves this milestone will no doubt be achieved, however with current system algorithms requiring a 5 cm intracorporeal clearance space for safe use of instruments, the retroperitoneal route will evade the current iteration of the Versius™ system.

Intuitive Surgical on the other hand have developed a Da Vinci SP system designed to drive laparoendoscopic single site surgery (LESS). Fang et al. recently presented their experience with single port RP-RAPN in 7 patients. Although safe and feasible this technique remains very much in the infancy of its journey. All patients were carefully selected to be performed off-clamp and the overall safety, cost effectiveness and perceived benefit to patients remains unanswered as yet [38].

Key Points

- Retroperitoneal robot assisted partial nephrectomy is increasingly establishing itself in the armamentarium of the management of small renal masses
- It displays advantages of the transperitoneal route with regard to shorter length of stay, quicker patient convalesence and being more affordable
- Retoperitoneal robot assisted partial nephrectomy is associated with a steep learning curve

- In experienced hands most small renal masses apart from anterior hilar masses can be managed successfully via the retroperitoneum
- Retroperitoneal surgery has been shown to be safe and efficacious in complex masses and patients with high BMI
- Intraoperatively management of the pre-renal and peri-renal fat are vital in optimising field of vision and space
- New generations and miniaturisation of robotic surgical systems should enable ongoing progress in the retroperitoneal RAPN
- Ultimately the choice of approach should be based on the surgeon's experience and expertise.

References

1. Clayman RV, et al. Laparoscopic nephrectomy: initial case report. J Urol. 1991;146(2):278–82.
2. Gill IS, Delworth MG, Munch LC. Laparoscopic retroperitoneal partial nephrectomy. J Urol. 1994;152(5 Pt 1):1539–42.
3. Gettman MT, et al. Robotic-assisted laparoscopic partial nephrectomy: technique and initial clinical experience with DaVinci robotic system. Urology. 2004;64(5):914–8.
4. Sukumar S, Rogers CG. Robotic partial nephrectomy: surgical technique. BJU Int. 2011;108(6 Pt 2):942–7.
5. Ghani KR, et al. Robotic retroperitoneal partial nephrectomy: a step-by-step guide. BJU Int. 2014;114(2):311–3.
6. Spaliviero M, et al. Intravenous mannitol versus placebo during partial nephrectomy in patients with normal kidney function: a double-blind, clinically-integrated, Randomized Trial. Eur Urol. 2018;73(1):53–9.
7. Omae K, et al. Mannitol has no impact on renal function after open partial nephrectomy in solitary kidneys. Int J Urol. 2014;21(2):200–3.
8. Le B, et al. Comparative analysis of vascular bulldog clamps used in robot-assisted partial nephrectomy. J Endourol. 2013;27(11):1349–53.
9. Sukumar S, et al. Robotic partial nephrectomy using robotic bulldog clamps. JSLS. 2011;15(4):520–6.
10. McClintock TR, et al. Can selective arterial clamping with fluorescence imaging preserve kidney function during robotic partial nephrectomy? Urology. 2014;84(2):327–32.
11. Komninos C, et al. Renal function is the same 6 months after robot-assisted partial nephrectomy regardless of clamp technique: analysis of outcomes for off-clamp, selective arterial clamp and main artery clamp techniques, with a minimum follow-up of 1 year. BJU Int. 2015;115(6):921–8.
12. Paulucci DJ, et al. Selective arterial clamping does not improve outcomes in robot-assisted partial nephrectomy: a propensity-score analysis of patients without impaired renal function. BJU Int. 2017;119(3):430–5.
13. Benway BM, et al. Robotic partial nephrectomy with sliding-clip renorrhaphy: technique and outcomes. Eur Urol. 2009;55(3):592–9.
14. Sammon J, et al. Barbed suture for renorrhaphy during robot-assisted partial nephrectomy. J Endourol. 2011;25(3):529–33.
15. Williams RD, et al. Has sliding-clip Renorrhaphy eliminated the need for collecting system repair during robot-assisted partial nephrectomy? J Endourol. 2017;31(3):289–94.
16. Peyton CC, et al. Urinary leak following partial nephrectomy: a contemporary review of 975 cases. Can J Urol. 2020;27(1):10118–24.

17. Porpiglia F, et al. Transperitoneal vs retroperitoneal minimally invasive partial nephrectomy: comparison of perioperative outcomes and functional follow-up in a large multi-institutional cohort (the RECORD 2 project). Surg Endosc. 2021;35(8):4295–304.
18. Hughes-Hallett A, et al. Robot-assisted partial nephrectomy: a comparison of the transperitoneal and retroperitoneal approaches. J Endourol. 2013;27(7):869–74.
19. Gin GE, et al. Comparison of perioperative outcomes of retroperitoneal and transperitoneal minimally invasive partial nephrectomy after adjusting for tumor complexity. Urology. 2014;84(6):1355–60.
20. Choo SH, et al. Transperitoneal versus retroperitoneal robotic partial nephrectomy: matched-pair comparisons by nephrometry scores. World J Urol. 2014;32(6):1523–9.
21. Kim EH, et al. Retroperitoneal robot-assisted partial nephrectomy for posterior renal masses is associated with earlier hospital discharge: a single-institution retrospective comparison. J Endourol. 2015;29(10):1137–42.
22. Sharma P, et al. Is surgeon intuition equivalent to models of operative complexity in determining the surgical approach for nephron sparing surgery? Indian J Urol. 2016;32(2):124–31.
23. Maurice MJ, et al. Robotic partial nephrectomy for posterior tumors through a retroperitoneal approach offers decreased length of stay compared with the Transperitoneal approach: a propensity-matched analysis. J Endourol. 2017;31(2):158–62.
24. Stroup SP, et al. Comparison of retroperitoneal and transperitoneal robotic partial nephrectomy for Pentafecta perioperative and renal functional outcomes. World J Urol. 2017;35(11):1721–8.
25. Laviana AA, et al. Retroperitoneal versus transperitoneal robotic-assisted laparoscopic partial nephrectomy: a matched-pair, bicenter analysis with cost comparison using time-driven activity-based costing. Curr Opin Urol. 2018;28(2):108–14.
26. Arora S, et al. Retroperitoneal vs Transperitoneal robot-assisted partial nephrectomy: comparison in a multi-institutional setting. Urology. 2018;120:131–7.
27. Harke NN, et al. Retroperitoneal versus Transperitoneal robotic partial nephrectomy: a multicenter matched-pair analysis. Eur Urol Focus. 2021;7(6):1363–70.
28. Paulucci DJ, et al. A multi-institutional propensity score matched comparison of Transperitoneal and retroperitoneal partial nephrectomy for cT1 posterior tumors. J Laparoendosc Adv Surg Tech A. 2019;29(1):29–34.
29. Abaza R, Gerhard RS, Martinez O. Feasibility of adopting retroperitoneal robotic partial nephrectomy after extensive transperitoneal experience. World J Urol. 2020;38(5):1087–92.
30. Mittakanti HR, et al. Transperitoneal vs. retroperitoneal robotic partial nephrectomy: a matched-paired analysis. World J Urol. 2020;38(5):1093–9.
31. Xia L, et al. Transperitoneal versus retroperitoneal robot-assisted partial nephrectomy: a systematic review and meta-analysis. Int J Surg. 2016;30:109–15.
32. McLean A, et al. Trans-peritoneal vs. retroperitoneal robotic assisted partial nephrectomy in posterior renal tumours: need for a risk-stratified patient individualised approach. A systematic review and meta-analysis. J Robot Surg. 2020;14(1):1–9.
33. Malki M, et al. Retroperitoneal robot-assisted partial nephrectomy in obese patients. J Laparoendosc Adv Surg Tech A. 2019;29(8):1027–32.
34. Tanaka K, et al. Comparison of the transperitoneal and retroperitoneal approach in robot-assisted partial nephrectomy in an initial case series in Japan. J Endourol. 2013;27(11):1384–8.
35. Marconi L, Challacombe B. Robotic partial nephrectomy for posterior renal Tumours: retro or Transperitoneal approach? Eur Urol Focus. 2018;4(5):632–5.
36. Sri D, et al. Robotic-assisted partial nephrectomy (RAPN) and standardization of outcome reporting: a prospective, observational study on reaching the "trifecta and Pentafecta". J Robot Surg. 2021;15:571–7.
37. Thomas BC, et al. Preclinical evaluation of the Versius surgical system, a new robot-assisted surgical device for use in minimal access renal and prostate surgery. Eur Urol Focus. 2021;7(2):444–52.
38. Fang AM, et al. Single-port robotic partial and radical nephrectomies for renal cortical tumors: initial clinical experience. J Robot Surg. 2020;14(5):773–80.

Transperitoneal Robotic Partial Nephrectomy

Christopher Anderson, Jens-Uwe Stolzenburg, Arman Tsaturyan, Mohannad Alsulami, Vinodh-Kumar-Adithyaa Arthanareeswaran, Evangelos Liatsikos, and Panagiotis Kallidonis

Introduction

The management of low stage renal cell carcinoma (RCC) has evolved over the last 20 years from radical nephrectomy to nephron-sparing surgery. Partial nephrectomy has been proven to provide comparable oncological results with significant preservation of renal tissue. Nephron-sparing surgery is now accepted as a standard of care for most T1a renal masses. Open partial nephrectomy is still considered the standard of care for localized tumours according to the European Association of Urology guidelines [1–3]. Nonetheless, the increasing experience and expertise in minimally invasive procedures allow the efficient and safe performance laparoscopic partial nephrectomy (LPN) and robot-assisted partial nephrectomy (RAPN) rendering them as alternatives to open surgery [3].

Laparoscopic partial nephrectomy provides similar oncological outcomes with benefits in terms of faster postoperative recovery, reduced blood loss, and postoperative pain compared to open surgery. Similarly, the RAPN offers the advantages of minimally invasive approach along with a wider range of movement,

---

Christopher Anderson and Jens-Uwe Stolzenburg contributed equally with all other contributors.

C. Anderson
Department Urology, St Georges University Hospital NHS Foundation Trust, London, UK

J.-U. Stolzenburg · V.-K.-A. Arthanareeswaran
Department of Urology, University Hospital of Leipzig, Leipzig, Germany

A. Tsaturyan · M. Alsulami · E. Liatsikos
Department of Urology, University Hospital of Patras, Patras, Greece

P. Kallidonis (✉)
Department of Urology, University Hospital of Patras, Patras, Greece

Department of Urology, University of Patras Medical School, Patras, Greece

C. Anderson, M. Afshar (eds.), *Renal Cancer*,
https://doi.org/10.1007/978-3-030-84756-2_15

three-dimensional (3D) and more magnified vision, and the camera controlled by the primary surgeon Those advantages can make a significant difference to intracorporeal suturing or fine tissue dissection [1, 4]. Regardless of the approach, partial nephrectomy is associated with several technical challenges. Technical expertise is mandatory for the functional and oncological efficacy of the procedure [5–7].

Nephrometry Scoring of Renal Anatomy and Tumour Complexity

The Nephrometry scoring systems of renal surgical anatomy are of importance for proper selection of the intraoperative technical approach and prediction of perioperative outcomes. The RENAL (radius, exophytic/endophytic, nearness, anterior/posterior and location) and PADUA (Preoperative Aspects and Dimensions Used for Anatomic) represented the initially adopted scoring systems [8, 9]. The interpretation of the these requires significant expertise; which itself determines the outcomes [10]. In 2016, the ABC (Arterial Based Complexity) scoring system was introduced [11]. The main reported advantages of the latter were ease of use and good correlation with perioperative morbidity. Nevertheless, all of the scoring systems possess similar potential in predicting perioperative outcomes such as ischemia time or estimated blood loss [12].

Selection of the Surgical RAPN Approaches

Transperitoneal RAPN has been embraced by urologists globally as it assures wider working space and adequate freedom of movement for robotic arm as well as easier identification of anatomical landmarks and access to the renal hilum. It remains the main modality of choice for patients subjected to RAPN. The results of the Transatlantic Robotic Nephron-sparing surgery study group showed that more than 70% of cases were operated using transperitoneal approach [13]. RAPN was successfully completed in 635 patients, only 25 experiencing major complications (Clavien-Dindo >2) [13]. It was also associated with excellent long-term oncological outcomes. As such, the 5-year and 7-year cumulative death incidence rate following RAPN was 1.8%. Local recurrence and distant metastasis was observed in less than 5%, proving the safety of the procedure [14]. Its most recent advancement was the single-port RAPN. Although initial results indicated that a single-port approach could be safely implemented in urological robotic surgery practice, further studies are required [15, 16].

Recently, the feasibility of retroperitoneal RAPN was reported in the literature [17, 18]. Positive findings in terms of decreased operative time and length of hospital stay were reported for posterior renal tumours undergoing retroperitoneal RAPN. In the meantime, no impact of the approach on the negative tumour margins, postoperative complications and renal function were observed [17, 18]. While the retroperitoneal RAPN might be beneficial for posterior renal tumours, its effectiveness for small renal masses in all renal locations must be proven. Thus, one cannot be prescriptive about which surgical approach to use and it should be based on the surgeon's preference and expertise.

Intraoperative Localization of Renal Lesions

The intraoperative localisation of renal masses is important to ensure safe excision with negative margins. While the margins of exophytic tumours can be visualized with relative ease enabling accurate excision, endophytic tumours pose more challenges for the surgeons. To overcome this issue, endoscopic ultrasound was introduced in conventional laparoscopy and thereafter successfully implemented in robotic surgeries. Several "drop-in" probes for RAPN have been proposed as well as contrast-enhanced ultrasonography (CEUS) [6]. With the ultrasound picture imposed on the console screen, the surgeon has the possibility to control the movement of the ultrasound robotic probe. This gives the surgeon complete autonomy in controlling the movement of the ultrasound probe.

In recent years, new modalities for intraoperative tumour localization have been proposed.; namely, fluorescence imaging using indocyanine green (ICG) and the intraoperative augmented reality with the use of hyper accuracy 3 dimensional (3D) reconstruction [19, 20] (Fig. 1). The fluorescence imaging with ICG allowed the successful differentiation of lesions from the normal kidney parenchyma in 73–100% of cases. Nonetheless, its effectiveness was not proven in completely endophytic tumours due to the presence of overlaying normal kidney tissue [20].A common application of immunofluorescence is its use in selective arterial clamping: by selectively clamping segmental branches the ischaemic area containing the tumour can be easily identified as the normal unclamped kidney area will be perfused and shine brighly with fluorescence. In contrast, the 3D augmented reality guidance demonstrated superior perioperative outcomes in comparison to 2D

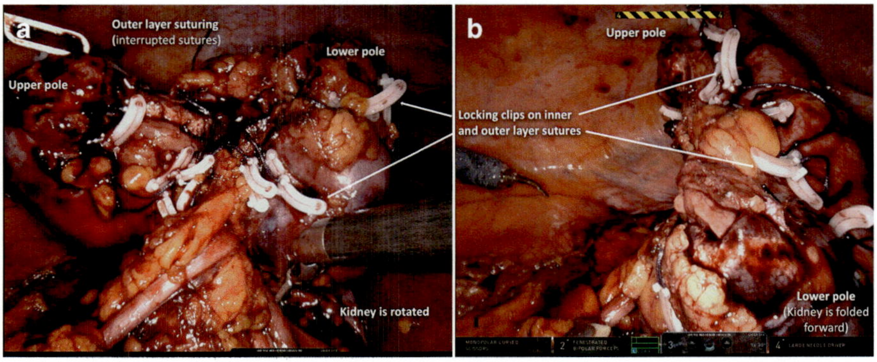

Fig. 1 (**a**) Intrarenal kidney tumour on right kidney. Renal hilar structures are looped. (**b**) 3D reconstruction (Source: www.innersightlabs.com) of the kidney with intrarenal tumor (green)

ultrasound guidance. A higher rate of tumour enucleation with a reduced rate of collecting system violation and ischemia were reported with its use [19]. Consequently, a lower rate of surgery-related complications was noted. Further investigations of the current advancements with a larger cohort of patients are awaited.

Clamping Technique

One of the main challenges during partial nephrectomy remains proper control of intraoperative bleeding and proper excision of the tumour (Fig. 2). The surgery can be performed using either off-clamp (zero ischemia) or on-clamp (warm or cold ischemia) technique (Fig. 2). There is much debate as to whether selective arterial clamping (SAC) or complete hilar clamping is more beneficial in sparing kidney function. In the most recent study of a large cohort of patients with solitary kidney the SAC was shown to be as safe as full clamping. However, no further advantages were reported with its use [21]. Similarly, Paulucci et al. found that SAC did not carry better outcomes in terms of positive surgical margins, complication rates or intermediate term renal function compared to main renal artery clamping [22].

The off-clamp technique offers theoretical advantages in that no impairment in kidney blood supply is expected during the procedure. Nonetheless, the studies evaluating the off- and on-clamp techniques did not reveal any significant differences in terms of renal function preservation between the 2 approaches [23–25]. Moreover, no benefit in estimated glomerular filtration rate was reported in patients with chronic kidney disease stage 3–5 using off-clamp [26]. Despite similar outcomes, off-clamp technique seems to be more challenging, demanding more effort and prolonging operative time [24]. Interestingly, the data from the ongoing randomized controlled CLOCK (CLamp vs Off Clamp the Kidney during robotic partial nephrectomy) trial

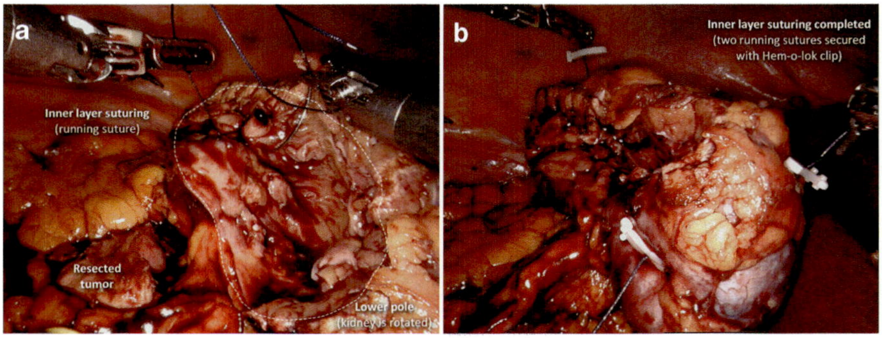

Fig. 2 (**a**) Introperative ultrasound showing the intraparenchymal kidney tumour. Inset: 3D reconstruction (Source: www.innersightlabs.com). (**b**) Tumour resection following bulldog clamping of the renal artery and vein. Renal vein is clamped in this case because of central tumour. Inset: The main and upper pole renal arteries are looped together. The renal arteries are not skeletonized to avoid intima damage

showed a 40% transition rate from off-clamp to on-clamp technique [27]. Consequently, renal mass diameter and complexity of renal anatomy were the identified predicting factors of technique transition. While 20–30 min of warm ischemia is considered safe for renal tissue [28], a shorter duration of warm ischemia should be preferred. Recent large series showed that early-unclamping of the renal pedicle was feasible and did not increase the 30-day complication rate following RAPN [29].

Tumour Excision and Renorrhaphy

Any proposed surgical technique for partial nephrectomy should follow the common rules of the "trifecta" of assuring adequate oncological outcomes (negative margins), preventing the development of peri- and postoperative complications and maximum preservation of postoperative renal function (Fig. 2). There is an ongoing debate regarding the most appropriate tumour resection technique during partial nephrectomy [30]. The initially introduced approach for tumour resection included the wide excision of the lesion along with surrounding normal kidney tissue. The main argument for the excision of normal parenchyma is the avoidance of positive surgical margins (PSM) following the resection. Nonetheless, the wider excision increases the risk of collecting system violation and bleeding [31]. Tumour enucleation (TE) has been intensively advocated during the last decade. It is achieved via blunt dissection along the pseudocapsule of the tumour which represents a less vascularized region. The drawback of the technique is the possibility of inadequate resection in case of tumours that invade the pseudocapsule or beyond [32]. In one study, the presence of peritumoral pseudocapsule was described in 95% of cases, whereas its invasion was apparent in 20%. Even when invasion of the tumour pseudocapsule was present, PSMs were documented in only 2.4% of the cases. This observation suggests that RAPN with TE is an oncologically safe procedure [33]. In a recent systematic review and meta-analysis comparing the wide excision of the tumour and TE, the authors found no differences of PSM, loco-regional recurrence (LRR) of renal recurrence (RR) [30]. Overall, 33 studies were selected, 28 included retrospective studies, 4 prospective and 1 prospective randomized controlled. RAPN was performed in eight studies and only 1 of them was conducted prospectively [30]. While oncological outcomes were similar in both the groups, TE seemed to possess lower rates of perioperative complications and improved kidney function [34].

Renorrhaphy Techniques

Once the lesion is successfully removed, renal reconstruction is required. The aim of renorrhaphy is assurance of accurate closure of the renal lesion bed, the collecting system and achievement of hemostasis. This is critical for minimizing postoperative bleeding as well as avoiding urinary leak. In several series, the use of fibrin sealants and hemostatic agents in addition to the renorrhaphy were studied. None of the used agents significantly reduced perioperative bleeding. Their use could be safely omitted if proper suturing is achieved [35–37]. Care should be taken to limit the extent of the suturing; thereby minimizing the area of potential devascularization and preserving postoperative kidney function [38].

Currently, a two-layer closure of the renal defect is advocated in most of the studies. Thereby, a first layer is used to close the collecting system and suture medullary vessels, while a second layer is used to approximate renal cortex (Fig. 3). Surgeons differ in their choice of suture material for the first layer and use monofilament or barbed sutures. With a monofilament suture the suture tension is increased by traction on both ends after completion as the suture will glide through the tissues (Fig. 4). However barbed sutures likely maintain their traction at the time the suture is placed.

In modified techniques with early unclamping, the second layer is performed with a re-perfused kidney. In addition, some series reported satisfactory results with only one-layer (inner layer) suturing technique. Its potential benefits are; shorter warm ischemia time and better visualization of arterial bleeding with targeted suturing of the bleeding tissue [39].

In 2009, "sliding-clip renorrhaphy" was introduced by Benway et al. [40]. It was found to be safe and efficient in comparison with tied-suture; with the shorter learning curve. The second layer renorrhaphy can be accomplished using a single or a double layer medullary knotless suture. Most commonly surgeons use the barbed suture V-Loc™ (Covidien). Others have also used the Lapra-Ty (Ethicon) clips and cortical suture [40]. In case of knotless suture, continuous suturing of the kidney medulla is performed leaving the end of the suture on the renal capsule. Clips are placed on entry and exit point of the suture. Furthermore, traditional interrupted and continuous suturing techniques with or without bolsters can be utilized [41]. Sliding-clip single layer renorrhaphy was further reported to be equally effective compared to double layer suturing [42]. Although the separate closure of the

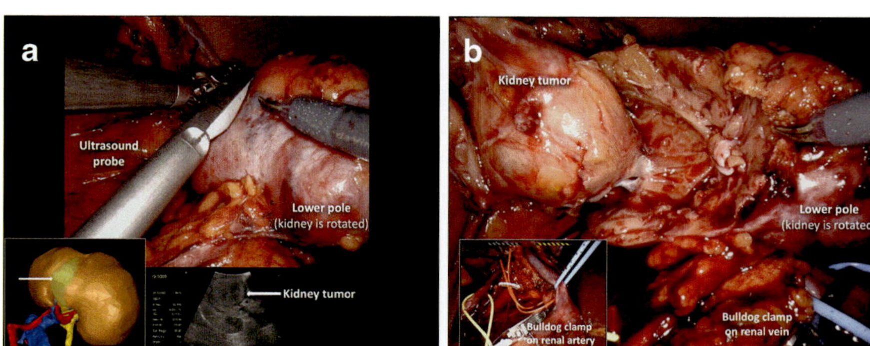

Fig. 3 (**a**) Inner layer suturing of the tumour bed with Polysorb 2–0, V-20 needle. (**b**) The direction of the needle is outside to inside the parenchyma followed by running suture for haemostasis and finally inside to outside which is secured by Hem-o-loc clips as shown in the image on the right

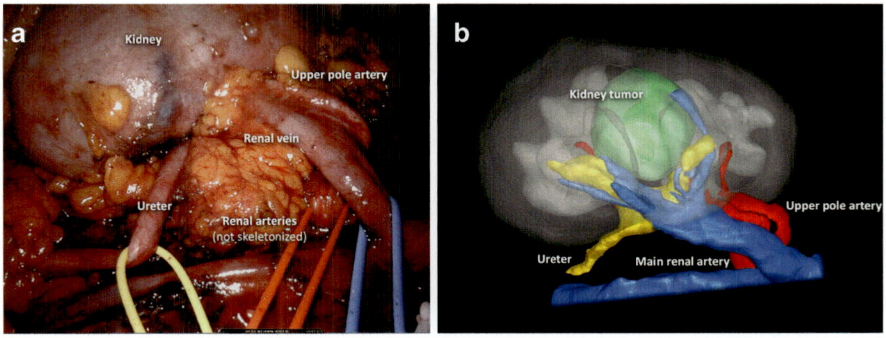

Fig. 4 (**a**) The outer layer suturing is performed in this case by using interrupted sutures (Polysorb 2–0, V-20 needle). The direction of the needle is from outside to inside and inside to outside for every suture. (**b**) The sutures are secured using Hem-o-loc clips. The inner and outer layer sutures are re-tensioned before final locking on both sides with Hem-o-loc clips

collecting system was omitted during the latter, it did not result in a higher rate of the urinary leak (Fig. 3).

During renorraphy there is variation in surgeon choice of the suture materials. In one study,an easier renal suturing was proposed using barbed suture material [43]. In a recent systematic review, the running barbed suture was associated with a shorter operative ischemia time [44]. An additional advantage of postoperative renal function was reported with single-layer suturing technique [39]. The latter might be important in patients with chronic kidney disease or solitary kidney where every nephron counts.

In summary, transperitoneal approach remains the most utilized technique for RAPN. It allows for a greater working space, the use of four robotic arms without clashing, and has anatomical landmarks that most minimally invasive surgeons are familiar with. Thorough preoperative knowledge of renal vascular and tumor anatomy improves the prediction of perioperative outcomes. Intraoperative ultrasound enhances the ability to delineate tumour anatomy. Tumour enucleation could be successfully performed in tumours with existing pseudocapsule. The performed renorrhaphy techniques should be safe and assure adequate hemostasis and collecting system repair, at the same time minimizing the ischemia of the normal kidney tissue.

Key Points

- Nephrometry scoring systems should be used for better prediction of perioperative outcomes.
- None of the existing scoring system has superiority over the other and experience and thorough understanding of tumour anatomy is beneficial
- Endoscopic robotic ultrasound is an effective tool for delineating renal masses intraoperatively and planning excision.

- Innovations such as Intraoperative augmented reality using hyper accuracy 3D reconstruction might be very useful for the localization of complex renal tumors.
- The transperitoneal RAPN remains the most commonly used surgical approach for all renal tumours despite their localization
- The role of selective versus full clamping as well as zero ischemia is still unclear.
- Warm ischemia time limited to 20 min may assure preservation of renal function even in patients with chronic kidney disease or solitary kidney.
- Tumor enucleation could be safely performed in cases where pseudocapsule is present.
- Adequate renal reconstruction with minimal involvement of normal kidney tissue is essential
- Two layer suturing reconstruction with sliding clip renorraphy remain the standard techniques of reconstruction

References

1. Azhar RA, Gill IS, Aron M. Robotic nephron-sparing surgery for renal tumors: current status. Indian J Urol. 2014;30(3):275–82.
2. Sanchez A, Feldman AS, Hakimi AA. Current Management of Small Renal Masses, including patient selection, renal tumor biopsy, active surveillance, and thermal ablation. J Clin Oncol. 2018;36(36):3591–600.
3. Ljungberg B, Albiges L, Bensalah K, Bex A, Giles RH, Hora M, et al. EAU guidelines on renal cell carcinoma. European association of. Urology. 2020;
4. Palep JH. Robotic asissted minimally invasive surgery. J Minim Access Surg. 2009;5(1):1–7.
5. Goonewardene SS, Brown M, Challacombe B. Robotic partial nephrectomy and early unclamping: an evolving paradigm. J Robot Surg. 2017;11(1):93–4.
6. Dias BH, Larcher A, Dell'Oglio P, Montorsi F, El Khoury F, D'Hondt F, et al. What's new in robotic partial nephrectomy. Arch Esp Urol. 2019;72(3):283–92.
7. Cacciamani GE, Medina LG, Gill T, Abreu A, Sotelo R, Artibani W, et al. Impact of surgical factors on robotic partial nephrectomy outcomes: comprehensive systematic review and meta-analysis. J Urol. 2018;200(2):258–74.
8. Ficarra V, Novara G, Secco S, Macchi V, Porzionato A, De Caro R, et al. Preoperative aspects and dimensions used for an anatomical (PADUA) classification of renal tumours in patients who are candidates for nephron-sparing surgery. Eur Urol. 2009;56(5):786–93.
9. Kutikov A, Uzzo RG. The R.E.N.A.L. nephrometry score: a comprehensive standardized system for quantitating renal tumor size, location and depth. J Urol. 2009;182(3):844–53.
10. Monn MF, Gellhaus PT, Masterson TA, Patel AA, Tann M, Cregar DM, et al. R.E.N.A.L. Nephrometry scoring: how well correlated are urologist, radiologist, and collaborator scores? J Endourol. 2014;28(8):1006–10.
11. Spaliviero M, Poon BY, Karlo CA, Guglielmetti GB, Di Paolo PL, Beluco Corradi R, et al. An arterial based complexity (ABC) scoring system to assess the morbidity profile of partial nephrectomy. Eur Urol. 2016;69(1):72–9.
12. Alvim RG, Audenet F, Vertosick EA, Sjoberg DD, Touijer KA. Performance prediction for surgical outcomes in partial nephrectomy using Nephrometry scores: a comparison of arterial based complexity (ABC), RENAL, and PADUA systems. Eur Urol Oncol. 2018;1(5):428–34.

13. Casale P, Lughezzani G, Buffi N, Larcher A, Porter J, Mottrie A, et al. Evolution of robot-assisted partial nephrectomy: techniques and outcomes from the transatlantic robotic nephron-sparing surgery study group. Eur Urol. 2019;76(2):222–7.
14. Bertolo R, Garisto J, Dagenais J, Sagalovich D, Stein R, Fareed K, et al. Transperitoneal robot-assisted partial nephrectomy with minimum follow-up of 5 years: oncological and functional outcomes from a single institution. Eur Urol Oncol. 2019;2(2):207–13.
15. Kaouk J, Aminsharifi A, Sawczyn G, Kim S, Wilson CA, Garisto J, et al. Single-port robotic urological surgery using purpose-built single-port surgical system: single-institutional experience with the first 100 cases. Urology. 2020;
16. Fang AM, Saidian A, Magi-Galluzzi C, Nix JW, Rais-Bahrami S. Single-port robotic partial and radical nephrectomies for renal cortical tumors: initial clinical experience. J Robot Surg. 2020;14(5):773–80.
17. McLean A, Mukherjee A, Phukan C, Veeratterapillay R, Soomro N, Somani B, et al. Transperitoneal vs. retroperitoneal robotic assisted partial nephrectomy in posterior renal tumours: need for a risk-stratified patient individualised approach. A systematic review and meta-analysis. J Robot Surg. 2020;14(1):1–9.
18. Paulucci DJ, Beksac AT, Porter J, Abaza R, Eun DD, Bhandari A, et al. A multi-institutional propensity score matched comparison of Transperitoneal and retroperitoneal partial nephrectomy for cT1 posterior tumors. J Laparoendosc Adv Surg Tech A. 2019;29(1):29–34.
19. Porpiglia F, Checcucci E, Amparore D, Piramide F, Volpi G, Granato S, et al. Three-dimensional augmented reality robot-assisted partial nephrectomy in case of complex Tumours (PADUA >/=10): a new intraoperative tool overcoming the ultrasound guidance. Eur Urol. 2019;
20. Hekman MCH, Rijpkema M, Langenhuijsen JF, Boerman OC, Oosterwijk E, Mulders PFA. Intraoperative imaging techniques to support complete tumor resection in partial nephrectomy. Eur Urol Focus. 2018;4(6):960–8.
21. Badani KK, Kothari PD, Okhawere KE, Eun D, Hemal A, Abaza R, et al. Selective clamping during robot-assisted partial nephrectomy in patients with a solitary kidney: is it safe and does it help? BJU Int. 2020;125(6):893–7.
22. Paulucci DJ, Rosen DC, Sfakianos JP, Whalen MJ, Abaza R, Eun DD, et al. Selective arterial clamping does not improve outcomes in robot-assisted partial nephrectomy: a propensity-score analysis of patients without impaired renal function. BJU Int. 2017;119(3):430–5.
23. Anderson BG, Potretzke AM, Du K, Vetter J, Figenshau RS. Off-clamp robot-assisted partial nephrectomy does not benefit short-term renal function: a matched cohort analysis. J Robot Surg. 2018;12(3):401–7.
24. Anderson BG, Potretzke AM, Du K, Vetter JM, Bergeron K, Paradis AG, et al. Comparing off-clamp and on-clamp robot-assisted partial nephrectomy: a prospective randomized trial. Urology. 2019;126:102–9.
25. Shah PH, George AK, Moreira DM, Alom M, Okhunov Z, Salami S, et al. To clamp or not to clamp? Long-term functional outcomes for elective off-clamp laparoscopic partial nephrectomy. BJU Int. 2016;117(2):293–9.
26. Beksac AT, Okhawere KE, Rosen DC, Elbakry A, Dayal BD, Daza J, et al. Do patients with stage 3-5 chronic kidney disease benefit from ischaemia-sparing techniques during partial nephrectomy? BJU Int. 2020;125(3):442–8.
27. Antonelli A, Cindolo L, Sandri M, Annino F, Carini M, Celia A, et al. Predictors of the transition from off to on clamp approach during ongoing robotic partial nephrectomy: data from the CLOCK randomized clinical trial. J Urol. 2019;202(1):62–8.
28. Thompson RH, Lane BR, Lohse CM, Leibovich BC, Fergany A, Frank I, et al. Every minute counts when the renal hilum is clamped during partial nephrectomy. Eur Urol. 2010;58(3):340–5.
29. Delto JC, Chang P, Hyde S, McAnally K, Crociani C, Wagner AA. Reducing Pseudoaneurysm and urine leak after robotic partial nephrectomy: results using the early unclamping technique. Urology. 2019;132:130–5.
30. Minervini A, Campi R, Sessa F, Derweesh I, Kaouk JH, Mari A, et al. Positive surgical margins and local recurrence after simple enucleation and standard partial nephrectomy for malignant

renal tumors: systematic review of the literature and meta-analysis of prevalence. Minerva Urol Nefrol = The Italian journal of urology and nephrology. 2017;69(6):523–38.
31. Gupta GN, Boris RS, Campbell SC, Zhang Z. Tumor enucleation for sporadic localized kidney cancer: pro and con. J Urol. 2015;194(3):623–5.
32. Minervini A, Carini M. Tumor enucleation is appropriate during partial nephrectomy. Eur Urol Focus. 2019;5(6):923–4.
33. Minervini A, Campi R, Di Maida F, Mari A, Montagnani I, Tellini R, et al. Tumor-parenchyma interface and long-term oncologic outcomes after robotic tumor enucleation for sporadic renal cell carcinoma. Urol Oncol. 2018;36(12):527.e1–e11.
34. Takagi T, Kondo T, Tachibana H, Iizuka J, Omae K, Yoshida K, et al. Comparison of surgical outcomes between resection and enucleation in robot-assisted laparoscopic partial nephrectomy for renal tumors according to the surface-Intermediate-Base margin score: a propensity score-matched study. J Endourol. 2017;31(8):756–61.
35. Peyronnet B, Oger E, Khene Z, Verhoest G, Mathieu R, Roumiguie M, et al. The use of hemostatic agents does not prevent hemorrhagic complications of robotic partial nephrectomy. World J Urol. 2015;33(11):1815–20.
36. Maurice MJ, Ramirez D, Kara O, Malkoc E, Nelson RJ, Caputo PA, et al. Omission of hemostatic agents during robotic partial nephrectomy does not increase postoperative bleeding risk. J Endourol. 2016;30(8):877–83.
37. Cohen J, Jayram G, Mullins JK, Ball MW, Allaf ME. Do fibrin sealants impact negative outcomes after robot-assisted partial nephrectomy? J Endourol. 2013;27(10):1236–9.
38. Porpiglia F, Bertolo R, Amparore D, Fiori C. Nephron-sparing suture of renal parenchyma after partial nephrectomy: which technique to go for? Some best practices. Eur Urol Focus. 2019;5(4):600–3.
39. Shatagopam K, Bahler CD, Sundaram CP. Renorrhaphy techniques and effect on renal function with robotic partial nephrectomy. World J Urol. 2020;38(5):1109–12.
40. Benway BM, Wang AJ, Cabello JM, Bhayani SB. Robotic partial nephrectomy with sliding-clip renorrhaphy: technique and outcomes. Eur Urol. 2009;55(3):592–9.
41. Kaouk JH, Hillyer SP, Autorino R, Haber GP, Gao T, Altunrende F, et al. 252 robotic partial nephrectomies: evolving renorrhaphy technique and surgical outcomes at a single institution. Urology. 2011;78(6):1338–44.
42. Williams RD, Snowden C, Frank R, Thiel DD. Has sliding-clip Renorrhaphy eliminated the need for collecting system repair during robot-assisted partial nephrectomy? J Endourol. 2017;31(3):289–94.
43. Sammon J, Petros F, Sukumar S, Bhandari A, Kaul S, Menon M, et al. Barbed suture for renorrhaphy during robot-assisted partial nephrectomy. J Endourol. 2011;25(3):529–33.
44. Bertolo R, Campi R, Klatte T, Kriegmair MC, Mir MC, Ouzaid I, et al. Suture techniques during laparoscopic and robot-assisted partial nephrectomy: a systematic review and quantitative synthesis of peri-operative outcomes. BJU Int. 2019;123(6):923–46.

Lymph Node Dissection in Renal Cancer and Upper Tract Urothelial Cancer

Pieter J. le Roux

Lymph Node Dissection in Renal Cell Carcinoma

Introduction

The role of lymph node dissection (LND) in the treatment of renal cell carcinoma (RCC) is controversial. LND is accepted as the most reliable staging procedure to detect lymph node involvement but any therapeutic benefit remains unproven. Many urological surgeons have abandoned routine LND at time of nephrectomy due to a lack of proven benefit in cancer control and the increased use of laparoscopic surgery which makes LND a challenging and time consuming exercise. Robotic assisted surgery enables minimally invasive LND comparable to what can be achieved with open surgery. The widespread application of cross-sectional imaging has led to stage migration with increased diagnosis of early stage, low risk disease, where the incidence of nodal spread is negligible and where LND has no therapeutic or staging benefit. A subset of high risk patients may benefit from LND.

Guidelines

The 2019 update of the EAU guidelines in the management of renal cancer advises against LND in patients with clinically negative nodes [1]. The guidelines state that LND was not associated with reduced risk of distant metastases, cancer specific mortality or all-cause mortality. LND also did not improve oncological outcomes for patients at high risk of nodal involvement. LND can be considered for staging

P. J. le Roux (✉)
Consultant Urological Surgeon, St George's Hospital, London, UK
e-mail: pieter.leroux@nhs.net

C. Anderson, M. Afshar (eds.), *Renal Cancer*,
https://doi.org/10.1007/978-3-030-84756-2_16

purposes. Resection of visibly enlarged nodes on preoperative imaging and palpable nodes found at time of surgery is recommended where this is technically feasible.

Evidence

The only published prospective randomised trial of nephrectomy with and without LND enrolled 772 patients with clinically node negative disease. Patients were randomised to nephrectomy alone versus nephrectomy plus regional lymphadenectomy [2]. EORTC 30881 did not show any benefit in cancer control for patients treated with LND and nephrectomy but the majority of patients in the trial had low-stage tumours with a very low risk of nodal involvement where LND was unlikely to be beneficial. Precise information regarding the template used for LND and the number of nodes removed were lacking and the number of high risk patients was too small to assess the benefit of LND. The trial could not answer the question of where and to what extent LND should be performed. It is possible that these results may not be applicable to all RCC patients.

EORTC 30881 included only cT1-3N0M0 cases according to the 1978 TNM classification. Today 70% of the cases enrolled in this trial would be classified as cT1abN0M0. The trial provides level one evidence that LND has no therapeutic benefit in low risk patients. In addition the risk of occult nodal metastases is so low that LND also has no staging role in these patients. This is in keeping with the findings of numerous retrospective series as shown in Table 1 [3–5].

Some observational studies have reported a survival benefit for LND with radical nephrectomy and it has been argued that a more extensive dissection might confer a survival advantage [6]. In subsets of patients with clinically isolated N1M0 disease long term survival has been observed after LND [7–11]. However several modern observational studies have failed to demonstrate a survival benefit with LND in both non-metastatic and metastatic settings [4, 12, 13]. Bhindi et al. conducted a systematic review and meta-analysis of 51 unique studies and reported that the current literature does not support a therapeutic benefit for LND in either M0 or M1 renal carcinoma. The authors note that high-risk M0 patients warrant further study since a subset of patients with isolated nodal metastases experience long term survival after surgical resection [14].

Blute et al. proposed a protocol for LND based on metastatic risk. In a series of 1652 patients undergoing radical nephrectomy for clinical M0 clear cell RCC 93% were pN0 and 7% were node positive. Multivariable analysis demonstrated that the presence of nuclear Grade 3 or 4, presence of sarcomatoid components, tumour size more than or equal to 10 cm, tumour stage pT3 or pT4, and presence of coagulative tumour necrosis were independent predictors of regional lymph node involvement at time of nephrectomy [15]. Crispin et al. presented similar data with stage, grade, coagulative necrosis and sarcomatoid differentiation being strong predictors of lymph node involvement, and proposed that patients with larger masses might benefit from LND, at least for staging purposes. The likelihood of lymph node

Table 1 Papers published in the last 20 years assessing the effect of LND on survival

References	Study design	Number of patients	Patients included	LND definition and extension[a]	Measured outcomes	Effect of LND
Feuerstein et al.	Retrospective, single institution, controlled for confounders	524	≥7 cm TanyNanyMany	Mixed, non-standardized	Overall survival	No survival difference
Feuerstein et al.	Retrospective, single institution	258	M1	Mixed, non-standardized 0–3 nodes (30%) 4–7 (21%) ≥8 (49%)	Overall survival	No survival difference
Capitanio et al.	Retrospective, single institution, controlled for confounders	1983	TanyNanyMany	Mixed, non-standardized: No LND (56%) Hilar LND (18%): 3.1 (3) Side-specific LND (15%): 10 (8) Extended LND (9%): 15 (13)	Cancer-specific survival; Metastatic progression	Protective effect in increasing the number of nodes removed in patients with pT2a–pT2b or pT3c–pT4 or tumour size >10 cm or when sarcomatoid features were found
Bekema et al.	Systematic review, post hoc analyses of a prospective randomized	645 + 213[b]	TanyNanyMany cT3N0M0[b]	Mixed, non-standardized, unknown number of nodes removed	Cancer-specific survival; other causes survival	No robust evidence to suggest superior oncologic outcomes
Capitanio et al.	Retrospective, single institution, controlled for confounders	44	pT4	Extended: 12 (8)	Cancer-specific survival	Protective effect in increasing the number of nodes removed

(continued)

Table 1 (continued)

References	Study design	Number of patients	Patients included	LND definition and extension[a]	Measured outcomes	Effect of LND
Whitson et al.	Retrospective, population based cohort, controlled for confounders	9586	TanyNanyMany	Mixed, non-standardized, unknown number of nodes removed	Cancer-specific survival	Increased disease-specific survival with extent of lymphadenectomy in pN1 cases
Blom et al.	Prospective randomized	732	T1-3N0M0	Limited, non-standardized, unknown number of nodes removed	Cancer-specific survival; other causes survival	No benefit in terms of survival for patients treated with LND
Vasselli et al.	Retrospective, single institution	154	M1	Non-standardized, unknown number of nodes removed	Overall survival	Indirect low evidence suggesting a potential effect of LND in preparation of adjuvant interleukin regimen
Schafhauser et al.	Retrospective, single institution	1035	T1-4NanyM0	No LND (29%) Removal of lymphadenopathy only (19%): 6 Systematic LND (51%): 18	Overall survival	Patients treated with systematic lymphadenectomy had the least favorable tumor stage but better survival relative to patients not treated with LND

[a]Mean (median) number of nodes removed when available
[b]Systematic review with post hoc analyses of level 1b evidence

involvement increased with the number of risk factors involved [16]. Neither of these studies assessed the impact of LND on survival.

Capitanio et al. evaluated whether the number of lymph nodes removed may affect cancer-specific survival or progression free survival in specific scenarios. After a mean follow up of 7 years the number of nodes removed showed an independent protective effect in patients with larger tumours [9]. Feuerstein et al. did not find a reduction in overall or recurrence free survival in patients with tumours more than or equal to 7 cm whether they underwent LND or not [4]. A subanalysis of the prospective EORTC trial looking at clinical T3 tumours only reported a 15% overall survival benefit at 5 years for the patients who underwent LND and nephrectomy versus nephrectomy alone [17].

More often than not lymph node involvement signifies metastatic disease whether this is visible on imaging at the time or not. There is considerable argument for lymph node involvement to be reclassified as such.

Anatomical Considerations and Surgical Templates

The lymphatic drainage of the kidneys is highly variable. The retroperitoneal lymph nodes are an extensive network of lymphatics between the first and fifth lumbar vertebrae. These nodes serve as the primary landing sites for renal lymph and have unpredictable interconnections before reaching the thoracic duct. The efferent lymphatic vessels from the right kidney drain into the paracaval, precaval, retrocaval and interaortocaval nodes. From the left kidney efferent lymphatic vessels drain into the para-aortic, preaortic, retroaortic and interaortocaval nodes [16]. On both sides posterior lymphatic vessels can pass through the crus of the diaphragm and connect with the thoracic duct without passing through any lymph nodes.

Crispin et al. reported on 169 consecutive high risk patients who underwent LND at the time of radical nephrectomy in a single institution. Of these 169 patients 64 (38%) had lymph node metastases. All patients with nodal metastases had involvement of the primary lymphatic landing sites for each kidney. Of the 64 patients with nodal involvement 29 (45%) had no metastases identified in the perihilar lymph nodes. No patient with a right sided tumour had involvement of the para-aortic nodes without involvement of the other retroperitoneal nodes and no patient with a left-sided tumour had involvement of the paracaval nodes without involvement of the para-aortic or interaortocaval nodes [16].

There is no prospective study comparing limited versus extended LND in RCC for positive node detection, cancer control or surgical safety. There are no validated agreed templates for LND in RCC and most studies delineate only the presence or absence of a surgeon-related LND. Even EORTC 30881 could not inform to what extent LND should be performed since information regarding the location and number of lymph nodes removed were lacking [2]. Based on anatomical studies and indirect evidence Capitanio et al. propose for the right kidney the removal of paracaval, retrocaval and precaval nodes from the adrenal vein to the level of the inferior

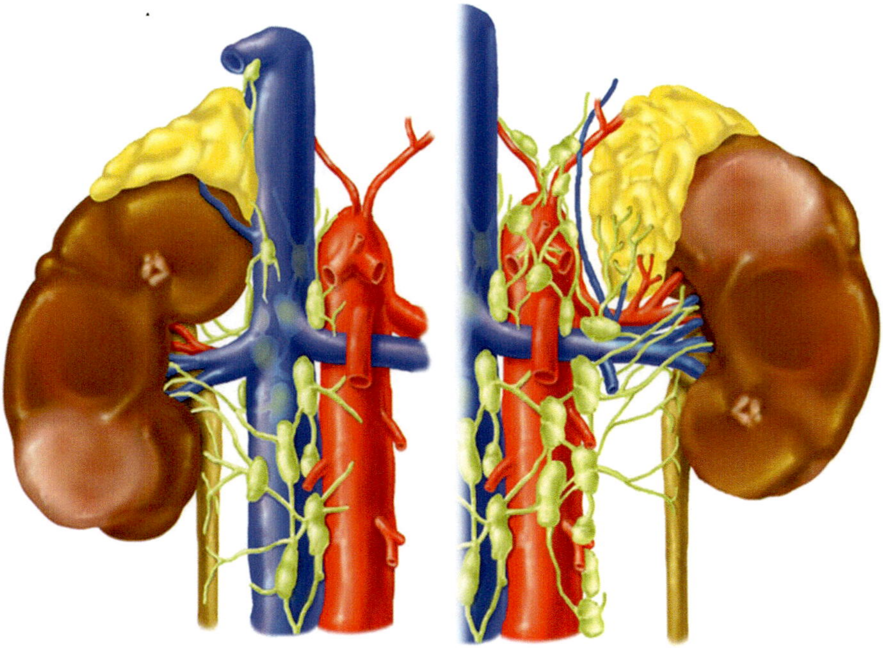

Fig. 1 LND might include, on the right side, para-, retro- and precaval nodes from the adrenal vein to the level of the inferior mesenteric artery. On the left, para-aortic and preaortic nodes from the crus of the diaphragm to the inferior mesenteric artery should be removed. Interaortocaval nodes should be removed as well when extended LND is sought. With permission from: Capitanio U, Leibivich BC (2017) The rationale and the role of lymph node dissection in renal cell carcinoma. World J Urol 35:497–506

mesenteric artery. For the left side the para-aortic and pre-aortic nodes from the level of the crus of the diaphragm to the inferior mesenteric artery should be removed. The interaortocaval nodes should also be removed for both left and right sided tumours if an extended LND is sought [10]. (See Fig. 1).

Salvage Lymph Node Dissection

Isolated regional lymphadenopathy during the follow up after surgery for RCC presents a dilemma due to lack of data in support of observation versus resection or systemic therapy. Retroperitoneal nodal recurrences are usually associated with systemic progression and distant metastases. In this scenario surgery is seldom indicated and patients are treated with systemic therapy if appropriate. If lymph node involvement appears to be truly isolated and this is confirmed by a trial of time, then salvage LND is indicated in selected patients if technically feasible. Similar to the concept of surgical resection of a solitary metastases this may delay disease progression and defer the start time of systemic therapy in some patients.

Imaging

Clinical node status is based on cross sectional imaging with CT or MRI and palpation at the time of surgery. Cross sectional imaging is not able to detect small metastases in nodes of normal shape or size. Studer et al. showed that histologically positive nodes were found in only 42% of patients with enlarged nodes at preoperative CT, with a false negative rate of 4.1% [18]. Abnormally enlarged nodes may be due to RCC metastases, reactive change, sarcoidosis or other malignancy such as lymphoma. Radiological features such as nodal size, contrast uptake, lack of hilar fat and restricted diffusion on MRI may increase sensitivity and specificity of cross sectional imaging. Lymph nodes more than 2 cm in diameter are more likely to be metastatic. Positron emission tomography (PET) CT with fluorine- 18 fluorodeoxyglucose (FDG) is seldom helpful.

Sentinel node biopsy has been proposed for RCC but is hampered by the extremely variable pattern of renal lymphatic drainage. Bex et al. investigated the feasibility of intratumoural injection with a radioisotope labelled nanocolloid (Technesium 99) on the day before surgery and intra-operative scintigraphy with the use of a gamma camera. Six of 8 patients demonstrated sentinel nodes on scintigraphy [19].

Molecular and Genetic Markers

Molecular and genetic markers have the potential to replace clinical characteristics and cross sectional imaging in determining which patients if any might benefit from LND. Turajlic et al. analysed 575 primary and 335 metastatic biopsies in a landmark study of matched primary and metastatic biopsies in 100 clear cell renal cell carcinoma (ccRCC) cases. Metastatic competence was heavily influenced by chromosome complexity with chromosome 9p loss a highly selected event driving metastases and ccRCC related mortality. Distinct patterns of metastatic spread were observed, including rapid progression to multiple sites seeded by primary tumours of monoclonal structure. Lymph node metastases were characterised by poor prognosis and very frequent 9p loss (21 of 22 cases) indicating that lymphatic and haematogenous spread require comparable metastatic competence [20]. These findings are consistent with the frequent presentation of lymph node metastases with visceral metastases and lack of proof of therapeutic benefit of LND in RCC.

Lymph Node Dissection in Upper Tract Urothelial Carcinoma

Upper tract urothelial carcinoma (UTUC) is a rare malignancy with a poor prognosis comprising 5–10% of urothelial malignancies. Lymph node dissection (LND) in the surgical management of muscle invasive urothelial carcinoma of the bladder is well-established but the role of LND in UTUC is controversial due to a lack of high quality evidence. The potential lymphatic drainage covers a wide area and is dependent on the laterality, the site, and the extent of the disease. Templates for LND in UTUC are not universally defined or validated. LND provides the most accurate staging tool for UTUC. The existing data consists mainly of retrospective level 3 evidence indicating improved staging and potential improved survival for some patients, particularly those with muscle invasive or locally advanced disease. Despite this the uptake of LND in UTUC by urological surgeons remain low outside of a specialist centres [21].

The EAU guidelines for treatment of UTUC updated in 2017 state that LND is not required for pTa and pT1 disease due to the low incidence of nodal involvement in superficial disease, with lymph node involvement of 2.2% for T1 versus 16% for T2–4 tumours [22]. The likelihood of lymph node involvement is directly related to T stage and likely to be under reported in retrospective data. It is often not possible to accurately stage patients pre-operatively with imaging and limited tissue biopsies provided by ureterorenoscopy. The guidelines state that it is not possible to standardise the indications or templates for LND.

The lymphatic drainage varies greatly for the renal pelvis and the different segments of the ureter. The potential wide area for LND could contribute to an unacceptable increase in perioperative morbidity. Matin et al., following on from the work of Kondo et al., performed a mapping study of lymph node metastases in UTUC [23, 24]. Matin et al. showed that upward migration of lymphatic metastases from UTUC of the distal ureter to the paracaval and para-aortic regions and downward migration from mid ureter to the iliac nodes were common events. Templates for LND in UTUC as proposed by Kondo et al. and Matin et al. are illustrated in Fig. 2.

Standardised dissection templates based on tumour location may improve lymph node yield and need to be evaluated for safety and potential clinical benefit, preferable in multi-centre prospective trials. Until such data and accompanying guidelines are available the utilisation of LND in UTUC will remain highly variable and at the discretion of local units and surgeons.

Key Points

- Lymphatic drainage from the kidneys is highly variable
- No role for LND in low risk localised disease
- LND can provide valuable staging information in intermediate and high risk cases
- Lymph node involvement usually signifies metastatic disease and carries a poor prognosis
- Some high risk patients may benefit from LND

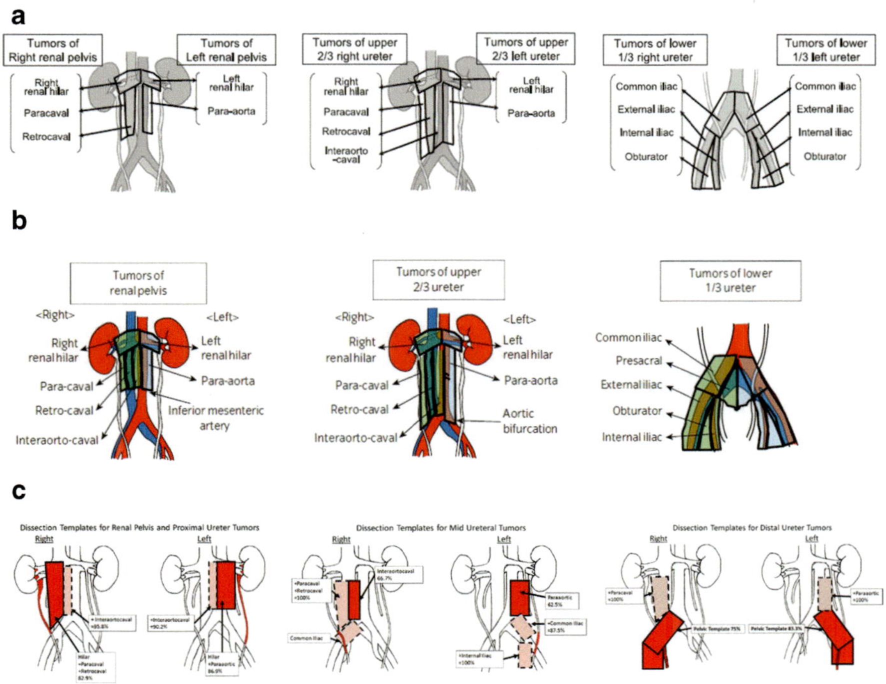

Fig. 2 Comparison of lymph node dissection templates according to tumor location between Kondo et al. (**a**, **b**) and Matin et al. (**c**). With permission from: Seisen T, Shariat SF, Cussenot O, Peyronnet B, Renard-Penna R, Colin P et al. (2017) Contemporary role of lymph node dissection at the time of radical nephroureterectomy for upper tract urothelial carcinoma. World J Urol 35: 535–548

References

1. Ljungberg B, Albiges L, Abu-Ghanem Y, Bensalah K, Dabestani S, Fernandez-Pello S, et al. European Association of Urology guidelines on renal cell carcinoma: the 2019 update. Eur Urol. 2019;75:799–810.
2. Blom JH, van Poppel H, Marechal JM, Jacqmin D, Schroder FH, de Prijck L, Sylvester R. Radical nephrectomy with and without lymph-node dissection: final results of the European Organisation for Research and Treatment of Cancer (EORTC) randomised phase 3 trial 30881. Eur Urol. 2009;55(1):28–34.
3. Capitanio U, Leibivich BC. The rationale and the role of lymph node dissection in renal cell carcinoma. World J Urol. 2017;35:497–506.
4. Feuerstein MA, Kent M, Bazzi WM, Bernstein M, Russo P. Analysis of lymph node dissection in patients with >=7cm renal tumours. World J Urol. 2014;32:1513–6.
5. Gershman B, Thompson RH, Modeira DM, et al. Lymph node dissection is not associated with improved survival among patients undergoing cytoreductive nephrectomy for metastatic renal cell carcinoma: a propensity score based analysis. J Urol. 2017;197(3 pt 1):574–9.
6. Whitson JM, Harris CR, Reese AC, Meng MV. Lymphadenectomy improves survival of patients with renal cell carcinoma and nodal metastases. J Urol. 2011;185:1615–20.

7. Boorjian SA, Crispin PL, Lohse CM, Leibovich BC, Blute MI. Surgical resection of isolated retroperitoneal lymph node recurrence of renal cell carcinoma following nephrectomy. J Urol. 2008;180:99–103.
8. Gershman B, Modeira DM, Thompson RH, et al. Renal cell carcinoma with isolated lymph node involvement: long term natural history and predictors of oncologic outcomes following surgical resection. Eur Urol. 2017;72:300–6.
9. Capitanio U, Suardi N, Matloob R, Roscigno M, Abdollah F, Di Trapani E, et al. Extent of lymph node dissection at nephrectomy affects cancer-specific survival and metastatic progression in specific sub-categories of patients with renal cell carcinoma (RCC). BJU Int. 2014;114(2):210–5.
10. Capitanio U, Becker F, Blute ML, Mulders P, Patard JJ, Russo P, Studer UE, Van Poppel H. Lymph node dissection in renal cell carcinoma. Eur Urol. 2011;60(nr. 6):1212–20.
11. Herrlinger A, Schrott KM, Schott G, Sigel A. What are the benefits of extended dissection of the regional lymph nodes in the therapy of renal cell carcinoma. J Urol. 1991;146(1224):1227.
12. Gershman B, Thompson RH, Modeira DM, et al. Lymph node dissection is not associated with improved survival among patients undergoing cytoreductive nephrectomy for metastatic renal cell carcinoma: a propensity score based analysis. J Urol. 2017;197(3 pt 1):574–9.
13. Feuerstein MA, Kent M, Bernstein M, Russo P. Lymph node dissection during cytoreductive nephrectomy: a retrospective analysis. Int J Urol. 2014;21(874):879.
14. Bhindi B, Wallis CJD, Boorjian S, Thompson RH, Farrell A, Kim S. The role of lymph node dissection in the management of renal cell carcinoma: a systematic review and meta-analysis. BJU Int. 2018;121:684–98.
15. Blute ML, Leibovich BC, Cheville JC, Lohse CM, Zincke H. A protocol for performing extended lymph node dissection using primary tumor pathological features for patients treated with radical nephrectomy for clear cell renal cell carcinoma. J Urol. 2004;172:465–9.
16. Crispin PL, Breau RH, Allmer C, Lohse CM, Cheville JC, Leibovich BC, Blute ML. Lymph node dissection at the time of radical nephrectomy for high-risk clear cell renal cell carcinoma: indications and recommendations for surgical templates. Eur Urol. 2011;59:18–23.
17. Bekema HJ, Maclennan S, Imamura M, Lam TB, Stewart F, Scott N, et al. Systemic review of adrenalectomy and lymph node dissection in locally advanced renal cell carcinoma. Eur Urol. 2013;64:799–810.
18. Studer UE, Scherz S, Scheidegger J, et al. Enlargement of regional lymph nodes in renal carcinoma is often not due to metastases. J Urol. 1990;144:243–5.
19. Bex A, Vermeeren L, de Windt G, Prevoo W, Horenblas S, Olmos RA. Feasibility of sentinel node detection in renal cell carcinoma: a pilot study. Eur J Nucl Med Mol Imaging. 2010;37:1117–23.
20. Turajlic S, Xu H, Litchfield K, Rowan A, Chambers T, Lopez J, et al. Tracking cancer evolution reveals constrained routes to metastases: TRACERx renal. Cell. 2018;173:581–94.
21. Seisen T, Shariat SF, Cussenot O, Peyronnet B, Renard-Penna R, Colin P, et al. Contemporary role of lymph node dissection at the time of radical nephroureterectomy for upper tract urothelial carcinoma. World J Urol. 2017;35:535–48.
22. Roupre M, Babjuk M, Comperat E, Zigeuner R, Sylvester R, Burger M, et al. European Association of Urology guidelines on upper urinary tract urothelial carcinoma: 2017 update. Eur Urol. 2018;73(1):111–22.
23. Matin SF, Sfakianos JP, Espiritu PN, Coleman JA, Spiess PE. Patterns of lymphatic metastases in upper tract urothelial carcinoma and proposed dissection templates. J Urol. 2015;194(6):1567–74.
24. Kondo T, Nakazawa H, Ito F, Hashimoto Y, Toma H, Tanabe K. Primary site and incidence of lymph node metastases in urothelial carcinoma of upper urinary tract. Urology. 2007;69:265–9.

Metastatic Renal Cancer: Systemic Therapy

Wing Kin Liu, Mehran Afshar, and Lisa Pickering

Background

Over the past 15 years the management of metastatic renal cell carcinoma (mRCC) has changed considerably from cytokine therapy alone, to a broad range of options encompassing targeted therapies against vascular endothelial growth factor (VEGF) and its receptor, to immune checkpoint inhibitors (ICIs) and now combinations of these treatments. The protein receptor tyrosine kinase inhibitors (TKIs) are themselves a heterogeneous group, incorporating including drugs that target the vascular endothelial growth factor receptor, the MET and AXL receptors and the mammalian target of rapamycin (mTOR). However, despite these advances that have led to improvements in prognosis, survival duration and quality of life, the majority of patients with mRCC will progress on these treatments and hence questions are raised regarding the best sequence or combination of treatments to optimize outcomes.

Introduction

Renal cell carcinoma (RCC) is one of the ten most common cancers in men and women accounting for up to 4% of all new cancer presentations and 2.5% of cancer mortality internationally [1]. Most RCC patients will present with localized disease

W. K. Liu · L. Pickering (✉)
Royal Marsden Hospital & Institute of Cancer Research, London, UK
e-mail: Wingkin.Liu@stgeorges.nhs.uk; Lisa.Pickering@rmh.nhs.uk

M. Afshar
Royal Marsden Hospital & Institute of Cancer Research, London, UK

Department Uro-Oncology, St Georges University Hospital NHS Foundation Trust, London, UK
e-mail: mehran.afshar@stgeorges.nhs.uk

C. Anderson, M. Afshar (eds.), *Renal Cancer*,
https://doi.org/10.1007/978-3-030-84756-2_17

which can be treated with curative intent such as surgery or radio-ablation. However 25–40% of these patients will relapse with distant disease and 20–25% of RCC patients will present with de-novo metastasis [2]. The majority of mRCC presents as clear cell histology [3] with other sub-types including papillary types 1 and 2, chromophobe, translocation and medullary cancers. Although there have been notable advances in new treatments for mRCC the 5 year survival for these patients is still poor [4, 5].

Nevertheless, recent advances in mRCC treatment have improved the prognosis of mRCC patients. The Memorial Sloan Kettering Cancer Center (MSKCC) criteria were developed in the cytokine era looking at performance status, lactate dehydrogenase levels, serum calcium, hemoglobin and time from initial diagnosis to systemic treatment in a validated prognostic model that categorized patients into favorable, intermediate and poor risk groups [6]. Following this the International Metastatic RCC Database Consortium (IMDC) criteria evolved to define the same three risk categories and included performance status, hemoglobin, calcium, and time from initial diagnosis to systemic therapy in addition to neutrophil and platelet counts [7]. This was found to be a more accurate model for predicting mRCC prognosis in the context of oral VEGF-directed treatments such as sunitinib. However with the advent of immunotherapy this may change again [8].

Tyrosine Kinase Inhibitors in the First Line Setting

VEGF receptor TKI monotherapy has been the standard of care for initial treatment of mRCC since 2007 until very recently with the advent of ICIs. A landmark randomized trial of 750 patients comparing sunitinib (an oral anti-VEGF receptor therapy) with interferon-alpha showed a superior median progression free survival (PFS) of 11 vs 5 months ($p < 0.001$). Follow up data showed improved median overall survival (OS) (26.4 vs 21.8 months) ((Hazard ratio for death (HR) 0.82, $p = 0.051$)) [9, 10]. Subsequently pazopanib (another oral anti-VEGF receptor therapy) was shown in a randomized phase 3 study to be superior to placebo in treatment naive mRCC patients or cytokine pre-treated patients. In the treatment naive group median PFS was 11.1 months compared with 2.8 months in the placebo group (HR 0.40, $p < 0.001$) [11]. The COMPARZ trial compared sunitinib and pazopanib in an international non-inferiority trial. Pazopanib was found to be non-inferior to sunitinib with a median PFS of 8.3 versus 9.5 months for sunitinib (HR 1.05, 0.90–1.22) [12]. Pazopanib was also found to have a reduced incidence of CTCAE (Common Terminology Criteria for Adverse Events) grade three fatigue, hand-foot syndrome and thrombocytopenia when compared with sunitinib. This improved toxicity profile was later supported by the PISCES trial which looked at 169 patients randomized between sunitinib and pazopanib in either sequence in a double blind, crossover, patient preference study. 70% of patients preferred pazopanib, reporting less fatigue and better quality of life although some patients preferred sunitinib [13].

Other TKIs approved for first line use in mRCC include tivozanib and cabozantinib. Tivozanib was shown in a randomized phase 3 trial to have a superior PFS to the oral anti-VEGF receptor therapy sorafenib of 11.9 vs 9.1 months (HR 0.80, p = 0.042) in favorable and intermediate risk patients. However the final OS data showed a better median OS for sorafenib (29.3 vs 28.8 months; HR 1.25, 0.954–1.624, p = 0.105) [14]. In the randomized phase 2 CABOSUN trial cabozantinib was compared with sunitinib in intermediate and poor risk patients. The primary median PFS was 8.6 versus 5.3 months (HR 0.48, p = 0.0008) and median OS was 26.6 versus 21.2 months (HR 0.80, 0.53–1.21), favoring cabozantinib. In this study 13% were Eastern Cooperative Oncology Group (ECOG) performance status 2, and 37% had bone metastases [15]. On the back of these data it has been suggested that cabozantinib may be beneficial for mRCC patients with bone metastasis which can cause morbid sequelae [16]. Both treatments are now licensed for treatment naive mRCC along with sunitinib, pazopanib and tivozanib.

Tyrosine Kinase Inhibitors Beyond the First Line Setting

After progression on first line oral anti-VEGF directed therapy current licensed options include axitinib and cabozantinib (two anti-VEGF directed therapy agents) and the oral TKI combination lenvatinib with the mTOR inhibitor everolimus.

AXIS was a phase 3 randomized trial which enrolled 723 patients to receive axitinib or sorafenib. PFS was superior at 6.7 months with axitinib compared with 4.7 months with sorafenib (HR 0.67, p < 0.0001). This lead to axitinib being licensed by the Food Drug Association (FDA) in January 2012 as a second line treatment for mRCC [17].

The oral anti-VEGF directed therapy cabozantinib demonstrated a beneficial PFS and OS in the randomized phase three trial METEOR. This trial evaluated 658 VEGF refractory patients who received cabozantinib or the mTOR inhibitor everolimus. Cabozantinib showed an improved PFS from 3.9 to 7.4 months (HR 0.51, 0.41–0.62, p < 0.0001). OS improved from 17.1 to 21.4 months with cabozantinib versus everolimus (HR 0.67, 0.58–0.86, p = 0.0002) [18, 19].

The oral TKI combination lenvatinib and everolimus is also highly active in mRCC. This combination was evaluated in a randomized phase 2 trial of 152 patients with VEGF-refractory mRCC. This showed a prolonged PFS of (14.6 vs 5.5 months; HR 0.40, 0.24–0.68, p = 0.0005) when compared with everolimus alone. However, when compared with lenvatinib alone PFS was not prolonged (7.4 months; HR 0.66, 0.30–1.10, p = 0.12) perhaps suggesting a synergistic effect of oral TKI and a mTOR inhibitor. Median OS was 25.5 months with the combination versus 15.4 months with everolimus (HR 0.51, p = 0.024) [20].

Everolimus can also be used as monotherapy based on results from the RECORD-1 trial which compared the use of everolimus versus best supportive care in patients with mRCC [21]. The median PFS was 4.9 months for everolimus versus 1.9 months for placebo (HR 0.32, P < 0.001) Serious adverse events with everolimus include an increased risk of infections, dyspnea and fatigue. 14 of 274 (5%) patients receiving everolimus developed a pneumonitis of which 4 patients had a grade 3 toxicity.

Immune Checkpoint Inhibitors

The advent of immunotherapy has profoundly changed the management of treatment naive mRCC and also in subsequent lines of therapy. Checkmate-025 was a phase 3 study evaluating the efficacy of anti-programmed cell death 1 (PD-1) inhibitor nivolumab in 821 previously treated mRCC patients versus everolimus. Median OS was 25 versus 19.6 months favoring nivolumab (HR 0.73, P = 0.002) regardless of PD-L1 expression. Grade 3–4 treatment-related adverse events were also lower with nivolumab compared with everolimus. Of patients who received nivolumab (n = 406) 19% experienced a grade 3/4 adverse event compared with 37% patients who received everolimus (n = 397). Also subsequent quality of life studies have shown preference towards nivolumab [22].

In the first line setting Checkmate 214 evaluated the combination of nivolumab and ipilimumab compared with sunitinib. Median OS was not reached in the combination arm versus 26 months with sunitinib (HR 0.63, p < 0.001) [23]. Median PFS was numerically longer at 11.6 vs 8.4 months but did not reach statistical significance.(HR 0.82, p = 0.03) Impressively the combination arm had a complete response rate of 9% compared with 1% for sunitinib. This is particularly important as mRCC requiring systemic therapy is generally thought to be incurable and so duration of complete response will be of particular interest.

An exploratory sub-analysis of this trial found that patients who were IMDC favorable risk had a median PFS favoring sunitinib (15.3 vs 25.1 months) with a hazard ratio favoring sunitinib (HR 1.45, p = 0.27) The benefit of the combination arm in OS was independent of PD-L1 expression but more pronounced in patients with PD-L1 > 1% compared with those patients with PD-L1 < 1%. (HRs for death 0.45 and 0.73, respectively). Treatment related adverse events leading to discontinuation was 22% in the combination arm compared with 12% in the sunitinib group. These results lead to the FDA approval of ipilimumab plus nivolumab for the treatment of intermediate and poor risk treatment naive mRCC and subsequently European Medicines Agency (EMA) approval in 2019.

A follow up study showing survival outcomes for Checkmate 214 at 42 months showed that in the IMDC intermediate and high risk group median OS was 47.0 months in the nivolumab and ipilimumab group compared with 26.6 months in the sunitinib group. (HR 0.66, p < 0.0001) For IMDC favorable patients median OS was not reached for either arm however the hazard ratio for death was 1.19 and OS probabilities were similar (70% with nivolumab + ipilimumab compared with 73% with sunitinib) [24]. This raises important questions regarding the preferred treatment of choice for treating IMDC favorable risk mRCC patients first line.

Immunotherapy Plus Tyrosine Kinase Inhibitor Combinations

More recently, the options for management of mRCC have changed once again with the advent of combination ICI + TKI treatment therapies. A randomized phase 3 study of first line axitinib and pembrolizumab (Anti-PD-1 ICI) in 861 mRCC patients showed an impressive median PFS of 15.1 months in the pembrolizumab plus axitinib group versus 11.1 months in the sunitinib group (HR 0.69, P < 0.001). The objective response rate was 59.3% in the pembrolizumab plus axitinib group and 35.7% in the sunitinib group (P < 0.001) The benefit of the combination, particularly improved OS was found irrespective of PD-L1 status [25].

A separate randomized phase 3 study of 886 patients compared the combination of avelumab (anti PD-L1) and axitinib with sunitinib. Among the PD-L1 positive tumors the median PFS was 13.8 months with avelumab plus axitinib, as compared with 7.2 months with sunitinib (HR 0.61, P < 0.001); in the overall population, the median PFS was 13.8 months, as compared with 8.4 months (HR P < 0.001). Among the patients with PD-L1–positive tumors, the objective response rate was 55.2% with avelumab plus axitinib and 25.5% with sunitinib [26]. It is important to note that despite the improved ORR and PFS OS is not currently statistically different between the two treatment arms hence follow up data is required.

CLEAR is an international randomized phase 3 trial which compared the oral TKI lenvatinib plus pembrolizumab or everolimus with sunitinib in treatment naive mRCC. The combination lenvatinib plus pembrolizumab demonstrated an impressive median PFS of 23.9 months vs 9.2 months against sunitinib (HR 0.39, P < 0.001) compared with a median PFS of 14.7 months for the lenvatinib plus everolimus combination. Median OS was significantly longer with lenvatinib plus pembrolizumab than with sunitinib (HR 0.66, P = 0.05) but not with lenvatinib plus everolimus than with sunitinib (HR 1.15, P = 0.30) [27]. With a median PFS of 23.9 months this is currently the highest median PFS demonstrated in the treatment of first line mRCC however long term survival outcome data is still required as median OS was not reached in the treatment arms.

Checkmate 9ER has also recently been published comparing the combination nivolumab plus cabozantinib against sunitinib. This randomized phase 3 trial demonstrated a median PFS of 16.6 months with nivolumab plus cabozantinib vs 8.3 months with sunitinib (HR 0.51, P < 0.01) OS at 12 months was 85.7% with nivolumab plus cabozantinib compared with 75.6% with sunitinib (HR 0.6, P = 0.001) Median OS was not reached in either arms [28].

Discussion

The management of mRCC has changed rapidly in the past ten years with new combination treatments being developed. The combinations of nivolumab plus ipilimumab, pembrolizumab plus axitinib, avelumab plus axitinib, pembrolizumab plus axitinib and nivolumab plus cabozantinib have shown superior PFS compared with sunitinib. All these combinations, with the exception of avelumab plus axitinib, have also shown improved overall survival compared with sunitinib in the trial populations. There is no trial comparison between these combinations, all have shown manageable toxicity and all are subject to further follow-up. Thus, collectively they constitute an important step forwards in the initial management of mRCC.

In practice the question of which treatment is best for a treatment naive mRCC patients currently involves weighing up a range of clinico-pathological factors. There is however increasing interest in the potential use of biomarkers to guide optimal treatment selection. Initially it was hypothesized that the use of PD-L1 expression may determine the subset of patients most likely to benefit from ICIs. The IMmotion 151 trial evaluated the combination of the anti-angiogenic drug bevacizumab plus the anti PD-L1 immune checkpoint inhibitor atezolizumab. Although this combination option is no longer being developed for use in mRCC, it showed improved PFS for both the PD-L1 positive and the intention to treat population [29, 30]. Also, the combination of nivolumab and ipilimumab showed improved survival regardless of PD-L1 expression however the OS benefit was higher for PD-L1–positive patients (HR 0.45) compared with PD-L1–negative patients (HR 0.73). IMDC favorable risk patients are more likely to be PD-L1 negative than intermediate and poor risk mRCC patients [31].

One study of 823 mRCC patients identified molecular subsets associated with differential clinical outcomes to angiogenesis blockade alone or with a checkpoint inhibitor [32]. They found seven molecular subsets with distinct angiogenesis, immune cell-cycle, metabolism and stromal molecular patterns. Somatic mutations in PBRM1 and KDM5C associated with high angiogenesis and AMPK/fatty acid oxidation gene expression, while CDKN2A/B and TP53 alterations associated with increased cell-cycle and anabolic metabolism. These findings could potentially stratify mRCC patients who are more likely to respond to VEGF blockade alone or in combination with anti PD-L1. However, despite the obvious attraction of using biomarkers to predict treatment benefit, these approaches require further analysis and validation before this approach could be recommended in routine practice.

A further important factor in selecting treatment and potentially choosing between regimens is their ability to induce complete response and particularly the likelihood of achieving durable complete response. Complete response rates for nivolumab plus ipilimumab, pembrolizumab plus axitinib, lenvatinib plus pembrolizumab and nivolumab plus cabozantinib were 9.0%, 5.8% 16.1% and 8.0% respectively [23, 25, 27, 28]. Extended survival data will determine how long these complete responses last and is of particular interest given this tantalizing possibility is the closest current surrogate for cure from metastatic RCC.

It is important to bear in mind that the majority of the previously mentioned clinical trials were conducted in patients with the most common histological subtype of clear cell mRCC, some of whom had sarcomatoid features. Other sub-types including papillary types 1 and 2, chromophobe, translocation and medullary cancers are sometimes collectively termed 'non-clear cell RCC' despite their clinico-pathological heterogeneity. Clinical trials are more limited in each of these less common sub-types although trials have shown some activity of both molecularly targeted tyrosine kinase inhibitors and ICIs. Given the relative paucity of robust evidence licensed treatment profiles may vary in these sub-types.

By using an immune checkpoint inhibitor and an anti-VEGFR directed therapy there is a higher chance of achieving early disease control as demonstrated by progression free survival and response rates. By targeting renal cancer with different mechanisms of action patients with rapidly progressing symptomatic disease may benefit from this rapid response to treatment as demonstrated by the high PFS and response rates reported in recently published clinical trials [25, 27, 28]. However slowly progressing or IMDC favorable risk mRCC patients may not need such rapid control. Long term follow-up survival data will be key in assessing this group of patients and other considerations such as toxicities of treatment may be important in choosing therapy.

Conclusion

Combination treatments, whether two ICIs or an ICI plus TKI, now constitute a new standard of care for first -line treatment of mRCC in most settings due to their superior response rates, PFS and initial survival data. TKI and ICI monotherapy are likely still to play a role in the management of some mRCC patients particularly in those who are considered not fit enough to perhaps tolerate the side effects of combination therapy. Since it is unlikely that we will see head to head clinical trials comparing these new therapies, extended survival data and improved biomarker research will be key to determine the subset of patients most likely to benefit from either ICIs, oral VEGF treatments or both in combination.

As the use of combination treatments increases clinicians will need to select which subsequent therapies to use. At present in most cases that will be an alternate TKI. Clinicians will also need to become more familiar with managing the increased side effects of combination therapies, as ICI and oral VEGF toxicities differ. As more front-line combination therapies are developed for mRCC patients we hope for improving survival outcomes whilst also minimizing toxicities of treatments as further research continues for a potential cure.

Key Points

1. Renal Cell Carcinoma (RCC) is one of the top ten common cancers accounting for 4% of new cancer presentations.
2. The predominant histology in RCC is clear cell carcinoma (some of which have sarcomatoid features). Other types include papillary types 1 and 2, chromophobe, translocation and medullary cancers.
3. The current treatment options for metastatic renal cell carcinoma are oral VEGF-directed treatments and immune checkpoint inhibitors(ICIs).
4. Prognostic scores for metastatic renal cell carcinoma include Memorial Sloan Kettering Cancer Center (MSKCC) criteria and International Metastatic RCC Database Consortium (IMDC).
5. VEGF receptor TKI monotherapy e.g. sunitinib has been the standard of care for initial treatment of metastatic RCC until recently.

6. There have been several new published studies showing promising outcomes for combination oral-VEGF directed treatments and ICIs.
7. Combination treatments are now standard of care for treatment naive metastatic RCC.
8. There is a need to identify biomarkers to assess metastatic RCC patients most likely to respond to these treatments.
9. As combination treatments increase in prevalence clinicians will need to become more comfortable with managing treatment related toxicities.

References

1. Ferlay J, Steliarova-Foucher E, Lortet-Tieulent J, Rosso S, Coebergh JWW, Comber H, et al. Cancer incidence and mortality patterns in Europe: estimates for 40 countries in 2012. Eur J cancer (Oxford, Engl). 2013 Apr;49(6):1374–403.
2. Dabestani S, Thorstenson A, Lindblad P, Harmenberg U, Ljungberg B, Lundstam S. Renal cell carcinoma recurrences and metastases in primary non-metastatic patients: a population-based study. World J Urol. 2016 Aug;34(8):1081–6.
3. Shuch B, Amin A, Armstrong AJ, Eble JN, Ficarra V, Lopez-Beltran A, et al. Understanding pathologic variants of renal cell carcinoma: distilling therapeutic opportunities from biologic complexity. Eur Urol. 2015 Jan;67(1):85–97.
4. Siegel RL, Miller KD, Jemal A. Cancer statistics, 2017. CA Cancer J Clin. 2017 Jan;67(1):7–30.
5. Howlader N, Noone AM, Krapcho M, Miller D, Brest A, Yu M, Ruhl J, Tatalovich Z, Mariotto A, Lewis DR, Chen HS, KA FEJC, editors. SEER Cancer Statistics Review (CSR) 1975–2017. Bethesda, MD: National Cancer Institute; 2017.
6. Mekhail TM, Abou-Jawde RM, Boumerhi G, Malhi S, Wood L, Elson P, et al. Validation and extension of the memorial Sloan-Kettering prognostic factors model for survival in patients with previously untreated metastatic renal cell carcinoma. J Clin Oncol Off J Am Soc Clin Oncol. 2005 Feb;23(4):832–41.
7. Heng DYC, Xie W, Regan MM, Harshman LC, Bjarnason GA, Vaishampayan UN, et al. External validation and comparison with other models of the international metastatic renal-cell carcinoma database consortium prognostic model: a population-based study. Lancet Oncol. 2013 Feb;14(2):141–8.
8. Noe A, de Bruijn RE, Blank C, Horenblas S, Haanen J, Bex A. Comparison of pre-treatment MSKCC and IMDC prognostic risk models in patients with synchronous metastatic renal cell carcinoma treated in the era of targeted therapy. World J Urol. 2016 Aug;34(8):1067–72.
9. Motzer RJ, Hutson TE, Tomczak P, Michaelson MD, Bukowski RM, Rixe O, et al. Sunitinib versus interferon alfa in metastatic renal-cell carcinoma. N Engl J Med. 2007 Jan;356(2):115–24.
10. Motzer RJ, Hutson TE, Tomczak P, Michaelson MD, Bukowski RM, Oudard S, et al. Overall survival and updated results for sunitinib compared with interferon alfa in patients with metastatic renal cell carcinoma. J Clin Oncol Off J Am Soc Clin Oncol. 2009 Aug;27(22):3584–90.
11. Sternberg CN, Davis ID, Mardiak J, Szczylik C, Lee E, Wagstaff J, et al. Pazopanib in locally advanced or metastatic renal cell carcinoma: results of a randomized phase III trial. J Clin Oncol. 2010 Feb;28(6):1061–8.
12. Motzer RJ, Hutson TE, Cella D, Reeves J, Hawkins R, Guo J, et al. Pazopanib versus sunitinib in metastatic renal-cell carcinoma. N Engl J Med. 2013 Aug;369(8):722–31.
13. Escudier B, Porta C, Bono P, Powles T, Eisen T, Sternberg CN, et al. Randomized, controlled, double-blind, cross-over trial assessing treatment preference for pazopanib versus sunitinib in patients with metastatic renal cell carcinoma: PISCES study. J Clin Oncol Off J Am Soc Clin Oncol. 2014 May;32(14):1412–8.

14. Motzer RJ, Nosov D, Eisen T, Bondarenko I, Lesovoy V, Lipatov O, et al. Tivozanib versus sorafenib as initial targeted therapy for patients with metastatic renal cell carcinoma: results from a phase III trial. J Clin Oncol Off J Am Soc Clin Oncol. 2013 Oct;31(30):3791–9.
15. Choueiri TK, Halabi S, Sanford BL, Hahn O, Michaelson MD, Walsh MK, et al. Cabozantinib versus Sunitinib as initial targeted therapy for patients with metastatic renal cell carcinoma of poor or intermediate risk: the Alliance A031203 CABOSUN trial. J Clin Oncol Off J Am Soc Clin Oncol. 2017 Feb;35(6):591–7.
16. Escudier B, Powles T, Motzer RJ, Olencki T, Arén Frontera O, Oudard S, et al. Cabozantinib, a new standard of care for patients with advanced renal cell carcinoma and bone metastases? Subgroup analysis of the METEOR trial. J Clin Oncol Off J Am Soc Clin Oncol. 2018 Mar;36(8):765–72.
17. Rini BI, Escudier B, Tomczak P, Kaprin A, Szczylik C, Hutson TE, et al. Comparative effectiveness of axitinib versus sorafenib in advanced renal cell carcinoma (AXIS): a randomised phase 3 trial. Lancet (London, England). 2011 Dec;378(9807):1931–9.
18. Choueiri TK, Escudier B, Powles T, Tannir NM, Mainwaring PN, Rini BI, et al. Cabozantinib versus everolimus in advanced renal cell carcinoma (METEOR): final results from a randomised, open-label, phase 3 trial. Lancet Oncol. 2016 Jul;17(7):917–27.
19. Motzer RJ, Escudier B, Powles T, Scheffold C, Choueiri TK. Long-term follow-up of overall survival for cabozantinib versus everolimus in advanced renal cell carcinoma. Br J Cancer. 2018 May;118(9):1176–8.
20. Motzer RJ, Hutson TE, Glen H, Michaelson MD, Molina A, Eisen T, et al. Lenvatinib, everolimus, and the combination in patients with metastatic renal cell carcinoma: a randomised, phase 2, open-label, multicentre trial. Lancet Oncol. 2015 Nov;16(15):1473–82.
21. Motzer RJ, Escudier B, Oudard S, Hutson TE, Porta C, Bracarda S, et al. Phase 3 trial of everolimus for metastatic renal cell carcinoma: final results and analysis of prognostic factors. Cancer. 2010 Sep;116(18):4256–65.
22. Cella D, Grünwald V, Nathan P, Doan J, Dastani H, Taylor F, et al. Quality of life in patients with advanced renal cell carcinoma given nivolumab versus everolimus in CheckMate 025: a randomised, open-label, phase 3 trial. Lancet Oncol. 2016 Jul;17(7):994–1003.
23. Motzer RJ, Tannir NM, McDermott DF, Aren Frontera O, Melichar B, Choueiri TK, et al. Nivolumab plus Ipilimumab versus Sunitinib in advanced renal-cell carcinoma. N Engl J Med. 2018 Apr;378(14):1277–90.
24. Motzer RJ, Escudier B, McDermott DF, Arén Frontera O, Melichar B, Powles T, et al. Survival outcomes and independent response assessment with nivolumab plus ipilimumab versus sunitinib in patients with advanced renal cell carcinoma: 42-month follow-up of a randomized phase 3 clinical trial. J Immunother Cancer. 2020 Jul;8(2):e000891.
25. Rini BI, Plimack ER, Stus V, Gafanov R, Hawkins R, Nosov D, et al. Pembrolizumab plus Axitinib versus Sunitinib for advanced renal-cell carcinoma. N Engl J Med. 2019 Mar;380(12):1116–27.
26. Motzer RJ, Penkov K, Haanen J, Rini B, Albiges L, Campbell MT, et al. Avelumab plus Axitinib versus Sunitinib for advanced renal-cell carcinoma. N Engl J Med. 2019 Mar;380(12):1103–15.
27. Motzer R, Alekseev B, Rha S-Y, Porta C, Eto M, Powles T, et al. Lenvatinib plus Pembrolizumab or Everolimus for advanced renal cell carcinoma. N Engl J Med. 2021 Feb;384(14):1289–300.
28. Choueiri TK, Powles T, Burotto M, Escudier B, Bourlon MT, Zurawski B, et al. Nivolumab plus Cabozantinib versus Sunitinib for advanced renal-cell carcinoma. N Engl J Med. 2021 Mar;384(9):829–41.
29. McDermott DF, Huseni MA, Atkins MB, Motzer RJ, Rini BI, Escudier B, et al. Publisher correction: clinical activity and molecular correlates of response to atezolizumab alone or in combination with bevacizumab versus sunitinib in renal cell carcinoma. Nat Med. 2018;24(6):749–57. https://doi.org/10.1038/s41591-018-0053-3.
30. Rini BI, Powles T, Atkins MB, Escudier B, McDermott DF, Suarez C, et al. Atezolizumab plus bevacizumab versus sunitinib in patients with previously untreated metastatic renal cell carcinoma (IMmotion151): a multicentre, open-label, phase 3, randomised controlled trial. Lancet (London, England). 2019 Jun;393(10189):2404–15.

31. Lalani A-KA, McGregor BA, Albiges L, Choueiri TK, Motzer R, Powles T, et al. Systemic treatment of metastatic clear cell renal cell carcinoma in 2018: current paradigms, use of immunotherapy, and future directions. Eur Urol. 2019 Jan;75(1):100–10.
32. Motzer RJ, Banchereau R, Hamidi H, Powles T, McDermott D, Atkins MB, et al. Molecular subsets in renal cancer determine outcome to checkpoint and angiogenesis blockade. Cancer Cell. 2020 Dec;38(6):803–817.e4.

Metastatic Renal Cancer: Radiotherapy

V. Khoo and D. Lim-Joon

Introduction

Radiotherapy is widely used for metastatic renal cell cancer (mRCC) in many different clinical scenarios. This is despite the traditional assumption that mRCC is a relatively radioresistant disease. However, the radiosensitivity spectrum of mRCC is wide and depending on the biological dose that can be delivered, secondary to the tissue constraints of the adjacent surrounding normal organs, radiotherapy can provide good palliation and local control [1].

Conventional low dose hypofractionated radiotherapy is most often used for simple palliation of symptoms such as pain or bleeding. Higher doses of radiotherapy have also been used to provide local control for metastatic lesions where growth constraint is needed to prevent local complications such as obstruction or organ invasion [2]. More recently, sophisticated radiation methods such as stereotactic ablative radiotherapy (SABR), also known as stereotactic body radiation therapy (SBRT), have been used to provide higher biological doses for improved local control and longer disease control with the potential for disease eradiation at the local site. There is a developing rationale for SABR as emerging data suggests that the

V. Khoo (✉)
Oncology Urology Unit, Royal Marsden Hospital & Institute of Cancer Research, London, UK

St. George's Hospital, London, UK

Monash University, Clayton, VIC, Australia

University of Melbourne, Parkville, VIC, Australia
e-mail: VincentPA.Khoo@rmh.nhs.uk; Vincent.Khoo@rmh.nhs.uk

D. Lim-Joon
Olivia Newton-John Cancer Wellness & Research Centre, Melbourne, Australia
e-mail: daryl.limjoon@austin.org.au

C. Anderson, M. Afshar (eds.), *Renal Cancer*,
https://doi.org/10.1007/978-3-030-84756-2_18

apparent radioresistance of RCC can be overcome by the biological effect of using the very high dose per fraction schema of SABR. These ultra-high fractional doses can activate vascular apoptotic pathways that is not usually affected by conventional dose-fractionation Schemes [3]. These data outline the translocation of ASMase and formation of the pro-apoptotic ceramide pathway for endothelial apoptosis. With RCC being vascular tumours, this would be one mechanism for a greater tumouricidal kill. Furthermore cell survival curves studies with human RCC lines have demonstrated a lower α/β ratio that also favours the use of larger dose per fraction or hypofractionation [4, 5]. Radiotherapy can be used alone or in combination with other local and systemic therapies such as surgery and immunotherapy respectively. The rationale and merit of using different methods of radiotherapy for these different clinical situations will be discussed.

Conventional Palliative Radiotherapy

Bone metastasis are common in mRCC with approximately one-third of cases being present at diagnosis and a subsequent one-third presenting during the course of the disease [6]. Radiotherapy is an effective treatment in providing pain relief for symptomatic lesions particularly in metastatic bony disease where it can also prevent bone fractures and support bone remineralization [7]. Conventional palliative radiotherapy regimes usually use short duration low dose hypofractionation regimes such as a single fraction of 8 Gy, 16 Gy in 2 fractions, 20 Gy in 5 daily fractions or 30Gy in 10 daily fractions. A meta-analysis of palliative radiotherapy trials for bone metastases comparing single fraction versus multiple fractions documented that both single and multiple fraction radiotherapy regimes provided equivalent pain relief [8]. These findings have resulted in many radiotherapy centres embracing the 8 Gy single fraction regime for bone palliation given that it would be both pragmatic in terms of resource allocation and convenient for the patient. However the re-treatment rates were 2.6 fold greater in those patients receiving single fractions [8]. Thus it is reasonable to consider using multiple fraction regimes in mRCC where better disease control is needed as survival in mRCC has been substantially lengthen with more effective modern systemic therapy using targeted agents and immunotherapy [9]. Another option is the use of SABR/SBRT which will be discussed later in this chapter.

Conventional palliative radiotherapy has been reported to provide palliation relief in 60–73% of patients suffering from symptomatic bony metastasis [8, 10–12] with complete symptomatic responses in 13–24% of cases [8, 13]. Most of these reports are not histology specific and usually include a heterogenous mix of solid tumours. There are few prospective reports of studies evaluating bony metastasis solely from mRCC using modern measures of pain assessment and benefit such as quality of life. A prospective non-randomized study of 31 mRCC patients reported a decrease in site-specific pain in 83% and complete response in 13% of cases [13]. These assessments were based on patient questionnaires. The median duration of response was

3 months. Quality of life (QOL) measures were improved in 33% but prolonged improvements in QOL was limited by the development of other metastasis and systemic disease progression. Another 90 patient study of both metastatic melanoma and mRCC cases reported a response rate of 65% that lasted for nearly 60% of their patients remaining lifetime [14]. For widespread bony metastatic disease, the use of bisphosphonate therapy with zoledronic acid or Denosumab has been shown to significantly reduce skeletal related events (SREs) in patients and increase time to first SRE [15, 16]. This can also be considered in combination with radiotherapy.

Conventional palliative radiotherapy is also used commonly to prevent or limit neurological impairment such as in spinal cord compression and nerve root or plexus invasion. In the management of spinal cord compression, a prospective randomised trial reported that the combination of initial direct decompressive surgical resection followed by post-operative radiotherapy improved survival and maintenance of ambulation compared with radiotherapy alone [17]. There were significantly more patients in the surgery and radiotherapy treatment arm able to walk after treatment compared to the radiotherapy arm (84% vs 57% respectively). The radiation dose used in this randomised trial was 30 Gy in 10 fractions. An ambulatory status at diagnosis and limited metastatic disease are favourable prognostic factors in those patients able to undergo surgery. This randomised trial enrolled a range of different solid cancers where lung and prostate cancer represented a large majority of the cases. Nevertheless, this same principle will apply to mRCC patients suffering from malignant spinal cord compression.

Stereotactic Radiotherapy

Stereotactic radiotherapy aims to deliver a series of highly conformally shaped beams localised to the tumour lesion with image guidance for high precision targeting [18]. The use of multiple overlapping beams or arcs often with intensity modulation enables the target volume to receive a high concentration of dose with a very sharp dose fall-off just outside the target volume thus limiting irradiation of the neighbouring normal tissues and organs (see Fig. 1). In this manner stereotactic radiotherapy regimes can deliver a much higher biological effective dose (BED) compared to the BED from conventional curative fractionation or conventional palliative regimes [19]. The BED for tumour (using its biological α/β of 10Gy) in conventional palliative regimes is usually <40 compared to conventional curative regimes with BED between 75 and 96 whilst stereotactic BEDs are often >100 [20].

Stereotactic regimes use a very high dose per fraction with one to a small number of fractions. Typical stereotactic dose regimes vary between 15 and 24Gy in a single fraction to 48–60Gy in 3–5 fractions depending on the anatomical site and its dose constraints [21]. Stereotactic radiotherapy used for intra-cranial lesions are usually called stereotactic radiosurgery (SRS) and those used extra-cranially are called SABR or SBRT. These latter two terms, SABR or SBRT are often used interchangeably.

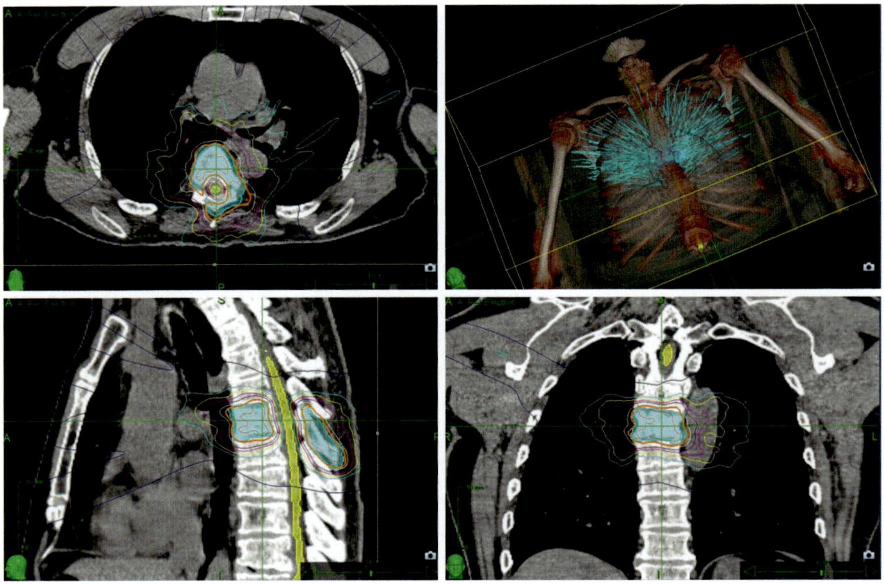

Fig. 1 This figure shows a typically stereotactic radiotherapy treatment of a thoracic vertebra from metastatic renal cell cancer. The upper left image shows the transverse view through the middle of the target volume highlighted in blue, the lower left shows the sagittal section and the lower right show the coronal section. The different coloured lines surrounding the target volume are the radiotherapy isodose lines. In the upper right image, the thorax, rib cage and spine of the patient are rendered to demonstrate the different beam orientations entering and exiting the thorax. Each blue line represents a beam direction

Radiotherapy plays in important role in the management of brain metastasis. Up to 10% of RCC patients will develop brain metastasis during the course of their illness [22] with multiple metastases in up to half of these cases [23]. The prognosis of these patients is dependent on many factors such as the number of brain metastasis (single versus multiple), whether they are surgically resectable or not, the presence of other metastasis, the rate of disease progression and the patient's performance status [1]. The choice of treatment(s) will depend on the prognostic factors previously mentioned. Untreated, these patients have a poor prognosis with a median survival time of approximately 1 month. The use of corticosteroids will only provide temporary relief of cerebral symptoms. Radiotherapy can improve the quality of life, local control and median survival time for these patients. It can also be used in combination with surgery.

Whole brain radiotherapy (WBRT) is usually given for palliation. It is effective in reducing the pressure effects of brain metastasis using the conventional palliative regimes outlined previously. WBRT is usually considered when there are several lesions scattered throughout both cerebral hemispheres, when the performance status is poor or when life expectancy is limited. SRS is usually considered for patients with better prognostic features and when the number of brain metastases are <4. Most trials in brain metastasis include only a small proportion of RCC cases. With the use of SRS delivering larger doses per fraction, the mRCC response outcomes are not thought to differ from other solid tumours.

Randomised trials for patients suffering from 1 to 3 brain metastases have reported that the addition of SRS or surgery to WBRT improves survival, enhances functional independence and limits long term steroid usage [24–26]. The addition of WBRT to either SRS or surgery has also been assessment for 1–4 brain metastases and showed improved intracranial control and reduced neurological deaths without influencing survival [27–30]. In general, the local control rates for treated lesions using SRS are improved compared to WBRT but there is a higher intra-cerebral recurrence rate elsewhere in the brain. Whilst the development of other intra-cerebral recurrence can impair neurocognitive function [28], it has also been recognized that WBRT is associated with early impairment of neurocognitive function long term [29, 31]. This aspect may be particularly pertinent for patients with mRCC given that longer survival from current modern effective systemic therapies. It would be reasonable to avoid WBRT in those patients expected to have a longer duration of disease control and life expectancy.

SABR/SBRT has also been reported to provide excellent local control with minimal morbidity in the treatment of extracranial lesions compared to conventional high dose fractionation regimes. A recent updated systemic review and meta-analysis evaluated the use of SABR/SBRT for patients with mRCC [32]. This meta-analysis found 28 studies with up to 1602 mutually exclusive patients in whom 3892 (1159 extracranial and 2733 intracranial) lesions were treated. This study reported that the 1-year local control rate was 89.1% for extracranial disease and 90.1% for intracranial disease with 1-year survival rates of 86.8% and 49.7% respectively. The incidence of any grade 3–4 toxicity for extracranial and intracranial treatments was 0.7% and 1.1% respectively. The authors surmised that SABR or SBRT can be considered to be safe and efficacious treatment in mRCC.

Key Points

- Radiotherapy can be delivered using different methods depending on the clinical situation and aim of the treatment.
- Conventional low dose hypofractionated radiotherapy is most often used for simple palliation of symptoms such as pain or bleeding. Higher doses of radiotherapy have also been used to provide local control for metastatic lesions where growth constraint is needed to prevent local complications such as obstruction or organ invasion
- Whilst conventional palliative radiotherapy is widely used, the rationale for SABR or SBRT is gaining recognition and acceptance.
- SABR/SBRT methods have demonstrated excellent local control rates with minimal toxicity and needs prospective evaluation in randomized trials.

- For the individual patient suffering from mRCC, the onus is on the treating physician to optimize their management and this would be best managed within a multi-disciplinary team setting with all members of the renal team where the treatment plan for the individual patient can be fully discussed and personalized to their clinical situation and specific needs.

References

1. Khoo V, Pyle L. Radiotherapy and supportive care. In: Eisen T, Christmas T, editors. Clinical progress in renal cancer. Oxford: Informa UK Ltd; 2007. p. 191–201.
2. Khoo V. Renal cancers: introduction. In: Patel U, editor. Carcinoma of the kidney. Contemporary issues in cancer imaging. Cambridge: Cambridge University Press; 2008. p. 1–16.
3. De Meerleer G, Khoo V, Escudier B, Joniau S, Bossi A, Ost P, et al. Radiotherapy for renal-cell carcinoma. Lancet Oncol. 2014;15(4):e170–7.
4. Ning S, Trisler K, Wessels BW, Knox SJ. Radiobiologic studies of radioimmunotherapy and external beam radiotherapy in vitro and in vivo in human renal cell carcinoma xenografts. Cancer. 1997;80(12 Suppl):2519–28.
5. Wilson D, Hiller L, Gray L, Grainger M, Stirling A, James N. The effect of biological effective dose on time to symptom progression in metastatic renal cell carcinoma. Clin Oncol (R Coll Radiol). 2003;15(7):400–7.
6. Wood SL, Brown JE. Skeletal metastasis in renal cell carcinoma: current and future management options. Cancer Treat Rev. 2012;38(4):284–91.
7. McDonald R, Ding K, Brundage M, Meyer RM, Nabid A, Chabot P, et al. Effect of radiotherapy on painful bone metastases: a secondary analysis of the NCIC clinical trials group symptom control trial SC.23. JAMA. Oncologia. 2017;3(7):953–9.
8. Chow E, Zeng L, Salvo N, Dennis K, Tsao M, Lutz S. Update on the systematic review of palliative radiotherapy trials for bone metastases. Clin Oncol (R Coll Radiol). 2012;24(2):112–24.
9. Escudier B, Porta C, Schmidinger M, Rioux-Leclercq N, Bex A, Khoo V, et al. Renal cell carcinoma: ESMO clinical practice guidelines for diagnosis, treatment and follow-up. Ann Oncol. 2019;30(5):706–20.
10. Ganju RG, TenNapel M, Mahan N, Zahra A, Shen X. The efficacy of conventionally fractionated radiation in the Management of Osseous Metastases from metastatic renal cell carcinoma. J Oncol. 2018;2018:6384253.
11. Sze WM, Shelley M, Held I, Mason M. Palliation of metastatic bone pain: single fraction versus multifraction radiotherapy - a systematic review of the randomised trials. Cochrane Database Syst Rev. 2004;2002(2):CD004721.
12. Wu JS, Wong R, Johnston M, Bezjak A, Whelan T. Cancer Care Ontario practice guidelines initiative supportive care G. Meta-analysis of dose-fractionation radiotherapy trials for the palliation of painful bone metastases. Int J Radiat Oncol Biol Phys. 2003;55(3):594–605.
13. Lee J, Hodgson D, Chow E, Bezjak A, Catton P, Tsuji D, et al. A phase II trial of palliative radiotherapy for metastatic renal cell carcinoma. Cancer. 2005;104(9):1894–900.
14. Huguenin PU, Kieser S, Glanzmann C, Capaul R, Lutolf UM. Radiotherapy for metastatic carcinomas of the kidney or melanomas: an analysis using palliative end points. Int J Radiat Oncol Biol Phys. 1998;41(2):401–5.
15. Henry DH, Costa L, Goldwasser F, Hirsh V, Hungria V, Prausova J, et al. Randomized, double-blind study of denosumab versus zoledronic acid in the treatment of bone metastases in patients with advanced cancer (excluding breast and prostate cancer) or multiple myeloma. J Clin Oncol. 2011;29(9):1125–32.

16. Rosen LS, Gordon D, Tchekmedyian NS, Yanagihara R, Hirsh V, Krzakowski M, et al. Long-term efficacy and safety of zoledronic acid in the treatment of skeletal metastases in patients with nonsmall cell lung carcinoma and other solid tumors: a randomized, phase III, double-blind, placebo-controlled trial. Cancer. 2004;100(12):2613–21.
17. Patchell RA, Tibbs PA, Regine WF, Payne R, Saris S, Kryscio RJ, et al. Direct decompressive surgical resection in the treatment of spinal cord compression caused by metastatic cancer: a randomised trial. Lancet. 2005;366(9486):643–8.
18. Tree AC, Khoo VS, Eeles RA, Ahmed M, Dearnaley DP, Hawkins MA, et al. Stereotactic body radiotherapy for oligometastases. Lancet Oncol. 2013;14(1):e28–37.
19. Aitken K, Tree A, Thomas K, Nutting C, Hawkins M, Tait D, et al. Initial UK experience of stereotactic body radiotherapy for extracranial Oligometastases: can we change the therapeutic paradigm? Clin Oncol (R Coll Radiol). 2015;27(7):411–9.
20. DiBiase SJ, Valicenti RK, Schultz D, Xie Y, Gomella LG, Corn BW. Palliative irradiation for focally symptomatic metastatic renal cell carcinoma: support for dose escalation based on a biological model. J Urol. 1997;158(3 Pt 1):746–9.
21. Hanna GG, Murray L, Patel R, Jain S, Aitken KL, Franks KN, et al. UK consensus on Normal tissue dose constraints for stereotactic radiotherapy. Clin Oncol (R Coll Radiol). 2018;30(1):5–14.
22. Siegel RL, Miller KD, Jemal A. Cancer statistics, 2020. CA Cancer J Clin. 2020;70(1):7–30.
23. Sheehan JP, Sun MH, Kondziolka D, Flickinger J, Lunsford LD. Radiosurgery in patients with renal cell carcinoma metastasis to the brain: long-term outcomes and prognostic factors influencing survival and local tumor control. J Neurosurg. 2003;98(2):342–9.
24. Andrews DW, Scott CB, Sperduto PW, Flanders AE, Gaspar LE, Schell MC, et al. Whole brain radiation therapy with or without stereotactic radiosurgery boost for patients with one to three brain metastases: phase III results of the RTOG 9508 randomised trial. Lancet. 2004;363(9422):1665–72.
25. Mintz AH, Kestle J, Rathbone MP, Gaspar L, Hugenholtz H, Fisher B, et al. A randomized trial to assess the efficacy of surgery in addition to radiotherapy in patients with a single cerebral metastasis. Cancer. 1996;78(7):1470–6.
26. Patchell RA, Tibbs PA, Walsh JW, Dempsey RJ, Maruyama Y, Kryscio RJ, et al. A randomized trial of surgery in the treatment of single metastases to the brain. N Engl J Med. 1990;322(8):494–500.
27. Aoyama H, Shirato H, Tago M, Nakagawa K, Toyoda T, Hatano K, et al. Stereotactic radiosurgery plus whole-brain radiation therapy vs stereotactic radiosurgery alone for treatment of brain metastases: a randomized controlled trial. JAMA. 2006;295(21):2483–91.
28. Aoyama H, Tago M, Kato N, Toyoda T, Kenjyo M, Hirota S, et al. Neurocognitive function of patients with brain metastasis who received either whole brain radiotherapy plus stereotactic radiosurgery or radiosurgery alone. Int J Radiat Oncol Biol Phys. 2007;68(5):1388–95.
29. Chang EL, Wefel JS, Hess KR, Allen PK, Lang FF, Kornguth DG, et al. Neurocognition in patients with brain metastases treated with radiosurgery or radiosurgery plus whole-brain irradiation: a randomised controlled trial. Lancet Oncol. 2009;10(11):1037–44.
30. Kocher M, Soffietti R, Abacioglu U, Villa S, Fauchon F, Baumert BG, et al. Adjuvant whole-brain radiotherapy versus observation after radiosurgery or surgical resection of one to three cerebral metastases: results of the EORTC 22952-26001 study. J Clin Oncol. 2011;29(2):134–41.
31. Brown PD, Jaeckle K, Ballman KV, Farace E, Cerhan JH, Anderson SK, et al. Effect of radiosurgery alone vs radiosurgery with whole brain radiation therapy on cognitive function in patients with 1 to 3 brain metastases: a randomized clinical trial. JAMA. 2016;316(4):401–9.
32. Zaorsky NG, Lehrer EJ, Kothari G, Louie AV, Siva S. Stereotactic ablative radiation therapy for oligometastatic renal cell carcinoma (SABR ORCA): a meta-analysis of 28 studies. Eur Urol Oncol. 2019;2(5):515–23.

Metastatic Tumours: Cytoreductive Nephrectomy

P. Brousil, David Manson-Bahr, and David Nicol

Introduction

Cytoreductive nephrectomy(CRN) is a term applied to the surgical removal of a primary renal cell carcinoma in a patient with established metastatic disease with the intention of potentially prolonging patient survival. It needs to be distinguished from palliative nephrectomy which may also be performed in the metastatic setting where the fundamental purpose is to alleviate symptoms—specifically pain and bleeding.

History

CRN Alone

CRN emerged as a concept based on observational reports of regression of metastatic disease after nephrectomy. These date back as early as 1917 [1] when a patients metastatic pulmonary disease spontaneously resolved following nephrectomy. Subsequent reports of nephrectomy with metastasectomy in the 1930s [2] provided further impetus to support the concept that metastatic disease could be

P. Brousil (✉)
Department of Urology, Epsom and St Helier University Hospitals NHS Trust, London, UK
e-mail: philip.brousil@nhs.net

D. Manson-Bahr
Department of Urology, Norfolk and Norwich University Hospitals, Norwich, UK
e-mail: David.Manson-Bahr@nnuh.nhs.uk

D. Nicol
Department of Urology, Royal Marsden Hospital & Institute of Cancer Research, London, UK
e-mail: David.nicol@rmh.nhs.uk

C. Anderson, M. Afshar (eds.), *Renal Cancer*,
https://doi.org/10.1007/978-3-030-84756-2_19

managed with surgery with a potential expectation of improving survival [3]. Many subsequent case reports and small institutional series appeared which supported the concept of both CRN and metastasectomy improving survival in patients with metastatic disease. The actual regression of metastatic disease following CRN was a feature in many reports. In some cases metastatic disease was confirmed by biopsy although many relied on the limited radiological investigations available and subjective interpretation of these. Nevertheless enthusiasm was sustained for CRN as an option for patients with metastatic disease in the absence of any other treatment for metastatic RCC [4–6]. Interestingly, 'immunological' factors were hypothesized as a potential mechanism to account for the systemic response to CRN for metastatic disease. Renal cell cancer is a heavily immunological cancer, and studies demonstrate inhibition or down-regulation of immune competence within the primary tumour and systemically, potentially contributing to progression of metastatic disease [7, 8]. Kawashima and colleagues demonstrated that the higher grade the tumour, the greater the consequent immune dysfunction [9]. Thus the effect of cytoreductive nephrectomy may be to remove the immunological 'sump' of the primary tumour, and well as attenuating the burden of proangiogenic factors the primary tumour secretes which may also potentiate the progression of disease [10]. The potential advantage of CRN was however limited to perhaps a subset of patients. It was not universally adopted given the potential morbidity and mortality of surgery in patients with limited life expectancy. A UK audit of national practice of CN in 2012 demonstrated a complication rate of 23% and 30 day mortality rate of 2% [11].

Cytoreductive Nephrectomy in Combination with Systemic Therapy

Systemic treatment of metastatic RCC emerged during the 1960s with utilisation of both chemotherapy and hormonal manipulation. Results were disappointing with both of these modalities [12, 13]. Consequently this sustained some level of support for CRN despite the fact that the metastatic regression described in case reports reflected anecdotal cases.

During the 1980s cytokine therapy, inducing upregulation of immunological response, emerged as a new and novel systemic therapy applicable to kidney cancer and other malignancies such as melanoma that were resistant to cytotoxic drugs. Both interferon-α and interleukin-2 were introduced with some success for patients with metastatic RCC [14, 15]. The toxicity of these agents, and particularly interleukin-2, was a concern which limited their uptake in many countries. CRN thus remained as an intervention of interest both alone and in combination with these cytokine therapies. The combination was supported by observations suggesting that responses at metastatic sites were more profound than with the primary tumour. CRN also appeared most applicable when the metastatic disease was limited and the primary tumour represented the majority of overall disease burden.

Subsequently two key identical randomised control trials, in North America (SWOG) [16] and Europe (EORTC) [17], published in 2001 established an evidence base for CRN in combination with systemic therapy (IFN). Participants in both studies had measureable metastatic disease, resectable primary tumours and Eastern Co-operative Oncology Group (ECOG) Performance Status 0 or 1. The basis for including performance status in this study was based on concerns that many patients with poorer performance status would not recovery sufficiently to receive systemic treatment following surgery [18].

These trials collectively demonstrated a survival advantage (13.6 months vs. 7.8 months) when CRN was combined with IFNα compared to IFNα alone. In the SWOG trial, when the patients were stratified by performance status, survival advantage was more dramatic in the ECOG 0 vs. the ECOG 1 group (5.7 vs. 2.1 months). This was not seen in the EORTC trial however.

These trials established initial CRN as the standard of care for appropriate patients with good performance status during the 'Interferon era'. They also influenced trial design and clinical practice for patients presenting with metastatic disease as newer and more effective therapeutic agents were introduced.

Tyrosine Kinase Inhibitor (TKI's) ERA

Shortly after the publication of the CRN trials, a new class of drugs—tyrosine kinase inhibitors (TKI's) emerged. These drugs targeted mediators of angiogenesis including vascular endothelial growth factor (VEGF)—many of which are regulated by the VHL gene which is mutated in clear cell renal cell carcinoma. Clinical trials showed these resulted in improved progression free survival, safety and quality of life compared to cytokine therapy [19]. Cytoreductive nephrectomy continued but TKI's replaced interferon as standard systemic therapy. Initial trials evaluating TKI's had included CRN as a preliminary to systemic therapy as this was viewed as standard practice. This retained CRN within the 'TKI era' management paradigm: In a large retrospective collaborative series, Choueiri and colleagues [20] demonstrated a 10 month survival advantage for those that had upfront surgery. Interestingly a sub-analysis with stratification by Karnofsky performance status (KPS) showed no appreciable benefit if the KPS was <80. The results were widely reproducible and reinforced with a systematic review published in 2016 [21].

The data was retrospective and soiled by selection basis, even though adjustments were made for prognostic factors. This led to two RCTs to evaluate CRN and its impact on patients presenting with metastatic disease treated with TKI's.

The CARMENA Trial

This trial comprised 450 patients enrolled over an 8 year period with a median follow-up of 51 months [22]. It compared the overall survival for patients receiving initial CRN followed by sunitinib (a TKI) to patients receiving sunitinib alone. Eligibility criteria was ECOG performance status 0 and 1, and a metastatic disease burden requiring systemic therapy. It was a non-inferiority study, and reported on an intention-to-treat basis.

The results were surprising: overall survival in the sunitinib only arm was 18 months compared to 13.9 months in the CRN arm, which reached statistical significance. This contrasted to the more favourable outcomes for initial CRN in systematic reviews of large volume retrospective series. A potential flaw of this study was the inclusion of poor risk stratified patients, previously shown not to benefit from CRN with IFN in the earlier RCT's. These patients comprised a significant proportion of the overall number.

Nevertheless the results have challenged the role of CRN in combination with TKI's with the lead author of this trial concluding that "cytoreductive nephrectomy is no longer the standard of care" [23].

This study and its conclusions remains a topic of debate. It has been suggested that several factors have meant that the results can not be generalised to the type of patient that would typically be selected for a CRN [24, 25]

1. Patient selection: a large proportion of these patients (>40%) had poor risk stratification on MSKCC criteria for survival [26]
2. Disease selection: the median number of metastatic sites was 2, with an estimated metastatic proportion of total disease of 40% (based on linear tumour measurements)
3. Completeness of reporting: TNM staging was only reported in 30% of the patients
4. Poor accrual of patients: 450 patients over 8 years amounts to 0.7 patients per centre per year. In the UK in 2012, there were c. 300 cytoreductive nephrectomies; France has a slightly larger population—at the authors own admission, many patients were excluded from the trial as 'too good for CARMENA'
5. Protocol violations: in the surgical arm, 7% did not undergo surgery whilst 18% did not receive sunitinib; whilst in the sunitinib only arm, 17% underwent subsequent nephrectomy, the majority of which were because of excellent systemic treatment response. As a result of this, the analysis of 'per protocol' outcomes in the supplementary data, in contrast to 'intention to treat', showed no difference in median survival

Despite criticism, the trial clearly indicates that for poor risk patients systemic treatment of their metastatic disease is the management priority and CRN is not indicated. The introduction of TKI's as an effective systemic treatment for metastatic RCC may have influenced practice independent of the CARMENA study which has only been recently reported. Poor risk patients may have proceeded to systemic therapy without CRN. This is a potential explanation for the apparent benefit of CRN seen in the large retrospective systematic reviews of outcomes with TKI treatment of metastatic RCC.

SURTIME

The SURTIME trial, another RCT published in 2018 [27] evaluated the timing of CRN in the patient with metastatic disease considered to require systemic therapy at presentation. Patients undergoing initial CRN followed by sunitinib were compared to those receiving sunitinib for 4 months who then underwent CRN if there was no progression of disease. Patients who underwent CRN in this group comprised those with either stable disease or regression on radiological parameters. Unfortunately only 100 patients were recruited compared to the 458 required for the aim of a superiority analysis. Patients with T3 or higher primary tumours, metastatic disease requiring systemic treatment, and no poor risk disease by Culp criteria were enrolled [28].

On analysis of enrolled patients there was no statistical difference in the primary endpoint (progression free status at 28 weeks). The trial did not have the power to demonstrate an overall superiority of survival on an intention-to-treat basis, although this was evident in the deferred nephrectomy group. This benefit was quite profound, with a median survival of 32.4 months compared to 15 months in those undergoing initial CRN. Caution is required in interpreting the results, as this endpoint was not part of the trial design, and that this benefit was not demonstrated in the per protocol analysis. A further point is that none of the patients in this trial had a metastatic disease burden that would be considered appropriate for initial surveillance, and therefore not typical of patients currently selected for cytoreductive nephrectomy.

This trial remains under significant discussion in reviews and other forums. A common conclusion has been that the results, which have limitations as a consequence of its termination, raise the suggestion that a trial of systemic therapy may serve as a 'litmus test' to select the appropriate patient who may benefit from CRN. Similarly the study suggests that patients who experience rapid progression with systemic therapy may avoid the morbidity of CRN as their outcome will remain poor.

Active Surveillance of Metastatic Kidney Cancer

Active surveillance of low volume asymptomatic metastatic disease as recurrence following initial radical nephrectomy has been adopted by many clinicians following the introduction of TKI's [29]. This is based on the observation that whilst metastatic disease can progress rapidly, it can also behave indolently with extended periods of stability or slow progression. Prospective studies have demonstrated no detriment to survival in patients with oligometastatic disease burdens who have TKI therapy until significant disease progression occurs [30, 31]. This is supported by the point that patients undergoing nephrectomy with initial curative intent but subsequently exhibit metastatic recurrence have effectively had a CRN. Clearly these patients have had sub-clinical metastases at diagnosis—with then slow progression before radiological detection. It logically follows that if a patient presents with low volume metastatic disease a CRN may be an appropriate initial intervention when the clinician is comfortable with surveillance and deferred systemic treatment.

With this approach, patients may avoid exposure to the toxicity of systemic treatment, from which a curative response is exceedingly rare, for significant periods of time. This management paradigm with CRN and deferred treatment should be considered for patients presenting with minimal metastatic burden as an option that is unlikely to impact on overall survival and reduce treatment related morbidity. This approach has been reported with a median time to progression of 12 months and time to systemic therapy of 14 months following CRN [32].

Impact of the Immuno-Oncology (IO) Era

The introduction IO drugs for metastatic kidney cancer has created further uncertainty with respect to the role of CRN. CRN clearly conferred a survival advantage, albeit modest, for good performance status patients for patients treated with IFN—a cytokine immune stimulant. Current IO agents are more specific in the effect and clearly rather more effective. It remains to be determined whether CRN will amplify the effects of these drugs in appropriate patients as it did with IFN—a rather crude and perhaps somewhat ineffective immunotherapy agent.

Currently nivolumab, ipilimumab and pembrolizumab are the most widely utilised of the many drugs available. These can be used alone, in combination with another IO drug or a TKI. As with the previous TKI trials, IO studies have included significant numbers of patients with prior nephrectomy. In CHECKMATE 214 [33], one of the initial studies demonstrating superiority of IO over TKI's—80% of patients had previous nephrectomy. Whilst TKI's appear to fundamentally be life prolonging—IO may result in profound responses and quite possibly complete responses in some patients.

Given both the efficacy and the mechanistic differences of IO agents with previous systemic treatments the role of CRN remains to be determined. Currently recent retrospective studies [34, 35] support the continued use of initial CRN although more trials are clearly needed and planned. Theoretically if 'priming' the immune system with the original tumour was important for a favourable response to IO treatment, an inferior response would be anticipated in patients undergoing initial CRN (prior to IO treatment) compared to CRN and TKI group. This has not been reported to date. The morbidity of IO may be substantial and overall it appears rather more toxic than TKIs. Thus management strategies that defer systemic therapy as long as possible may need to be considered. CRN is thus likely to continue as an initial step in patients with low volume metastatic disease as well as specific subsets of patients who require systemic therapy. Clinical trials will clearly be required to precisely define suitable patients.

Selecting the Candidate for Cytoreductive Nephrectomy

Metastatic RCC has a varied clinical course encompassing a spectrum from rapid progression to slow attenuated or intermittent progression. Evidence suggests that surgery has a limited role with the former but is likely to benefit the latter. Local management of tumour sites, including the primary disease, may prevent or delay the need for systemic treatments. CRN will thus remain as a treatment modality in patients with low volume metastatic disease likely to experience slow progression and patients who exhibit significant responses to systemic therapies. Case selection will be critical—which will require effective objective criteria to predict the pattern of progression and/or treatment response in individual patients.

Various tools have been developed including the MSKCC and the more recent IMDC risk stratification models [26, 36] to select patients for surgery. The parameters for IMDC are shown in Table 1

These models have been based on oncology tools developed to predict survival in patients who developed metastatic recurrence after initial nephrectomy who were treated with TKI's. These models include a number of parameters in patient selection for surgery including:

1. Good performance status
2. Expectation of slow progression of metastatic disease
3. Paraneoplastic syndrome indicating poor outcome (haematology disruption)

Several other major cancer centres have published more surgically orientated stratification models, including factors such as number of metastatic sites, specific metastatic sites (liver, bone, brain, lymph nodes), constitutional symptoms, degree of local progression, grade and necrosis within the tumour [28, 37–39]. In a pragmatic investigation [40] an external validation of ten prognostic models, including those previously mentioned was performed. Whilst the performance of all models was similar, none of these are particularly robust or provide tangible advantage in selecting patients for cytoreductive nephrectomy.

Plasma and genomic markers have also been studied to predict survival and systemic treatment response more generally in the metastatic patient. To date none have proven particularly effective although current research suggests that objective criteria are likely to be established through analysis of the genetic phenotypes of individual patients tumours which is discussed in a later section.

Other Indications for Cytoreductive Nephrectomy

There are specific clinical scenarios where nephrectomy, outside the criteria for a cytoreductive or palliative procedure, may be considered. RCC may be associated with intracaval tumour extension and attendant risks of caval obstruction, cardiac failure, hepatic congestion and Budd-Chiari syndrome, and recurrent pulmonary emboli. These factors can preclude patients from systemic treatment. Selected

Table 1 IMDC risk stratification criteria

IMDC risk factors	Risk stratification
1. Time from diagnosis to systemic therapy < 1 year 2. Karnofsky performance status < 80 3. Haemoglobin < low limit normal 4. Neutrophils > upper limit normal 5. Corrected calcium > upper limit normal 6. Platelets > upper limit normal	Favourable—0 risk factors Intermediate—1 or 2 risk factors Poor—3 or more risk factors

patients who are suitable candidates for surgery may be considered for CRN to facilitate their opportunities of receiving systemic therapy.

Bleeding and pain are future potential complications that may be avoided with initial surgery before systemic therapy has commenced. In the CARMENA study, only 3% of patients who commenced sunitinib without CRN subsequently required emergency nephrectomy for these reasons.

In contrast initial CRN may be beneficial for patients experiencing symptoms—although this would be regarded as a palliative procedure. A study investigating symptom control in metastatic RCC reported symptom resolution or improvement for local and systemic symptoms 43% and 71% respectively with CRN [41, 42]. For local symptoms, resolution was seen in 91%. The risk of surgery must of course be weighed against the control of symptoms which may possibly be achieved by other means. Major complications and mortality with palliative nephrectomy has been reported to be 10% and 3% respectively. There is also a concern that the morbidity of surgery or the delay and subsequent progression may obviate patients from receiving systemic therapy: this has been reported as 12% in some series, but up to 40% in others [43].

It is also uncertain whether nephrectomy will ameliorate paraneoplastic syndromes. Extremely limited evidence is available in the literature regarding improvement in paraneoplastic syndromes after CRN: 81% of patients normalised their calcium after surgery, but in this series of just 11 patients [44]. Anecdotally it has suggested that patients most likely to experience resolution or improvement of a paraneoplastic symptoms are those with a very large primary tumour burden and minimal volume metastatic disease.

Future Work

Defining patients who will benefit from CRN will remain an ongoing challenge as systemic therapies continue to evolve. Case selection currently is dependent on clinical features and patient performance status. These largely reflect the burden of disease and the physiological reserve of the patient in undergoing treatment both surgical and systemic. Objective information predicting the behaviour of an individual's tumour is likely to be far more useful.

Within the last 10 years, genomic analysis of RCC has made significant strides in understanding of key genetic mutations in RCC [41, 45]. Preliminary steps have been made in adding genomics parameters to existing risk stratification systems [46].

This work has been extended defining the protracted evolution of RCC which actually spans decades [47]. Progression encompasses sequences of mutations which define different patterns of tumour behaviour. Individual patients' primary disease consequently contains multiple discrete tumour clones—with metastatic disease evolving from a limited number of these [48].

Ultimately detailed genomic analysis of metastatic disease sites may define patients who will benefit clinically from a CRN as well as whether this should be prior to or after commencement of systemic therapy. Preliminary CRN may also be considered to allow a detailed genomic analysis of the clones within the primary to select the most appropriate systemic therapy for an individual patient, which might not be apparent from a biopsy.

Thus selection of patients for CRN may be driven by tumour specific genomic parameters rather than patient clinical features.

Conclusion

Whereas further trials are underway to produce high quality evidence for the use of cytoreductive nephrectomy in the IO era [49, 50], the same problems as those encountered with CARMENA and SURTIME may persist if inclusion criteria does not reflect current selection practice; the data may not be accepted as generalizable. Molecular profiling of metastatic vs primary tumours will allow us to appropriately classify the metastatic RCC patient at presentation and improve the accuracy of existing risk stratification models; we can then decide which deposit of cancer, for which treatment, and when we need to do it.

Currently, we must rely on good clinical judgement for patient selection for CRN with consideration of the following principles:

1. Decisions to be made on a patient by patient basis, with the help of a multidisciplinary team, in particular a consensus opinion between the medical oncologist and urologist
2. Consider which aspect of the disease forms the management priority for the patient, the primary, the individual metastasis or the systemic metastases, and treat those first
3. Heed the lessons of CARMENA—upfront surgery for multi-site metastases on poor risk patients does not improve outcomes
4. Surgery for symptoms and potential complications of the primary tumour remains apposite in maintaining quality of life for many patients

Key Points

1. Cytoreductive nephrectomy (CRN) is the surgical removal of a primary renal cell carcinoma in a patient with established metastatic disease with the intention of prolonging patient survival.
2. It was originally adopted after observation that removal of the primary tumour induced regression of metastatic disease, however this is a rare occurrence.
3. In some patients, CRN affords the patient potentially long periods of safe observation, sparing them systemic therapy until their indolent metastatic disease progresses.

4. Randomised controlled trials at the turn of the century demonstrated a survival advantage when given with immunotherapy drugs, such as interferon, compared to using interferon alone.
5. More recent randomised controlled trials have challenged this benefit with more effective targeted therapies available, however there have been problems generalising these findings to clinical practice.
6. As new systemic therapies emerge, the role of CRN may need to be repeatedly re-evaluated.
7. Choosing the appropriate candidate for CRN remains a key challenge. Scoring systems that use clinical factors and patient performance status to predict good outcome remain unreliable and good clinical judgement is still required.
8. Genetic understanding of renal cell carcinoma is developing rapidly and a more objective means of predicting appropriate candidates for cytoreductive nephrectomy will be available.

References

1. Bumpus H. The apparent disappearance of pulmonary metastasis in a case of hypernephroma following nephrectomy. J Urol. 1928;20(2):185–92.
2. Barney JD, Churchill E. Adenocarcinoma of the kidney with metastasis to the lung: cured by nephrectomy and lobectomy. J Urol. 1939;42(3):269–76.
3. Middleton R. Surgery for metastatic renal cell carcinoma. J Urol. 1967;97(6):973–7.
4. Snow RM, Schellhammer PF. Spontaneous regression of metastatic renal cell carcinoma. Urology. 1982;20(2):177–81.
5. Marcus SG, Choyke PL, Reiter R, Jaffe GS, Alexander RB, Linehan WM, et al. Regression of metastatic renal cell carcinoma after cytoreductive nephrectomy. J Urol. 1993;150(2 Pt 1):463–6.
6. Sakula A. Spontaneous regression of pulmonary metastases secondary to carcinoma of kidney. Br J Dis Chest. 1963;57:147–52.
7. Uzzo RG, Rayman P, Kolenko V, Clark PE, Cathcart MK, Bloom T, et al. Renal cell carcinoma-derived gangliosides suppress nuclear factor-kappaB activation in T cells. J Clin Invest. 1999;104(6):769–76.
8. Wang X, Lopez R, Luchtel RA, Hafizi S, Gartrell B, Shenoy N. Immune evasion in renal cell carcinoma: biology, clinical translation, future directions. Kidney Int. 2021;99(1):75–85.
9. Kawashima A, Kanazawa T, Kidani Y, Yoshida T, Hirata M, Nishida K, et al. Tumour grade significantly correlates with total dysfunction of tumour tissue-infiltrating lymphocytes in renal cell carcinoma. Sci Rep. 2020;10(1):6220.
10. Ono M. Molecular links between tumor angiogenesis and inflammation: inflammatory stimuli of macrophages and cancer cells as targets for therapeutic strategy. Cancer Sci. 2008;99(8):1501–6.
11. Jackson BL, Fowler S, Williams ST, British Association of Urological Surgeons (BAUS) - Section of Oncology. Perioperative outcomes of cytoreductive nephrectomy in the UK in 2012. BJU Int. 2015;116(6):905–10.
12. Hrushesky WJ, Murphy GP. Current status of the therapy of advanced renal carcinoma. J Surg Oncol. 1977;9(3):277–88.

13. Oevermann K, Buer J, Hoffmann R, Franzke A, Schrader A, Patzelt T, et al. Capecitabine in the treatment of metastatic renal cell carcinoma. Br J Cancer. 2000;83(5):583–7.
14. Quesada J. Role of interferons in the therapy of metastatic renal cell carcinoma. Urology. 1989;34(4, suppl):80–3.
15. Rosenberg SA, Yang JC, White DE, Steinberg SM. Durability of complete responses in patients with metastatic cancer treated with high-dose interleukin-2: identification of the antigens mediating response. Ann Surg. 1998;228(3):307–19.
16. Flanigan RC, Salmon SE, Blumenstein BA, Bearman SI, Roy V, McGrath PC, et al. Nephrectomy followed by interferon alfa-2b compared with interferon alfa-2b alone for metastatic renal-cell cancer. N Engl J Med. 2001;345(23):1655–9.
17. Mickisch GH, Garin A, van Poppel H, de Prijck L, Sylvester R, European Organisation for Research and Treatment of Cancer (EORTC) Genitourinary Group. Radical nephrectomy plus interferon-alfa-based immunotherapy compared with interferon alfa alone in metastatic renal-cell carcinoma: a randomised trial. Lancet. 2001;358(9286):966–70.
18. Walther MM, Alexander RB, Weiss GH, Venzon D, Berman A, Pass HI, et al. Cytoreductive surgery prior to interleukin-2-based therapy in patients with metastatic renal cell carcinoma. Urology. 1993;42(3):250–7. Discussion 7–8
19. Motzer RJ, Hutson TE, Tomczak P, Michaelson MD, Bukowski RM, Rixe O, et al. Sunitinib versus interferon alfa in metastatic renal-cell carcinoma. N Engl J Med. 2007;356(2):115–24.
20. Choueiri TK, Xie W, Kollmannsberger C, North S, Knox JJ, Lampard JG, et al. The impact of cytoreductive nephrectomy on survival of patients with metastatic renal cell carcinoma receiving vascular endothelial growth factor targeted therapy. J Urol. 2011;185(1):60–6.
21. Petrelli F, Coinu A, Vavassori I, Cabiddu M, Borgonovo K, Ghilardi M, et al. Cytoreductive nephrectomy in metastatic renal cell carcinoma treated with targeted therapies: a systematic review with a meta-analysis. Clin Genitourin Cancer. 2016;14(6):465–72.
22. Méjean A, Ravaud A, Thezenas S, Colas S, Beauval JB, Bensalah K, et al. Sunitinib alone or after nephrectomy in metastatic renal-cell carcinoma. N Engl J Med. 2018;379(5):417–27.
23. The ASCO Post. 2018 ASCO: Carmena trial compares nephrectomy plus adjuvant sunitinib vs sunitinib alone in metastatic RCC 2018. Available from: www.ascopost.com/news/58905.
24. Motzer RJ, Russo P. Cytoreductive nephrectomy - patient selection is key. N Engl J Med. 2018;379(5):481–2.
25. Flanigan RC. Re: Sunitinib alone or after nephrectomy in metastatic renal-cell carcinoma. Eur Urol. 2019;75(5):876–7.
26. Motzer RJ, Bacik J, Murphy BA, Russo P, Mazumdar M. Interferon-alfa as a comparative treatment for clinical trials of new therapies against advanced renal cell carcinoma. J Clin Oncol. 2002;20(1):289–96.
27. Bex A, Mulders P, Jewett M, Wagstaff J, van Thienen JV, Blank CU, et al. Comparison of immediate vs deferred cytoreductive nephrectomy in patients with synchronous metastatic renal cell carcinoma receiving sunitinib: the SURTIME Randomized Clinical Trial. JAMA Oncol. 2019;5(2):164–70.
28. Culp SH, Tannir NM, Abel EJ, Margulis V, Tamboli P, Matin SF, et al. Can we better select patients with metastatic renal cell carcinoma for cytoreductive nephrectomy? Cancer. 2010;116(14):3378–88.
29. Pickering LM, Mahgoub MO, Mukherji D. Is observation a valid strategy in metastatic renal cell carcinoma? Curr Opin Urol. 2015;25(5):390–4.
30. Rini BI, Dorff TB, Elson P, Rodriguez CS, Shepard D, Wood L, et al. Active surveillance in metastatic renal-cell carcinoma: a prospective, phase 2 trial. Lancet Oncol. 2016;17(9):1317–24.
31. Harrison MR, Costello BA, Bhavsar NA, Vaishampayan U, Pal SK, Zakharia Y, et al. Active surveillance of metastatic renal cell carcinoma: Results from a prospective observational study (MaRCC). Cancer. 2021;127(13):2204–12.
32. Bex A, Bruijn R, Noe A, Blank CU, Horenblas S, Haanen JBAG. Time to targeted therapy after cytoreductive nephrectomy (CN) and surveillance in patients with synchronous unresectable metastases of renal cell carcinoma (RCC). J Clin Oncol. 2016;34(2_suppl):604.

33. Motzer RJ, Tannir NM, McDermott DF, Arén Frontera O, Melichar B, Choueiri TK, et al. Nivolumab plus ipilimumab versus sunitinib in advanced renal-cell carcinoma. N Engl J Med. 2018;378(14):1277–90.
34. Bakouny Z, Xie W, Dudani S, Wells C, Gan CL, Donskov F, et al. Cytoreductive nephrectomy (CN) for metastatic renal cell carcinoma (mRCC) treated with immune checkpoint inhibitors (ICI) or targeted therapy (TT): A propensity score-based analysis. J Clin Oncol. 2020;38(6_suppl):608.
35. Ishihara H, Takagi T, Kondo T, Fukuda H, Tachibana H, Yoshida K, et al. Prognostic impact of systemic therapy change in metastatic renal cell carcinoma treated with cytoreductive nephrectomy. Jpn J Clin Oncol. 2021;51(2):296–304.
36. Heng DY, Xie W, Regan MM, Warren MA, Golshayan AR, Sahi C, et al. Prognostic factors for overall survival in patients with metastatic renal cell carcinoma treated with vascular endothelial growth factor-targeted agents: results from a large, multicenter study. J Clin Oncol. 2009;27(34):5794–9.
37. Leibovich BC, Cheville JC, Lohse CM, Zincke H, Frank I, Kwon ED, et al. A scoring algorithm to predict survival for patients with metastatic clear cell renal cell carcinoma: a stratification tool for prospective clinical trials. J Urol. 2005;174(5):1759–63. Discussion 63
38. Karakiewicz PI, Briganti A, Chun FK, Trinh QD, Perrotte P, Ficarra V, et al. Multi-institutional validation of a new renal cancer-specific survival nomogram. J Clin Oncol. 2007;25(11):1316–22.
39. Margulis V, Shariat SF, Rapoport Y, Rink M, Sjoberg DD, Tannir NM, et al. Development of accurate models for individualized prediction of survival after cytoreductive nephrectomy for metastatic renal cell carcinoma. Eur Urol. 2013;63(5):947–52.
40. Westerman ME, Shapiro DD, Tannir NM, Campbell MT, Matin SF, Karam JA, et al. Survival following cytoreductive nephrectomy: a comparison of existing prognostic models. BJU Int. 2020;126(6):745–53.
41. Sato Y, Yoshizato T, Shiraishi Y, Maekawa S, Okuno Y, Kamura T, et al. Integrated molecular analysis of clear-cell renal cell carcinoma. Nat Genet. 2013;45(8):860–7.
42. Alessandro L, Giuseppe F, Giuseppe R, Chiara R, Gianfranco B, Stefano A, Daniele C, Gianmarco C, Giuseppe B, Alberto B, Andrea S, Roberto B, Francesco M, Umberto C. Cytoreductive nephrectomy in metastatic patients with signs or symptoms: implications for renal cell carcinoma guidelines. Eur Urol. 2020;78(3):321–6. https://doi.org/10.1016/j.eururo.2020.05.014.
43. Bhindi B, Abel EJ, Albiges L, Bensalah K, Boorjian SA, Daneshmand S, et al. Systematic review of the role of cytoreductive nephrectomy in the targeted therapy era and beyond: an individualized approach to metastatic renal cell carcinoma. Eur Urol. 2019;75(1):111–28.
44. Walther MM, Patel B, Choyke PL, Lubensky IA, Vocke CD, Harris C, et al. Hypercalcemia in patients with metastatic renal cell carcinoma: effect of nephrectomy and metabolic evaluation. J Urol. 1997;158(3 Pt 1):733–9.
45. Cancer Genome Atlas Research Network. Comprehensive molecular characterization of clear cell renal cell carcinoma. Nature. 2013;499(7456):43–9. https://doi.org/10.1038/nature12222.
46. Voss MH, Reising A, Cheng Y, Patel P, Marker M, Kuo F, et al. Genomically annotated risk model for advanced renal-cell carcinoma: a retrospective cohort study. Lancet Oncol. 2018;19(12):1688–98.
47. Turajlic S, Xu H, Litchfield K, Rowan A, Horswell S, Chambers T, et al. Deterministic evolutionary trajectories influence primary tumor growth: TRACERx renal. Cell. 2018;173(3):595–610.e11.
48. Turajlic S, Xu H, Litchfield K, Rowan A, Chambers T, Lopez JI, et al. Tracking cancer evolution reveals constrained routes to metastases: TRACERx renal. Cell. 2018;173(3):581–94.e12.
49. Deferred cytoreductive nephrectomy in synchronous metastatic renal cell carcinoma: the NORDIC-SUN-Trial (NORDIC-SUN) clinicaltrials.gov: U.S. National Library of Medicine; 2019. Available from: https://clinicaltrials.gov/ct2/show/NCT03977571.
50. Comparing the outcome of immunotherapy-based drug combination therapy with or without surgery to remove the kidney in metastatic kidney cancer, the PROBE Trial (PROBE) clinicaltrials.gov: US National Library of Medicine; 2020. Available from: https://www.clinicaltrials.gov/ct2/show/NCT04510597.

Urothelial Cell Carcinoma of the Kidney and Other Non-clear Cell Renal Cell Carcinomas

Óscar Rodríguez Faba, Ferran Algaba, Alberto Breda, and Joan Palou

Urothelial Cell Carcinoma of the Kidney

Urothelial cell carcinomas (UCC) are the fourth most common tumors in developed countries. Bladder cancer (BC) represents 90–95% of all UCC, while upper urinary tract urothelial cell carcinoma (UUT-UCC) accounts for only 5–10% [1]. At diagnosis, UUT-UCC are located in the renal pelvis twice as often as in the ureter [2]. In a retrospective article published by Cosentino et al, concerning 450 patients, 76 (17%) presented concomitant primary UUT-UCC and BC. The location of primary UUT-UCC was in the calyx and/or renal pelvis in 25 patients (34%), in the upper ureter in 8 (11%), and in the lower ureter in 37 (49%). Concomitant BC was found in 10%, 18%, and 33% of patients with primary caliceal/renal pelvis, upper ureter, and lower ureter UUT-UCC, respectively. On multivariate analysis, location of UUT-UCC was the only factor predictive for concomitant BC [3]. Hereditary UUT-UCC represents 20% of all UUT-UCC and is associated with hereditary non-polyposis colorectal carcinoma. Balkan nephropathy, associated with the consumption of aristolochic acid and also phenacetin, has also been linked with UUT-UCC [4].

Diagnosis of UUT-UCC is based on a combination of laboratory imaging and endoscopic modalities. Positive urinary cytology is suggestive of high-grade UUT-UCC. Fluorescence in situ hybridization increases the sensitivity of urinary cytology but at the same time diminishes the specificity [5]. The highest imaging accuracy

Ó. Rodríguez Faba · A. Breda · J. Palou (✉)
Department of Urology, Fundació Puigvert, Autonomous University of Barcelona, Barcelona, Spain
e-mail: orodriguez@fundacio-puigvert.es; abreda@fundacio-puigvert.es; jpalou@fundacio-puigvert.es

F. Algaba
Department of Pathology, Fundació Puigvert, Autonomous University of Barcelona, Barcelona, Spain
e-mail: FAlgaba@fundacio-puigverts.es

C. Anderson, M. Afshar (eds.), *Renal Cancer*,
https://doi.org/10.1007/978-3-030-84756-2_20

for the diagnosis of UTUC is provided by multidetector computed tomography urography (CTU).

Fluorodeoxyglucose positron emission tomography/computed tomography has a higher sensitivity than CTU in the detection of metastases (85% vs. 50%) [6]. Endoscopy, specifically flexible ureteroscopy (URS), is an essential tool to obtain information about stage, grade, and tumor appearance [6]. Preoperative predictive models improve prediction and help decision making. Long-term smoking, preoperative hydronephrosis, and tumor location in the renal pelvis are predictive of more advanced disease [7]. High-risk tumors are associated with hydronephrosis, a tumor size of >2 cm, high-grade cytology, high-grade URS biopsy, multifocal disease, previous cystectomy for bladder cancer, and variant histology [1]. Radical nephroureterectomy is the treatment of choice for high-risk tumors and should be performed with lymphadenectomy and bladder cuff resection. Moreover, a single intravesical instillation of chemotherapy is recommended to reduce the likelihood of intravesical recurrence during follow-up. Kidney-sparing management should be offered as a primary treatment option to patients with low-risk tumors and patients with high-risk tumors in the distal ureter [1].

Non-clear Cell Renal Cell Carcinomas

Introduction

The majority of malignant renal tumors (85%) are renal cell carcinomas (RCC) arising from the different areas of tubular epithelium. Clear cell RCC (cc-RCC) accounts for 80% of renal tumors in adults while the remaining 20% are non-clear cell renal cell carcinomas (non-cc-RCC), which represent a heterogeneous group under continuous revision and with ongoing identification of new entities. Each of these subtypes presents different molecular features and also has a different clinical presentation and response to treatment. The 2016 WHO histological classification of RCC is based on genetic, molecular, and histological features [8]. Although papillary and chromophobe RCC represent 80% of non-cc-RCC [9], many other subtypes have been identified (Table 1) and these must be known because they are biologically distinct.

Multilocular Cystic Renal Neoplasm of Low Malignant Potential (MCRCC)

This neoplasm is a rare subtype of RCC. Most patients are asymptomatic and diagnosed accidentally. MCRCC represents 4% of all RCC and is more frequent in females between the 2nd and 7th decades of life. They cannot be distinguished from other complex cystic renal lesions by imaging. Final diagnosis is based on pathological features after surgical resection, as the cystic morphology is not always detected on biopsy [10]. CT scan with intravenous contrast shows the multiloculated morphology of this tumor. Microscopically it is composed of multiple cysts separated by thick

Table 1 Subtypes of non-cc-RCC

Multilocular cystic renal neoplasm of low malignant potential
Papillary renal cell carcinoma
Hereditary leiomyomatosis and RCC-associated renal cell carcinoma
Chromophobe renal cell carcinoma
Collecting duct carcinoma
Renal medullary carcinoma
MiT (microphthalmia-associated transcription factor) family translocation renal cell carcinoma
Succinate dehydrogenase-deficient renal cell carcinoma
Mucinous tubular and spindle cell carcinoma
Tubulocystic renal cell carcinoma
Acquired cystic disease-associated renal cell carcinoma
Clear cell papillary renal cell carcinoma
Renal cell carcinoma, unclassified

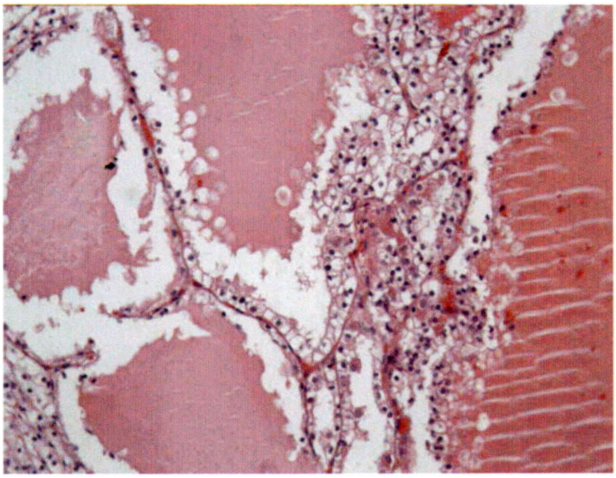

Fig. 1 Multilocular cystic renal neoplasm of low malignant potential

septa lined by a monolayer of clear cells, with the same characteristics as low-grade cc-RCC (LOH 3p) (Fig. 1). Tumors are positive for paired box gene 8 (PAX8), carbonic anhydrase IX (CAIX), cytokeratin (CK)7, and CK34βE12 [11]. A recent large series of MCRCC has confirmed its favorable prognosis, and for this reason it has been renamed as multilocular cystic renal neoplasm of low malignant potential [12].

Papillary RCC (pRCC)

This is the second most common type of RCC (10–15%). Two histological subtypes have been recognized for a long time (type 1 and type 2), but now it is recognized the heterogeneity of type 2 for this reason it is considered that the grading has more clinical impact in pRCC.:

Classical pRCC (former Type 1) often presents as multifocal disease characterized by papillae and tubular structures covered with small cells containing basophilic cytoplasm and small uniform oval nuclei [13] (Fig. 2). It is more frequently associated with *MET* or epidermal growth factor receptor *(EGFR)* mutations [14] and trisomies. Some morphological patterns as biphasic with squamous cells, vacuolated cells, reverse polarity are considered variants of the classical pRCC.

The former Type 2 is molecular heterogeneous neoplasm, contains papillae covered by large cells with eosinophilic cytoplasm and large spherical nuclei with prominent nucleoli [13] (Fig. 3). It often presents clinically as unique tumors with an aggressive phenotype. Molecular studies of this morphological variant have shown very different alterations; some are associated with *SETD2* mutations, *CDKN2A* mutations, or *TFE3* fusions [14] or with a fumarate hydratase (*FH*) mutation [9], so some of these tumors are currently being reclassified, reducing the number of cases considered to be high grade pure papillary RCC. Typical AMACR expression is present in both subtypes.

Hereditary Leiomyomatosis and Renal Cell Carcinoma-Associated RCC (HLRCC)

This is an autosomal dominant condition with an *FH* mutation that is characterized by the variable presentation of multiple cutaneous leiomyomas, uterine leiomyomas, and RCC [15]. It is also known as MCUL (multiple cutaneous and uterine leiomyomatosis) and Reed's syndrome, following first documentation of the condition by Reed in 1973 [16]. Initial studies suggested that histologically HLRCC tumors always have the morphology of type 2 papillary RCC, but recent studies have reported other histologies, including papillary, tubulopapillary, tubular, solid, and cystic tumors, as well as collecting-duct like carcinoma and sarcomatoid

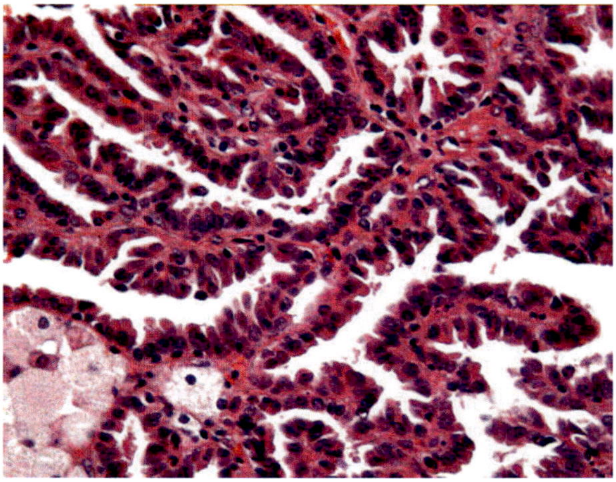

Fig. 2 Classical pRCC (former type 1)

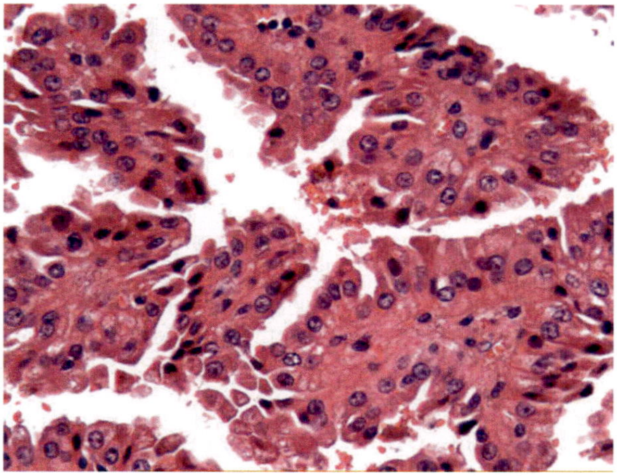

Fig. 3 The former Type 2 pRCC

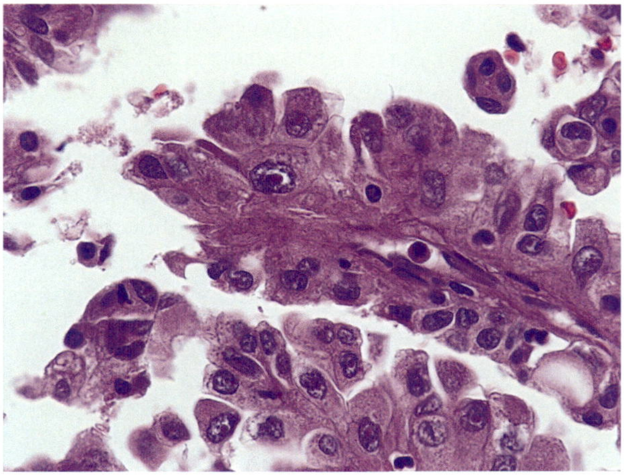

Fig. 4 Fumarate hydratase (FH) deficient carcinoma

differentiation [17]. The most typical morphological finding is the presence of large eosinophilic nucleoli with a halo around them that results in an appearance similar to that of a viral inclusion (Fig. 4). Most tumors are unilateral and solitary, and metastatic disease is often present [16]. The sporadic cases are frequent and the nomenclature is Fumarate hydratase (FH) deficient carcinoma.

Chromophobe Renal Cell Carcinoma (ChRCC)

This neoplasm is characterized by large cells with finely reticular cytoplasm, with a clear or eosinophilic aspect at hematoxylin and eosin staining (Fig. 5). ChRCC has diffuse positivity for cytokeratin 7 (CK7) and CD117 (c-kit) and displays more frequent chromosome loss. ChRCC has a good prognosis, with a low tendency to

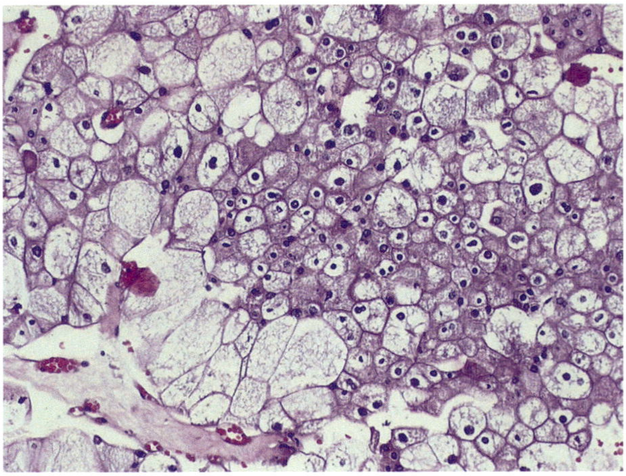

Fig. 5 Chromophobe renal cell carcinoma (ChRCC)

progress and metastasize. Only 1.3% of patients present distant metastasis at diagnosis and the 5- and 10-year cancer-specific survival (CSS) rates are 93% and 88.9% respectively [18]. Sarcomatoid changes and pT stage are independent predictors for aggressiveness of ChRCC [19, 20]. One important issue is the differential diagnosis with oncocytoma. Several findings suggest a close relationship between ChRCC and oncocytoma. First, both tumors share a phenotype of intercalated cells of the collecting duct system and mitochondrial DNA alterations. Second, some cases of coexistent oncocytoma and ChRCC, and oncocytic multifocal tubular transformation designated as "renal oncocytosis", have recently been reported. Third, oncocytic areas in ChRCC that have similar ultrastructural features to those of oncocytomas have been reported as "hybrid tumors".

Collecting Duct Carcinoma (CDC)

Collecting duct carcinoma, or Bellini duct carcinoma, is an aggressive RCC arising from the renal collecting tubules. At the time of diagnosis, about 50% of patients present metastases and these patients have poor outcomes. CDC is more likely to occur in the middle-aged to elderly. Integrase interactor-1 proteins (INI-1) is present [21].

Renal Medullary Carcinoma (RMC)

This is a highly aggressive malignancy very often associated with sickle cell anemia. It is characterized by undifferentiated cells with an interstitial polymorphonuclear infiltrate and with OCT 3/4 expression. Some authors consider it an undifferentiated form of collecting duct carcinoma.

MiT (Microphthalmia-Associated Transcription Factor) Family Translocation Renal Cell Carcinomas

Translocation-associated RCC (tRCC) is an uncommon subtype of RCC characterized by recurrent gene rearrangements involving the *TFE3* or *TFEB* loci. *TFE3* and *TFEB* are members of the microphthalmia transcription factor (MiT) family, which regulates differentiation in melanocytes and osteoclasts, and MiT family gene fusions activate unique molecular programs that can be detected immunohistochemically and by fluorescent in situ hybridization analysis [22]. tRCC is more frequent in young patients, less than 40 years old. Microscopically a papillary and solid or complex architecture with large clear cells and/or epithelioid cells and irregular calcifications is present [9]. The oncological outcomes of this tumor are poor and it is associated with an aggressive clinical behavior, especially in older adults [23].

Succinate Dehydrogenase-Deficient Renal Cell Carcinoma

This is a renal cell carcinoma recently recognized in the 2016 WHO classification [24]. It is associated with *SDH* gene germline mutations, also associated with paraganglioma/pheochromocytoma and gastrointestinal stromal tumors. The tumor is more frequent in young adults. The tumors are composed of solid nests or tubules and frequently show cystic change. The most distinctive histologic feature is the presence of cytoplasmic vacuoles or inclusions (Fig. 6). Loss of SDH subunit B immunostaining is needed for a definite diagnosis. The prognosis is good for low-grade tumors but worse for tumors with high-grade nuclei, sarcomatoid change, or coagulative necrosis. Long-term follow-up is indicated [25].

Mucinous Tubular and Spindle Cell Carcinoma (MTSRCC)

This is an uncommon variant of RCC characterized by an admixture of cuboidal cells in tubules and sheets of spindle cells, as well as variable amounts of mucinous stroma (Fig. 7). MTSRCC has a female predominance, with a mean age at diagnosis of 53 years. An association of MTSRCC with nephrolithiasis and end-stage renal disease has been reported [26]. Immunohistochemical markers, including CK7, CK19, EMA, vimentin, and AMACR, show positive expression in tumor cells. Patients with MTSRCC are likely to have an improved prognosis following surgery compared with patients with other renal cell carcinomas [27].

Tubulocystic Renal Cell Carcinoma (TCRCC)

This tumor is more frequent in males in the fifth or six decade of life. Macroscopically, it is a well-circumscribed and unencapsulated tumor with frequent cystic components (Bosniak III and IV). Microscopically, cystic formations of various diameters

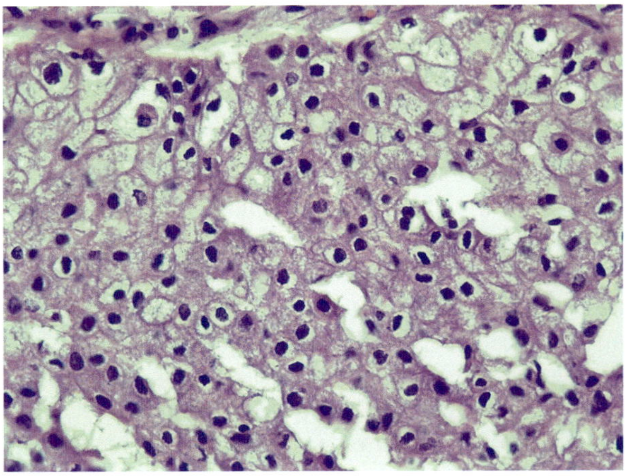

Fig. 6 Succinate dehydrogenase-deficient renal cell carcinoma

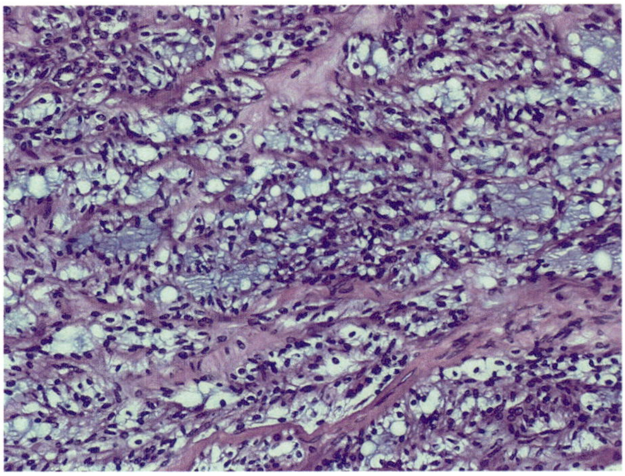

Fig. 7 Mucinous tubular and spindle cell carcinoma (MTSRCC)

coated by monolayer epithelium with a prominent nucleus, low grade, cells are identified (Fig. 8). Immunohistochemistry shows vimentin and α-methylacyl-CoA racemase (AMACR). At the molecular level, TCRCC shows gain in chromosome 17 (trisomy 17) [28]. TCRCC typically presents a clinically benign course, with only a few cases having presented progression and/or metastases [29]. There is no established targeted therapy in metastatic TCRCC, but a few case reports have suggested a partial response to sunitinib and everolimus [30].

Acquired Cystic Disease-Associated Renal Cell Carcinoma (ACD-RCC)

This type of RCC was described in patients with ACD of the kidney. It is the predominant subtype of RCC occurring in patients with ACD and end-stage renal disease [31]. Macroscopically, tumors are generally well circumscribed and show a

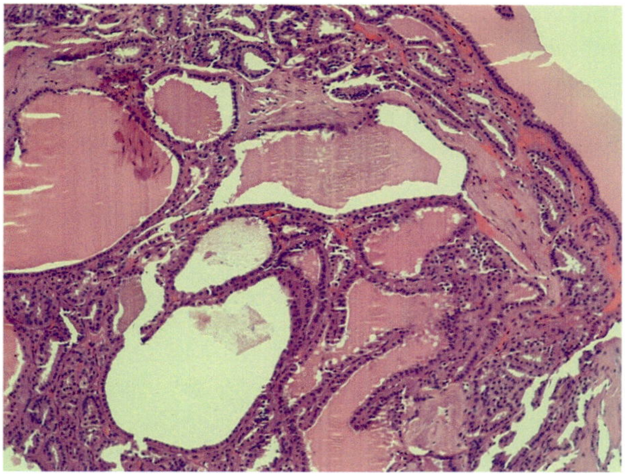

Fig. 8 Tubulocystic renal cell carcinoma (TCRCC)

brown, red-brown, or light brown color on the cut surface. Hemorrhage or necrosis is occasionally observed. Histologically the tumor consists of a microcystic or cribriform pattern of neoplastic cells with deeply eosinophilic to oncocytic cytoplasm on the background of oxalate crystal deposition [32]. A recent multi-institutional study analyzed 40 cases of ACD-RCC. Of the 36 patients (90%) with available follow-up information, four (11%) had adverse events: two patients developed a local recurrence, one had multiple visceral metastases and subsequently died of disease, and one developed metastases to regional lymph nodes only [33].

Clear Cell Papillary Renal Cell Carcinoma (CCP-RCC)

This neoplasm is composed of various proportions of papillary, tubular/acinar, cystic, and solid sheet-like or nested architectures with clear cytoplasm with an apical nucleus [34]. This tumor lacks the genetic abnormalities observed in pRCC or ccRCC [35]. Immunohistochemically, tumor cells generally show diffuse expression for cytokeratin 7 and CA9 (cup-shaped pattern), but are negative for AMACR, RCC Ma, and TFE3. Genetically, this tumor has no characteristics of clear cell RCC or papillary RCC. Prognostically, patients with CCP-RCC present a favorable behavior [35].

Renal Cell Carcinoma, Unclassified

Unclassified RCC, as defined by WHO 2016 Classification of RCC, is a diagnostic category, not an entity, used for renal tumors that do not fit into any of the well-recognized subtypes; it includes admixed patterns of more than one recognized subtype [8]. Clear cell, oncocytic/eosinophilic, and mucinous are the main cell types that may be seen in these tumors; papillary, pure sarcomatoid, nested, solid, tubular, and tubulopapillary architectures are also seen [36]. Underlying molecular alterations may guide treatment decisions in patients with unclassified RCCs, and the scope for precision medicine may be expected to expand in the future, although these targets need to be tested in clinical trials [37].

The Future of Non-clear Cell Renal Cell Carcinomas

Since the WHO 2016 Classification of RCC, new patterns of RCC have been recognized that do not coincide with those described so far. As a consequence, the literature includes "new" entities of non-cc-RCC [24]. Some of these new entities display molecular differences but in many cases it remains to be ascertained whether they represent true anatomoclinical entities. In spite of this, information on such new findings is important, since it assists in standardization of the defined entities and opens possibilities for finding new therapies.

References

1. Roupret M, Babjuk M, Comperat E, Zigeuner R, Sylvester RJ, Burger M, et al. European Association of Urology guidelines on upper urinary tract urothelial carcinoma: 2017 update. Eur Urol. 2018;73:111–22.
2. Favaretto RL, Shariat SF, Chade DC, Godoy G, Adamy A, Kaag M, et al. The effect of tumor location on prognosis in patients treated with radical nephroureterectomy at Memorial Sloan-Kettering Cancer Center. Eur Urol. 2010;58:574–80.
3. Cosentino M, Palou J, Gaya JM, Breda A, Rodriguez-Faba O, Villavicencio-Mavrich H. Upper urinary tract urothelial cell carcinoma: location as a predictive factor for concomitant bladder carcinoma. World J Urol. 2013;31:141–5.
4. Roupret M, Yates DR, Comperat E, Cussenot O. Upper urinary tract urothelial cell carcinomas and other urological malignancies involved in the hereditary nonpolyposis colorectal cancer (Lynch syndrome) tumor spectrum. Eur Urol. 2008;54:1226–36.
5. Reynolds JP, Voss JS, Kipp BR, Karnes RJ, Nassar A, Clayton AC, et al. Comparison of urine cytology and fluorescence in situ hybridization in upper urothelial tract samples. Cancer Cytopathol. 2014;122:459–67.
6. Tanaka H, Yoshida S, Komai Y, Sakai Y, Urakami S, Yuasa T, et al. Clinical value of 18F-fluorodeoxyglucose positron emission tomography/computed tomography in upper tract urothelial carcinoma: impact on detection of metastases and patient management. Urol Int. 2016;96:65–72.
7. Isbarn H, Jeldres C, Shariat SF, Liberman D, Sun M, Lughezzani G, et al. Location of the primary tumor is not an independent predictor of cancer specific mortality in patients with upper urinary tract urothelial carcinoma. J Urol. 2009;182:2177–81.
8. Moch H, Cubilla AL, Humphrey PA, Reuter VE, Ulbright TM. The 2016 WHO classification of tumours of the urinary system and male genital organs-part A: renal, penile, and testicular tumours. Eur Urol. 2016;70:93–105.
9. Escudier B, Porta C, Schmidinger M, Rioux-Leclercq N, Bex A, Khoo V, et al. Renal cell carcinoma: ESMO Clinical Practice Guidelines for diagnosis, treatment and follow-up dagger. Ann Oncol. 2019;30:706–20.

10. Palmeiro MM, Niza JL, Loureiro AL, Conceicao e Silva JP. Unusual renal tumour: multilocular cystic renal cell carcinoma. BMJ Case Rep. 2016; https://doi.org/10.1136/bcr-2016-214386.
11. Brimo F, Atallah C, Li G, Srigley JR. Cystic clear cell papillary renal cell carcinoma: is it related to multilocular clear cell cystic neoplasm of low malignant potential? Histopathology. 2016;68:666–72.
12. Tretiakova M, Mehta V, Kocherginsky M, Minor A, Shen SS, Sirintrapun SJ, et al. Predominantly cystic clear cell renal cell carcinoma and multilocular cystic renal neoplasm of low malignant potential form a low-grade spectrum. Virchows Arch. 2018;473:85–93.
13. Delahunt B, Eble JN. Papillary renal cell carcinoma: a clinicopathologic and immunohistochemical study of 105 tumors. Mod Pathol. 1997;10:537–44.
14. Cancer Genome Atlas Research Network, Linehan WM, Spellman PT, Ricketts CJ, Creighton CJ, Fei SS, et al. Comprehensive molecular characterization of papillary renal-cell carcinoma. N Engl J Med. 2016;374:135–45.
15. Launonen V, Vierimaa O, Kiuru M, Isola J, Roth S, Pukkala E, et al. Inherited susceptibility to uterine leiomyomas and renal cell cancer. Proc Natl Acad Sci U S A. 2001;98:3387–92.
16. Mehrtens S, Veitch D, Kulakov E, Perrett CM. A case of hereditary leiomyomatosis and renal cell carcinoma. Case Rep Dermatol Med. 2016;2016:3793986.
17. Wei MH, Toure O, Glenn GM, Pithukpakorn M, Neckers L, Stolle C, et al. Novel mutations in FH and expansion of the spectrum of phenotypes expressed in families with hereditary leiomyomatosis and renal cell cancer. J Med Genet. 2006;43:18–27.
18. Volpe A, Novara G, Antonelli A, Bertini R, Billia M, Carmignani G, et al. Chromophobe renal cell carcinoma (RCC): oncological outcomes and prognostic factors in a large multicentre series. BJU Int. 2012;110:76–83.
19. Amin MB, Paner GP, Alvarado-Cabrero I, Young AN, Stricker HJ, Lyles RH, et al. Chromophobe renal cell carcinoma: histomorphologic characteristics and evaluation of conventional pathologic prognostic parameters in 145 cases. Am J Surg Pathol. 2008; 32:1822–34.
20. Casuscelli J, Becerra MF, Seier K, Manley BJ, Benfante N, Redzematovic A, et al. Chromophobe renal cell carcinoma: results from a large single-institution series. Clin Genitourin Cancer. 2019;17(5):373–9.e4.
21. Seo AN, Yoon G, Ro JY. Clinicopathologic and molecular pathology of collecting duct carcinoma and related renal cell carcinomas. Adv Anat Pathol. 2017;24:65–77.
22. Magers MJ, Udager AM, Mehra R. MiT family translocation-associated renal cell carcinoma: a contemporary update with emphasis on morphologic, immunophenotypic, and molecular mimics. Arch Pathol Lab Med. 2015;139:1224–33.
23. Argani P, Reuter VE, Zhang L, Sung YS, Ning Y, Epstein JI, et al. TFEB-amplified renal cell carcinomas: an aggressive molecular subset demonstrating variable melanocytic marker expression and morphologic heterogeneity. Am J Surg Pathol. 2016;40:1484–95.
24. Trpkov K, Hes O. New and emerging renal entities: a perspective post-WHO 2016 classification. Histopathology. 2019;74:31–59.
25. Wang G, Rao P. Succinate dehydrogenase-deficient renal cell carcinoma: a short review. Arch Pathol Lab Med. 2018;142:1284–8.
26. Nouh MA, Kuroda N, Yamashita M, Hayashida Y, Yano T, Minakuchi J, et al. Renal cell carcinoma in patients with end-stage renal disease: relationship between histological type and duration of dialysis. BJU Int. 2010;105:620–7.
27. Sun N, Fu Y, Wang Y, Tian T, An W, Yuan T. Mucinous tubular and spindle cell carcinoma of the kidney: a case report and review of the literature. Oncol Lett. 2014;7:811–4.
28. Yang XJ, Zhou M, Hes O, Shen S, Li R, Lopez J, et al. Tubulocystic carcinoma of the kidney: clinicopathologic and molecular characterization. Am J Surg Pathol. 2008;32:177–87.
29. Bhullar JS, Thamboo T, Esuvaranathan K. Unique case of tubulocystic carcinoma of the kidney with sarcomatoid features: a new entity. Urology. 2011;78:1071–2.
30. Banerjee I, Yadav SS, Tomar V, Yadav S, Talreja S. Tubulocystic renal cell carcinoma: a great imitator. Rev Urol. 2016;18:118–21.

31. Foshat M, Eyzaguirre E. Acquired cystic disease-associated renal cell carcinoma: review of pathogenesis, morphology, ancillary tests, and clinical features. Arch Pathol Lab Med. 2017;141:600–6.
32. Kuroda N, Naroda T, Tamura M, Yorita K, Kojima F, Murata SI. Acquired cystic disease-associated renal cell carcinoma: a clinicopathological study of seven cases. Pol J Pathol. 2017;68:306–11.
33. Przybycin CG, Harper HL, Reynolds JP, Magi-Galluzzi C, Nguyen JK, Wu A, et al. Acquired cystic disease-associated renal cell carcinoma (ACD-RCC): a multiinstitutional study of 40 cases with clinical follow-up. Am J Surg Pathol. 2018;42:1156–65.
34. Gobbo S, Eble JN, Grignon DJ, Martignoni G, MacLennan GT, Shah RB, et al. Clear cell papillary renal cell carcinoma: a distinct histopathologic and molecular genetic entity. Am J Surg Pathol. 2008;32:1239–45.
35. Kuroda N, Tanaka A. Recent classification of renal epithelial tumors. Med Mol Morphol. 2014;47:68–75.
36. Perrino CM, Grignon DJ, Williamson SR, Idrees MT, Eble JN, Cheng L. Morphological spectrum of renal cell carcinoma, unclassified: an analysis of 136 cases. Histopathology. 2018;72:305–19.
37. Sirohi D, Smith SC, Agarwal N, Maughan BL. Unclassified renal cell carcinoma: diagnostic difficulties and treatment modalities. Res Rep Urol. 2018;10:205–17.

The Mental Health, Psychological and Quality of Life Related Impact of Renal Cancers

Asanga Fernando, Sahil Suleman, Joanne Butler, and Poorna Nagasinghe

Introduction

Radio-oncological, surgical and medical anti-cancer therapies have developed at pace and scale in recent years, yet there remains a huge unmet need for the effective and timely assessment, recognition and management of psychological and psychiatric illness in cancer care. This chapter provides an overview of these challenges specifically in regard to renal cancers. It is important to highlight that the cost of not adequately recognising or treating cancer related mental illness affects patients, carers and families. The authors advocate that clinicians using this book recognise the common problems discussed and where they can locally refer such patients for evidence based assessment and management.

Across all cancers, some 10% of patients will require formal psychological and mental health support within 1 year of being diagnosed with cancer. Alarmingly, some 73% of cancer patients with depression do not receive potentially effective care for their depression. Depression is under-recognised and undertreated in cancer patients at all stages of treatment. It is important to highlight that people with cancer at an increased risk of suicide compared with the age and sex matched general population. Renal cancers are no exception to having a profoundly interlinked mental health impact from diagnosis through to survivorship and end of life. The authors recognise that there needs to be a greater awareness of the intertwined nature of cancer and mental health co-morbidity, and that in order to effectively serve the

A. Fernando (✉) · S. Suleman · P. Nagasinghe
St Georges University NHS Foundation Trust, London, UK
e-mail: asanga.fernando@kcl.ac.uk; Sahil.Suleman@stgeorges.nhs.uk; Poorna.Nagasinghe@stgeorges.nhs.uk

J. Butler
South London & Maudsley NHS Foundation Trust, London, UK
e-mail: Joanne.Butler0@stgeorges.nhs.uk; Joanne.butler@slam.nhs.uk

C. Anderson, M. Afshar (eds.), *Renal Cancer*,
https://doi.org/10.1007/978-3-030-84756-2_21

needs of patients and carers, that there needs to be greater integration and better adaptation of mental health provision across clinical cancer care.

The Psychological Impact of Renal Cancer

Renal cancer brings with it a significant range of challenges in relation to adjustment and living with uncertainty around the treatment outcome, particularly when the risk of recurrence remains. The illness itself can threaten self-image, identity, family relationships and social roles. These psychosocial factors are a common part of the cancer experience and can have an impact on disease adjustment, quality of life and potentially survival outcomes.

The psychosocial impact of renal cancer extends beyond the impact of the diagnosis and into its management. Considering more closely patient perspectives of their care, a study surveying potential sources of frustration in patients with renal cell carcinoma found 71.5% of those surveyed reported emotional or practical sources of frustration in their care, with worsened frustration associated with non-clear cell histology. Particularly common themes included a fear of recurrence or progression (15.8%), distrust of the cancer care system (12.9%) and lack of appropriate information (9.8%). Focusing on those with metastatic renal cell carcinoma, screening for psychosocial distress identified the most common causes of distress ranged across physical and functional issues (e.g. fatigue, pain, sleep, mobility), practical issues (transport, finances) and emotional (ability of family to cope).

There is also some indication that psychosocial factors can impact on cancer outcomes. In a study in patients with renal cell carcinoma, survival outcomes were also notably improved for patients who reported both high positive affect and low depressive symptoms, with a 50% reduction in mortality relative to those reporting low positive affect and high depressive symptoms, even after controlling for prognostic risk.

The UK's National Institute for Health and Care Excellence (NICE) guidance for improving outcomes in urological cancers continues to emphasise the necessity for specialist mental health professionals such as clinical psychologists and liaison psychiatrists to remain closely linked to urology teams. Importantly, the proportion of patients affected by renal cancer reporting significant and relevant distress is much higher than those self-reporting a need for psychosocial support.

Health-Related Quality of Life and Living with Renal Cancer

With developments in treatment options and patients living with renal cancer living for longer, approaches have in recent years shifted towards attending to maximising health-related quality of life (HRQoL) for these patients.

The impact of psychosocial factors on health-related quality of life (HRQoL) in renal cancer is sizeable, and indeed these factors have been shown to be more closely linked to quality of life than disease-related factors. Early intervention and education for clinicians is therefore particularly pertinent, in light of the range of preventable and treatable psychosocial concerns that have been identified within the renal cancer population (e.g. depression, anxiety, sleep difficulties, fear of cancer recurrence and pain management) and the important role they play in impacting outcomes.

In addition to the broader psychological challenges that diagnosis and treatment may cause, the particular side effect profile of differing treatments bring their own specific challenges to HRQoL across a range of domains (e.g. physical, psychological, social, practical) and with varying chronicity. Aspects of the quality of life burden of living with renal cancer also differ in how visible or easily assessed they are by clinicians. Whilst some are more routinely considered in clinics (e.g. pain, mobility, nausea), many components of HRQoL can go unidentified in this population. For instance, patients with renal cancer commonly report poorer sexual functioning than in comparable chronically ill populations, which in turn carry a significant psychological impact. It is therefore important that clinicians routinely take a holistic approach (often with the use of validated tools) to assessing HRQoL to what is already a challenging illness and treatment profile.

The Psychological and Psychiatric Impact of Treatment

Surgical treatment of urological malignancies can cause anxiety and depression related to the adjuvant effects of the treatment such as hospital admissions, pain and psychophysical changes, including changes in body structure, urinary incontinence and sexual dysfunction [1]. Psychological distress can negatively impact the outcome of surgery, impeding post surgical recovery and rehabilitation. When compared to patients undergoing surgery for other urological malignancies, patients with kidney cancer have been shown to demonstrate higher levels of preoperative anxiety and depression [1].

Studies demonstrate that patients undergoing radical nephrectomy experience higher levels of anxiety, depression and a lower quality of life compared with patients who have more parenchyma spared though the evidence is far from conclusive.

Finally, despite the limited use of chemotherapeutic agents in the management of renal cell cancers, it is important to highlight that where they are used (primarily in the treatment of rarer transitional cell cancers), that older agents such as 5-Fluoro-Uracil (5FU) would require clinicians to be aware of the possible impact on low mood and cognitive impairment, and the clear need to check for possible pharmacological interactions.

The Clinical Assessment and Mental State Examination of the Renal Cancer Patient

Renal cancers have multiple symptoms stemming from disease and treatments. Reported prevalence of emotional distress in cancer patients varies widely across studies [2]. Psychological distress is significantly higher among females after diagnosis and throughout treatment for non-metastatic renal cell carcinoma (RCC) [3]. Symptoms that are most prominent among localised RCC are irritability, fatigue, worry and sleep disturbance [4].

Renal cancer patients are found to have comorbid anxiety, depression and post-traumatic stress symptoms in an increasing frequency [5]. Depressive symptoms are a key predictor of survival in renal cell carcinoma patients with potential links to dysregulation of cortisol and inflammatory biology [6]. A high prevalence of depressive and anxiety symptoms were reported among Chinese bladder and renal cancer patients in a cross sectional study [7].

There are different approaches to diagnose major depression in cancer patients [8]. Various different validated screening tools for depression amongst people with cancer have been reviewed [9, 10], and it is important to recognise that these, or indeed the widely used distress thermometer, which forms part of the holistic needs assessment used in UK cancer centres is not alone sufficient to identify major depression [11] and should not be a substitute for a detailed history and mental state examination.

Hodgkiss [11] highlights that screening only leads to better care if there are clear pathways to treatment once a psychiatric disorder is detected.

In assessment of a patient's mood [11], it is important to consider that the biological and somatic symptoms of depression and anxiety are often unreliable guides to mood in the cancer patient. Emphasis should be placed on the psychological symptoms of depression including hopelessness, helplessness and worthlessness, anhedonia (the loss of capacity to experience pleasure), and suicidal thoughts and plans.

Posttraumatic stress symptoms (PTSS) occur both independently and comorbid with depressive symptoms in patients with RCC [12]. Mixed anxiety and depression is associated with poorer psychosocial and treatment outcomes, worse quality of life, poorer adherence to treatment, slower recovery, greater suicide risk, and higher cost-utilization [13]. A large national cohort study in the UK, found patients with a urological malignancy are five times more likely to complete suicide compared to the general population [14].

Therefore it is paramount for clinicians to conduct a risk assessment bearing in mind that there is a high risk of completed suicide in cancer patients. Efforts should be made to explore the degree of intent, planning and preparation, whilst also considering other risks such as the risk of self-neglect, poor engagement with treatment and exploitation in the context of cognitive impairment.

A clinician should focus on completing a full bio-psycho-social clinical assessment that holistically review the needs of the patient [15]. This is likely to include a full psychiatric and physical health history, mental state examination, consideration of the risk factors and timeframes.

In the context of kidney cancer, appropriate assessment of cognitive function and mood should take place in those with renal cell cancer. Given that there is a possibility of brain metastases, brain imaging would be indicated in the presence of cognitive impairment on clinical examination. It is also appropriate to consider monitoring thyroid function tests given the possibility of clinical hypothyroidism particularly if vascular endothelial growth factor receptor (VEGFR) inhibitors are used.

Key Points

- Renal cancer patients may be affected by both psychological and psychiatric co-morbidity, for which effective, evidence based treatments exist.
- Across all cancers, some 10% of patients will require formal psychological and mental health support within 1 year of being diagnosed.
- The authors advocate for a Multi-disciplinary team (MDT) based approach to the assessment and management of psychological and mental health co-morbidity in cancer patients, with local access to counselling, psychology and psychiatry with expertise in managing cancer patients. Clinicians should familiarise themselves with evidence based, local referral pathways for cancer psychological support and mental healthcare.
- The authors highlight recognising the adverse impact of the CoVid-19 pandemic on cancer patients and the adverse impact that this has had on their cancer journeys and mental health.
- Service integration should also consider the opportunities for research and educational collaboration [14].
- Alarmingly, some 73% of cancer patients with depression do not receive potentially effective care for their depression
- Depression is under-recognised and under-treated in cancer patients at all stages of treatment.
- The psychosocial impact of renal cancer extends beyond the impact of the diagnosis and into its management.
- In assessment of a patient's mood emphasis should be placed on the psychological symptoms of depression including hopelessness, helplessness and worthlessness, anhedonia (the loss of capacity to experience pleasure), and suicidal thoughts and plans as biological symptoms of depression can be an unreliable marker of mood in the cancer patient.
- With developments in treatment options and patients living with renal cancer living for longer, there has been a greater emphasis on measuring and maximising health-related quality of life (HRQoL).

References

1. Pastore A, Maruccia S, Mir AB, Palleschi G, Carbone A, Bellonch NC, Palou J. Psychological distress in patients undergoing surgery for urological cancer: a prospective single centre cross-sectional study. Eur Urol Suppl. 2017;16(3). https://doi.org/10.1016/s1569-9056(17)30729-7.

2. Linden W, Vodermaier A, Mackenzie R, Greig D. Anxiety and depression after cancer diagnosis: prevalence rates by cancer type, gender, and age. J Affect Disord. 2012;141(2–3):343–51. https://doi.org/10.1016/j.jad.2012.03.025.
3. Ajaj R, Cáceres JOH, Berlin A, Wallis CJD, Chandrasekar T, Klaassen Z, Goldberg H. Gender-based psychological and physical distress differences in patients diagnosed with non-metastatic renal cell carcinoma. World J Urol. 2020. https://doi.org/10.1007/s00345-019-03057-2.
4. Harding G, Cella D, Robinson D, Mahadevia PJ, Clark J, Revicki DA. Symptom burden among patients with renal cell carcinoma (RCC): content for a symptom index. Health Qual Life Outcomes. 2007;5(1). https://doi.org/10.1186/1477-7525-5-34.
5. Li M, Wang L. The associations of psychological stress with depressive and anxiety symptoms among Chinese bladder and renal cancer patients: the mediating role of resilience. PLoS One. 2016;11(4). https://doi.org/10.1371/journal.pone.0154729.
6. Cohen L, Cole SW, Sood AK, Prinsloo S, Kirschbaum C, Arevalo JMG, Pisters L. Depressive symptoms and cortisol rhythmicity predict survival in patients with renal cell carcinoma: role of inflammatory signaling. PLoS One. 2012;7(8). https://doi.org/10.1371/journal.pone.0042324.
7. Yang Y-L, Liu L, Li M-Y, Shi M, Wang L. Psychological disorders and psychosocial resources of patients with newly diagnosed bladder and kidney cancer: a cross-sectional study. PLoS One. 2016;11(5). https://doi.org/10.1371/journal.pone.0155607.
8. Breitbart W, Bruera E, Chochinov H, Lynch M. Neuropsychiatric syndromes and psychological symptoms in patients with advanced cancer. J Pain Symptom Manage. 1995;10(2):131–41. https://doi.org/10.1016/0885-3924(94)00075-v.
9. Mitchell AJ, Bultz BD. Psychological assessment in psychopharmacology. In: Psychopharmacology in oncology and palliative care. Berlin: Springer; 2014. p. 49–67.
10. Vodermaier A, Linden W, Siu C. Screening for emotional distress in cancer patients: a systematic review of assessment instruments. J Natl Cancer Inst. 2009;101(21):1464–88.
11. Hodgkiss A. Biological psychiatry of cancer and cancer treatment. Oxford: Oxford University Press; 2016.
12. Thekdi SM, Milbury K, Spelman A, Wei Q, Wood C, Matin SF, Cohen L. Posttraumatic stress and depressive symptoms in renal cell carcinoma: association with quality of life and utility of single-item distress screening. Psychooncology. 2015;24(11):1477–84. https://doi.org/10.1002/pon.3758.
13. Brintzenhofe-Szoc KM, Levin TT, Li Y, Kissane DW, Zabora JR. Mixed anxiety/depression symptoms in a large cancer cohort: prevalence by cancer type. Psychosomatics. 2009;50(4):383–91. https://doi.org/10.1176/appi.psy.50.4.383.
14. Afshar M, Bardoli A, Tanner J-R, Macfarlane N, Pickering L, Anderson C, Patel P. Patients with urological malignancy are 5 times more likely to commit suicide: a large national cohort study. Eur Urol Suppl. 2018;17(2). https://doi.org/10.1016/s1569-9056(18)30920-5.
15. Bostwick JM, Pabbati C, Geske JR, Mckean AJ. Suicide attempt as a risk factor for completed suicide: even more lethal than we knew. Am J Psychiatry. 2016;173(11):1094–100. https://doi.org/10.1176/appi.ajp.2016.15070854.

Training in Minimal Invasive Surgery

Elio Mazzone, Sergi Beato, and Alexandre Mottrie

Introduction

Minimally invasive surgery (MIS) is a widespread approach in urology [1] (Fig. 1). However, the decision to use this approach relies on different factors. For instance, limited experience with minimally invasive approaches, economic reasons, lack of training and fear of complications can lead to choose an open operation instead of MIS. For many surgical procedures, MIS has been shown to offer advantages compared with open procedures such as decreased postoperative pain and morbidity, blood loss, shorter hospital stay, and better cosmetic results [2–4]. Moreover, surgical outcomes such as oncological control and functional results are non-inferior for MIS compared to open surgery.

To date, the laparoscopic approach is the gold standard for some surgical procedures such as radical nephrectomy or in rapidly expanding use like in radical prostatectomy, radical cystectomy or partial nephrectomy. Consequently, training in laparoscopic and robotic surgery is a rising topic of discussion in the literature [5, 6].

Historical training models such as Halsted [7] ("see one, do one, teach one") are outdated, and the learning methods for the new generations of surgeons require a change. However, this need for adequate training faces restrictions related with

E. Mazzone (✉)
Division of Oncology/Unit of Urology, URI, IRCCS Ospedale San Raffaele, Milan, Italy

Department of Urology, Onze Lieve Vrouw Hospital, Aalst, Belgium

ORSI Academy, Melle, Belgium

Vita-Salute San Raffaele University, Milan, Italy

S. Beato · A. Mottrie
Department of Urology, Onze Lieve Vrouw Hospital, Aalst, Belgium

ORSI Academy, Melle, Belgium

C. Anderson, M. Afshar (eds.), *Renal Cancer*,
https://doi.org/10.1007/978-3-030-84756-2_22

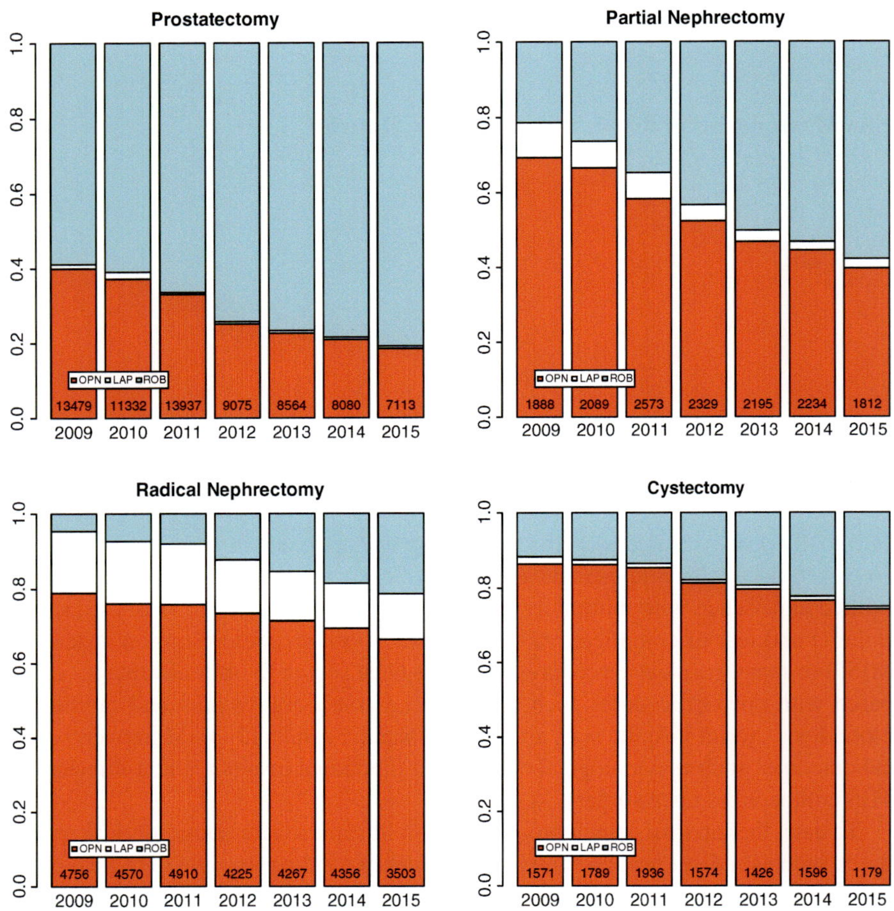

Fig. 1 Barplot reporting the distribution of surgical approach for major uro-oncological surgery performed in United States between 2009 and 2015 (data extracted from the National Inpatient Sample database)

reduced working hours and ethical considerations that increase the difficulty of achieving optimal training.

The time to achieve the necessary skills to perform a procedure and accomplish an optimal performance is known as the learning curve. Specifically, a learning curve is a graphical representation of the concept of the improvement of surgical outcomes with the increasing of surgical experience [8]. The surgical outcomes that are generally assessed in a learning curve are related to technical aspects (i.e. operative time, transfusion rate), complications, oncological and/or functional results. During this initial learning phase, the possibility of complications and worse postoperative outcomes is higher compared to more experienced surgeons [8, 9]. Based on this premise, multiple training methods have been proposed in order to reduce the length of the initial learning curve phase in MIS and to progressively increase trainee's responsibility with minimal impact on patient's outcome. The aim of the current chapter is to describe the most recent evidence on the different methods of training designated to improve surgical skills in MIS, particularly in robot-assisted urological surgery with a specific focus in robot-assisted partial nephrectomy (RAPN).

Initial Steps

In the first steps of training, it is essential to achieve basic knowledge [10]. The goal is to obtain good baseline knowledge of different techniques in MIS, to understand the environment of the operation room and to be introduced to the role of specific MIS characteristics, such as trocar placement or robot positioning. In this initial phase, in addition to this insight into surgical techniques and MIS characteristics, case observation, E-learning, courses and work-shops should be highlighted.

Case Observation

Observation of an experienced surgeon performing an MIS procedure is commonly practised during early stages of learning. This occurs despite there being limited evidence that it improves surgical ability. It does however allow familiarisation of the procedure and it offers an optimal model to imitate when performing the intervention. Moreover, it is an opportunity to ask questions to address gaps in knowledge. Although there is no evidence in the literature of its effectiveness, it is a recommended first step in multiple training models [11, 12].

E-Learning

The use of computer technology offers easy access to knowledge in a flexible way and without time or location restrictions, with the possibility of evaluating and obtaining instant feedback. E-learning helps to simplify education and has become another established methodology for acquiring knowledge [13, 14].

Courses and Workshops

Attending a course in a dedicated skills lab increases the motivation and attention of trainees and it can help to improve surgical skills faster. The attendance of accessible and periodic courses, aimed at improving specific skills, obtaining feedback and a concrete evaluation, has been shown to have a beneficial impact on the surgical performance of most participants [15, 16].

Simulation Training

The use of a simulator allows the surgeon to perform procedures in a controlled, safe environment without risk for patients. Moreover, it is also useful for familiarising with new technologies and instruments and for allowing the improvement of surgical psychomotor and visuospatial skills. It also allows the repetition of a task and can be interrupted as needed, providing an opportunity for immediate feedback. It has been reported that the early use of simulators may be associated with reduced training costs, by its impact on patient safety, and with error reduction. In other medical fields, such as interventional radiology or central venous catheter insertion, simulation training has evidenced to reduce complications [17–19]. This essential step has been demonstrated that could be retained over time, even if surgeons do not practice MIS for approximately 2 years [20]. Moreover, thanks to the application of standardized platforms with objective evaluation, the use of simulation training may be provide a record that a trainee has attained the prescribed level of proficiency and has achieved enough surgical skills for a determined procedure. This method has been introduced in different surgical examinations such as the ESU-initiated European Basic Laparoscopic Urological Skills (EBLUS) or the Fundamentals of Laparoscopic Surgery (FLS) [15, 21, 22]. Different simulation training models can be categorized into basic and advanced training models.

Basic Training Models

Basic training models enable the ability to improve basic laparoscopic skills such as two-dimensional vision, bimanual dexterity, and handling of instruments to minimise tremor. They include:

Virtual Reality

Virtual reality consists in a simulated model, designed by software, that can represent a complete urological procedure or an exercise to improve a specific technical skill. Virtual reality has the advantage of making the simulator easily accessible without the use of disposable material and with minimal supervision needed. It offers the possibility of analyzing and scoring performance of trainee's procedural skills using objective and transparent metrics. Despite the potential advantages, the main limitations are related to the high initial cost and the inability to achieve a realism comparable to a real-life case. However, the improvement of the graphic designs and the recreated feedback can turn virtual reality into the ideal method to improve technical skills in MIS [18, 21].

Box Trainer

The box trainer is a physical simulation of the surgical scenario of laparoscopic or robotic surgery. It requires the use of a camera, a monitor and laparoscopic trocars. Inside the box, the use of inanimate and synthetic models allows the trainee to develop basic or advanced laparoscopic skills such as visuospatial perception or suturing. Advantages of box trainers are low price, great flexibility, and availability, as well as being portable allowing, for example, the use at home [23]. On the other hand, the anatomic fidelity is low, and the correct representability of tissues texture is difficult to achieve. Several studies have highlighted its benefits, comparing the use of traditional training alone versus traditional training plus structured training on box trainers with significantly higher improvement in surgical skills [24, 25].

Advanced Training Models

Advanced training models are ideal for performing complex procedures in models that reproduce human anatomy and tissues. They include:

Animals

The use of live animals or part of their tissues represent an advanced model to perform complete urological procedures. Advantages of animal models are tissue texture, comparable to the human body, similar anatomy and, for live models, the opportunity to simulate intraoperative complications. On the other hand, they are expensive , as well as require specialized personnel, in addition to the ethical approvals when using live animals. Despite these limitations, it is the model preferred by experienced trainees in anonymous questionnaires because inanimate models such as virtual reality or box trainer are perceived as less stimulating [26]. For example, the use of the animal model is the last step before a supervised performance in clinical practice in some of the urological standardized curriculum for robotic surgery, both for radical prostatectomy and partial nephrectomy [12, 27].

Cadaver

With the modernization of preservation methods, the use of human cadavers can play an important role in surgical training. It allows us to perform procedures by real encounter anatomy. Similar to animal models, its use its limited by high cost and the requirement of centers with specific facilities [28].

Taken together, despite all these available simulation tools, there is no evidence of the superiority of any model over the others in skill acquisition [29]. There are also controversies about duration, tasks, facilities, mentoring and availability [16,

30]. In the light of these pieces of evidence, the need for structured training programs, as well as standardized evaluation methods, has become a priority in the field of robotic surgery. To achieve this goal, the European Association of Urology Robotic Urology Section (ERUS) has developed the structured and validated curricula in urology [11, 12]. Specifically, these curricula describe validated tools to increase preclinical exposure: initial steps consist of e-learning module and observation, next step composed with simulation-based training (virtual reality, and dry/wet lab) and finally a modular console training until full procedural performance is achieved. Amongst these curricula, a specific training program on robot-assisted partial nephrectomy (RAPN) was proposed with the aim of helping surgeons willing to start robotic renal cancer surgery [12] (Fig. 2). After the initial e-Learning phase and an intensive week of preclinical simulation-based training, this RAPN-specific pathway proceeds with a clinical modular training that is based on the

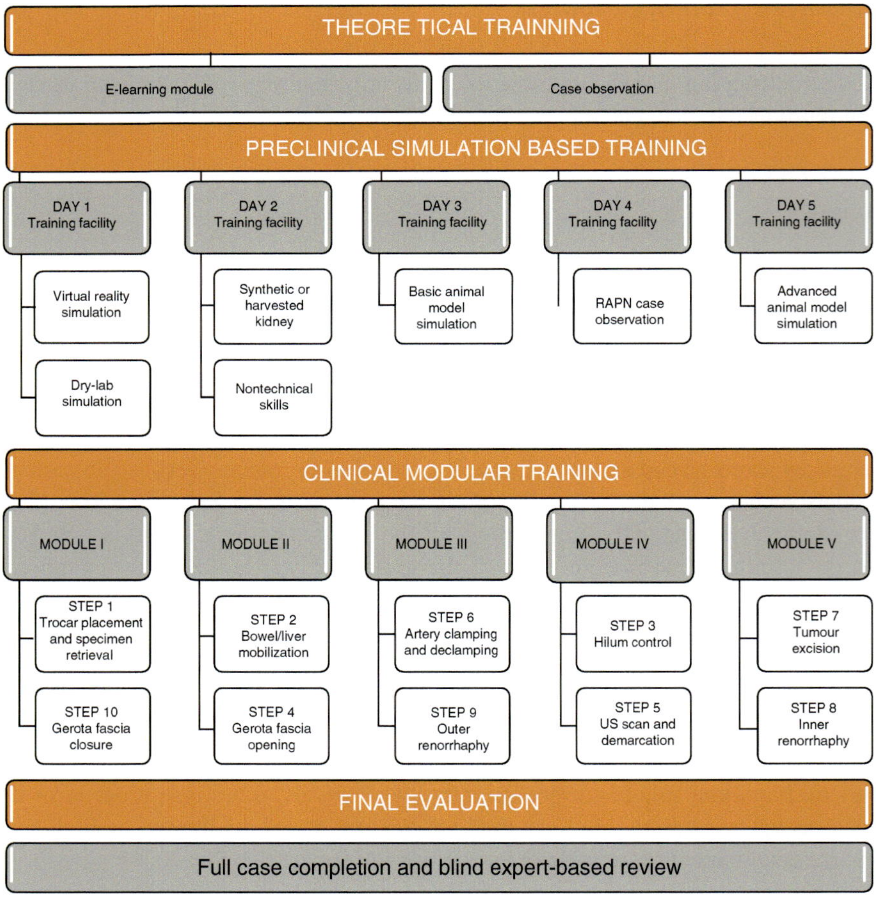

Fig. 2 Structure of the European Association of Urology Robotic Urology Section curriculum for robot-assisted partial nephrectomy defined by the modified Delphi consensus process

partition of a complete RAPN case in 10 fundamental steps, in order to divide the procedure into replicable modules to be learned [12]. Specifically, five modules including ten specific steps were proposed and ordered according to increasing level of step complexity after a Delphi consensus process. Of note, the RAPN curriculum course is the first training curriculum validated in a clinical setting, demonstrating that performing a supervised clinical modular training has no detrimental effect on patient outcomes compared to RAPN entirely performed by an experienced surgeon. This data demonstrate that the program allows a safe transition from the beginning of surgical experience through increasing responsibility to the independent completion of a full case [12]. Moreover, the effect of the ERUS simulation-based training on trainee's skills improvement was confirmed through virtual reality comparing exercise completion metrics before and after the course [11, 21].

Team Training And Cognitive/Non-technical Skills

Despite the critical importance of technical skill in the surgical field, other abilities are necessary when performing MIS procedures. Indeed, what also defines experienced surgeons are their non-technical skills which are categorized into cognitive skills and social skills [31]. The greater technical complexity of robotic surgical procedures requires adequate development of cognitive abilities, which include situational awareness, decision-making, and planning. Similarly, we have to highlight the importance of social skills that include communication, teamwork and leadership skills. For example, ineffective communication may contribute to >40% of errors during surgery [32, 33]. The development of other nontechnical skills such as teamwork, communication, leadership, situational awareness, and decision-making play an essential role in ensuring patient safety.

Similar to technical skills, the attendance of didactic sessions and practices in a controlled environment allow the improvement of these abilities. The use of decision-based simulation models has been shown to improve non-technical skills [34]. Also, team training can improve communication abilities, team integration, and decision-making process related to teamwork [35]. Despite these alternatives, there is conflicting evidence in the literature on this topic. Specifically, we can find contradictory results with studies showing superior task performance in a dyad team, but other studies show equivalent performances for both dyad team and individual training [36, 37].

Mentorship

Once the necessary knowledge and skills have been acquired, the end of the learning curve process should culminate in performing surgical procedures on patients. In this last phase, the role of the mentor becomes relevant [30]. The classic figure of the mentor already present in historical models [7] allows sharing knowledge and practical teaching "in situ" in order to complete the skills acquisition. In this context, modular teaching has become crucial, since it divides the procedure into several steps categorized according to the level of difficulty. By doing so, the required technical skills can be developed progressively until reaching the necessary level to be able to perform the entire procedure. Although the mentor is usually presented by an experienced surgeon from the same institution of the trainee, there are currently alternative models, such as a formal fellowship with an expert surgeon in the field. Similarly, tele mentoring also represents an alternative to classical mentorship. Through real-time video links, a mentor can provide guidance during a procedure despite being in another location. However, tele mentoring should still be considered as experimental and validation studies of its efficacy are needed [10, 38].

Current Nuances and Future Perspective

As the robotic technology advances, surgeons training has to be focused on machinery type, as well as on new surgery techniques. Uniquely, from a clinical standpoint, surgical training programmes have to accommodate for innovations in robot-assisted surgery (e.g. clinical availability of different robot-assisted surgical platforms) in order to guarantee virtually the same clinical outcomes among different centers. This added complexity underlines the fundamental need to design standardized and validated training programmes. Despite not having reached a final consensus on the optimal combination of training methods and technological improvements, the increase of opportunities to improve technical skills and the development of new methodologies for optimizing skills evaluation [15, 22, 39, 40], provide an optimistic scenario of future directions in MIS training.

References

1. Mazzone E, Mistretta FA, Knipper S, Tian Z, Larcher A, Widmer H, et al. Contemporary national assessment of robot-assisted surgery rates and total hospital charges for major surgical uro-oncological procedures in the United States. J Endourol. 2019;33(6):438–47.
2. Leow JJ, Reese SW, Jiang W, Lipsitz SR, Bellmunt J, Trinh Q-D, et al. Propensity-matched comparison of morbidity and costs of open and robot-assisted radical cystectomies: a contemporary population-based analysis in the United States. Eur Urol. 2014;66(3):569–76.
3. Yaxley JW, Coughlin GD, Chambers SK, Occhipinti S, Samaratunga H, Zajdlewicz L, et al. Robot-assisted laparoscopic prostatectomy versus open radical retropubic prostatectomy: early outcomes from a randomised controlled phase 3 study. Lancet Lond Engl. 2016;388(10049):1057–66.
4. Larcher A, Capitanio U, De Naeyer G, Fossati N, D'Hondt F, Muttin F, et al. Is robot-assisted surgery contraindicated in the case of partial nephrectomy for complex tumours or relevant comorbidities? A comparative analysis of morbidity, renal function, and oncologic outcomes. Eur Urol Oncol. 2018;1(1):61–8.

5. Birch DW, Bonjer HJ, Crossley C, Burnett G, de Gara C, Gomes A, et al. Canadian consensus conference on the development of training and practice standards in advanced minimally invasive surgery. Can J Surg. 2009;52(4):321–7.
6. Janetschek G. Standardized and validated training programs for robot-assisted laparoscopy: the challenge of the future. Eur Urol. 2019;75(5):786–7.
7. Romero P, Günther P, Kowalewski K-F, Friedrich M, Schmidt MW, Trent SM, et al. Halsted's "see one, do one, and teach one" versus Peyton's four-step approach: a randomized trial for training of laparoscopic suturing and knot tying. J Surg Educ. 2018;75(2):510–5.
8. Vickers AJ, Bianco FJ, Serio AM, Eastham JA, Schrag D, Klein EA, et al. The surgical learning curve for prostate cancer control after radical prostatectomy. JNCI J Natl Cancer Inst. 2007;99(15):1171–7.
9. Larcher A, Muttin F, Peyronnet B, De Naeyer G, Khene Z-E, Dell'Oglio P, et al. The learning curve for robot-assisted partial nephrectomy: impact of surgical experience on perioperative outcomes. Eur Urol. 2019;75(2):253–6.
10. Brunckhorst O, Volpe A, van der Poel H, Mottrie A, Ahmed K. Training, simulation, the learning curve, and how to reduce complications in urology. Eur Urol Focus. 2016;2(1):10–8.
11. Volpe A, Ahmed K, Dasgupta P, Ficarra V, Novara G, van der Poel H, et al. Pilot validation study of the European Association of Urology robotic training curriculum. Eur Urol. 2015;68(2):292–9.
12. Larcher A, De Naeyer G, Turri F, Dell'Oglio P, Capitanio U, Collins JW, et al. The ERUS curriculum for robot-assisted partial nephrectomy: structure definition and pilot clinical validation. Eur Urol. 2019; https://doi.org/10.1016/j.eururo.2019.02.031.
13. Evgeniou E, Loizou P. The theoretical base of E-learning and its role in surgical education. J Surg Educ. 2012;69(5):665–9.
14. Chumley-Jones HS, Dobbie A, Alford CL. Web-based learning: sound educational method or hype? A review of the evaluation literature. Acad Med J Assoc Am Med Coll. 2002;77(10 Suppl):S86–93.
15. Somani BK, Van Cleynenbreugel B, Gözen A-S, Skolarikos A, Wagner C, Beatty J, et al. Outcomes of European Basic Laparoscopic Urological Skills (EBLUS) examinations: results from European School of Urology (ESU) and EAU Section of Uro-Technology (ESUT) over 6 years (2013–2018). Eur Urol Focus. 2019; https://doi.org/10.1016/j.euf.2019.01.007.
16. Torres-de la Roche LA, Leicher L, Steljes I, Eidswick J, Larionov O, de Wilde MS, et al. Training and qualification in gynecological minimal access surgery: a systematic review. Best Pract Res Clin Obstet Gynaecol. 2019;59:2–11.
17. Achurra P, Lagos A, Avila R, Tejos R, Buckel E, Alvarado J, et al. Allowing new opportunities in advanced laparoscopy training using a full high-definition training box. Surg Innov. 2017;24(1):66–71.
18. Yang C, Kalinitschenko U, Helmert JR, Weitz J, Reissfelder C, Mees ST. Transferability of laparoscopic skills using the virtual reality simulator. Surg Endosc. 2018;32(10):4132–7.
19. Gallagher AG, Traynor O. Simulation in surgery: opportunity or threat? Ir J Med Sci. 2008;177(4):283–7.
20. Molinas CR, Campo R. Retention of laparoscopic psychomotor skills after a structured training program depends on the quality of the training and on the complexity of the task. Gynecol Surg. 2016;13(4):395–402.
21. Larcher A, Turri F, Bianchi L, Dell'Oglio P, Collins J, Capitanio U, et al. Virtual reality validation of the ERUS simulation-based training programmes: results from a high-volume training centre for robot-assisted surgery. Eur Urol. 2019;75(5):885–7.
22. Cullinan DR, Schill MR, DeClue A, Salles A, Wise PE, Awad MM. Fundamentals of laparoscopic surgery: not only for senior residents. J Surg Educ. 2017;74(6):e51–4.
23. Thinggaard E, Konge L, Bjerrum F, Strandbygaard J, Gögenur I, Spanager L. Take-home training in a simulation-based laparoscopy course. Surg Endosc. 2017;31(4):1738–45.

24. Supe A, Prabhu R, Harris I, Downing S, Tekian A. Structured training on box trainers for first year surgical residents: does it improve retention of laparoscopic skills? A randomized controlled study. J Surg Educ. 2012;69(5):624–32.
25. Clevin L, Grantcharov TP. Does box model training improve surgical dexterity and economy of movement during virtual reality laparoscopy? A randomised trial. Acta Obstet Gynecol Scand. 2008;87(1):99–103.
26. Shetty S, Zevin B, Grantcharov TP, Roberts KE, Duffy AJ. Perceptions, training experiences, and preferences of surgical residents toward laparoscopic simulation training: a resident survey. J Surg Educ. 2014;71(5):727–33.
27. Ahmed K, Khan R, Mottrie A, Lovegrove C, Abaza R, Ahlawat R, et al. Development of a standardised training curriculum for robotic surgery: a consensus statement from an international multidisciplinary group of experts. BJU Int. 2015;116(1):93–101.
28. Lim CP, Roberts M, Chalhoub T, Waugh J, Delgaty L. Cadaveric surgery in core gynaecology training: a feasibility study. Gynecol Surg. 2018;15(1)
29. Nagendran M, Toon CD, Davidson BR, Gurusamy KS, Cochrane Hepato-Biliary Group, editor. Laparoscopic surgical box model training for surgical trainees with no prior laparoscopic experience. Cochrane Database Syst Rev. 2014; https://doi.org/10.1002/14651858.CD010479.pub2.
30. De Win G, Everaerts W, De Ridder D, Peeraer G. Laparoscopy training in Belgium: results from a nationwide survey, in urology, gynecology, and general surgery residents. Adv Med Educ Pract. 2015;6:55–63.
31. Collins JW, Dell'Oglio P, Hung AJ, Brook NR. The importance of technical and non-technical skills in robotic surgery training. Eur Urol Focus. 2018;4(5):674–6.
32. Gawande AA, Zinner MJ, Studdert DM, Brennan TA. Analysis of errors reported by surgeons at three teaching hospitals. Surgery. 2003;133(6):614–21.
33. Lingard L, Espin S, Whyte S, Regehr G, Baker G, Reznick R, et al. Communication failures in the operating room: an observational classification of recurrent types and effects. Qual Saf Health Care. 2004;13(5):330–4.
34. Nguyen N, Watson WD, Dominguez E. Simulation-based communication training for general surgery and obstetrics and gynecology residents. J Surg Educ. 2019;76(3):856–63.
35. Andrew B, Plachta S, Salud L, Pugh CM. Development and evaluation of a decision-based simulation for assessment of team skills. Surgery. 2012;152(2):152–7.
36. Zheng B, Verjee F, Lomax A, MacKenzie CL. Video analysis of endoscopic cutting task performed by one versus two operators. Surg Endosc. 2005;19(10):1388–95.
37. Seal FB, He W, Pinzon D, Zheng B. Training of laparoscopic novices both individually and in dyads using a simulation task. J Robot Surg. 2020;14(1):29–33.
38. Schlachta CM, Nguyen NT, Ponsky T, Dunkin B. Project 6 Summit: SAGES Telementoring Initiative. Surg Endosc. 2016;30(9):3665–72.
39. Burden C, Fox R, Lenguerrand E, Hinshaw K, Draycott TJ, James M. Curriculum development for basic gynaecological laparoscopy with comparison of expert trainee opinions; prospective cross-sectional observational study. Eur J Obstet Gynecol Reprod Biol. 2014;180:1–7.
40. Fisher RA, Dasgupta P, Mottrie A, Volpe A, Khan MS, Challacombe B, et al. An over-view of robot assisted surgery curricula and the status of their validation. Int J Surg. 2015;13:115–23.

The Role of Big Data in Renal Cell Carcinoma Research and Management

Hosam Serag and Prashant Patel

Introduction

Great technological development has been achieved during the last decade in the fields of data generation and computational analysis, leading to the coining of terms such as "the big data era" [1]. The term "big data" has gained widespread use and can be defined as "large, diverse, complex, longitudinal, and/or distributed data sets generated from instruments, sensors, internet transactions, email, video, click streams, and/or all other digital sources available today and in the future" [2].

The analysis of Big Data exceeds the capabilities of humans alone, and their emergence has led to dependence on machines. Hence came the development of various methods that were grouped under the broad term of artificial intelligence (AI) [3]. The use of Big Data was introduced into various sciences, including medicine [4].

The main methods of AI utilized in medicine include machine learning (ML), natural language processing (NLP), deep learning, and artificial neural networks as well as computer vision. All these methods depend on identification of features and patterns from provided datasets, computing algorithms, then inferring models that can be used to support decision-making. Applications of AI in medicine include, though not limited to, analysis of electronic medical record (EMR) and medical imaging as well as precision medicine [5, 6].

The application of AI has extended to the field of urology, as is the case with several medical specialties, to improve the diagnosis of urological conditions and the prediction of outcome [7].

H. Serag
University Hospitals Birmingham NHS Foundation Trust, Birmingham, UK
e-mail: hosam.serag@uhb.nhs.uk

P. Patel (✉)
Institute of Cancer and Genomic Sciences, University of Birmingham, Birmingham, UK
e-mail: p.patel@bham.ac.uk

C. Anderson, M. Afshar (eds.), *Renal Cancer*,
https://doi.org/10.1007/978-3-030-84756-2_23

Renal cell carcinoma (RCC) ranks as the sixth and tenth most frequently diagnosed cancers in men and women, respectively [8]. The rate of newly diagnosed RCC cases has increased, partially due to the increase in incidental detection of renal masses during abdominal imaging [9].

This chapter summarizes the application of Big Data and AI in management of RCC. Big Data that are generated from radiological imaging (radiomics), histopathological examination (pathomics), and molecular subtyping (genomics) are fueled into techniques of AI that produce models which have the potential to improve management of RCC.

The use of Big Data techniques can help improve the diagnosis of RCC by differentiating it from other benign renal masses. The differentiation of histopathology subtypes and the grading of the tumor can impact the planning of treatment. This information enables prognostication of disease course and patients' outcomes. Another important, emerging aspect is precision medicine where the therapy is tailored according to individual patient's characteristics. Furthermore, Big Data techniques have been evaluated as methods to monitor and assess the effect of therapy.

Genomics in Renal Cell Carcinoma

Study of genome was facilitated by the advent of less costly genotype arrays and the large size of samples provided by biobanks. Studies have provided important insights into risk factors and the pathogenesis of kidney diseases [10, 11].

Multiple technologies are available to study the genome, such as whole-exome sequencing (WES) and whole-genome sequencing (WGS). Both WGS and WES provide information about substitutions, deletions, insertions, duplications, copy number changes, inversions, and translocations of the genome. However, genome sequencing is not widely used in clinical medicine. This is attributed to the vast amount of data provided by WGS that exceed the current human's ability to interpret. Moreover, it is difficult to assess the functional impact of genetic alterations, particularly those in the non-coding regions [12].

Some genes were identified to be related to RCC, including BR-CA1 associated protein-1 (BAP-1), protein polybromo-1 (PBRM1) or SET domain containing 2 enzyme (SETD2) and lysine-specific demethylase 5C (KDM5C) [13–15]. The PBRM1 mutation has been associated with favorable survival across all treatments. On the other hand, BAP1 loss and SETD2 have been linked to advanced stage of disease and poor survival [16].

The use of biomarkers and signatures that are derived from the expression of several genes has been assessed for the prediction of the overall survival of patients with clear cell RCC and their prognosis. Li et al. [17] created a risk score model based on 15 genes utilizing The Cancer Genome Atlas dataset. The model correlated well with the prognosis and survival, with the higher risk group having poorer prognosis and survival compared to the lower risk group. The risk groups were associated with tumor features the primary tumor size and grade.

Another model was developed by Li et al. [18] to predict stages of clear cell RCC samples, based also on datasets from The Cancer Genome Atlas. The model consisted of 23 genes and showed an accuracy of 81.2% and good discriminatory power (AUC 0.86); these results superseded state-of-the-art models that had an accuracy of 72.6% with an AUC of 0.81.

Radiomics in Renal Cell Carcinoma

Radiomics refer to the extraction of large amounts of high-dimensional quantitative features from radiological images that is used for decision support. Several quantitative features can be extracted from radiological images, including data pertaining to size, shape, morphology, and parenchymal heterogeneity [19]. The application of radiomics in RCC is an area of active research, with a plethora of studies published addressing the differentiation of RCC from benign lesions, grading, and assessment of response to therapy.

A recent systematic review and meta-analysis [20] which assessed radiomics in renal cancer included 57 studies (with a total number of 4590 patients). Out of the 57 included, 22 studies assessed models to differentiate benign from malignant lesions, 15 studies addressed the differentiation of subtypes, and 12 studies investigated treatment response and outcome prediction.

Differentiating Renal Cell Carcinoma from Benign Lesions

Studies have investigated pixel distribution and texture features analysis as quantitative methods that can be used to develop algorithms for the identification of differences between RCC and benign lesions [21].

Lipid-poor angiomyolipomas (AMLs) and oncocytomas are common renal neoplasms that are sometimes mistaken for RCC, resulting in unnecessary interventions [22–24].

Radiomic research showed that heterogeneity of the mass tends to be less in case of AMLs compared to RCC [25]. A meta-analysis by Ursprung et al. [20] was carried out based on data from ten studies using the random effects model. The summary effect size showed a diagnostic odds ratio of 5.89 (95% confidence interval 4.02–8.23, $p < 0.001$) for radiomics models differentiating lipid-poor AML from RCC, with moderate heterogeneity across the studies due to considerable variability in the radiomics features utilized.

Differences were also detected between RCC and oncocytomas, where the latter were found to be less heterogeneous than clear cell RCC, but more heterogeneous than papillary RCC and had more negatively skewed pixel histograms than RCC [26].

Assessment of Renal Cell Carcinoma Aggressiveness

Less aggressive management is recommended for early and more indolent types of RCC; thus, identification of tumor aggressiveness is required [27]. The nuclear grade is considered among the most important prognostic factors that impact treatment decision [28]. Unfortunately, determination of the nuclear grade on biopsy is challenging and is prone to sampling bias, as evidenced by upgrading of the nuclear grade at surgery in approximately 40% of cases [29]. Radiomics can help identify texture features of the more aggressive tumors.

Models were developed by ML from extracted texture features of computerized tomography (CT) images in previous studies. These models were able to differentiate high and low grades in lesions of clear cell RCC, with accuracy ranging from 0.73 to 0.93 [21, 30–34]. A model was developed by Schieda et al. [35] that identified high grade chromophobe RCC against low grade tumors as the former were found to be larger, higher in attenuation, and more heterogeneous at unenhanced CT. The model had an AUC of 0.84.

Moreover, Vendrami et al. [36] created a model that was derived from magnetic resonance (MR) imaging texture features. They reported that the addition of texture analysis to the conventional qualitative MR imaging features increased the probability of differentiating type I from the more aggressive type II of papillary RCC.

Another application of Big Data has combined radiomics with genetic profiling and is referred to as Radiogenomics, which correlates imaging features with the expression of specific genes [37–39]. Several CT and MR imaging features have been reported in association with gene expression in clear cell RCC, and these features and genes were in turn associated with survival of patients as well as metastasis and recurrence of RCC. Radiogenomics may be more valuable than genetic profiling. The high diversity of intratumoral mutation in clear cell RCC may not be reflected in the gene expression profile tested on a single biopsy sample. On the other hand, radiogenomics can enable inferring the gene expression profile from imaging features of the lesion [40].

Assessment of Response to Therapy

Radiomics can aid in the assessment of patients' response to chemotherapeutic agents, as response may involve changes in tumor characteristics other than the tumor size. Radiomics depend on extraction of the features of these changes, such as the tumor morphology, attenuation, and changes in enhancement [41, 42].

Pathomics in Renal Cell Carcinoma

The accurate grading of RCC, particularly the clear cell subtype, is of paramount importance to guide treatment and predict outcome of disease. However, the assignment of grade to these lesions is challenging and is a subjective procedure, rendering the diagnosis variable according to the observer's expertise. Several studies [30,

43, 44] have developed automated pathology systems using the techniques of AI, based on large datasets of images of tissue slides obtained from RCC lesions. These automated systems can provide an objective method of grading RCC with comparable accuracy to human pathologists.

Several differences exist across these developed systems, owing to the inherent variations in image processing of tissue slides, the types of features extracted, the used software as well as the classification and grading methods (2 or 4-tiered grades) [45].

Key Points

- The use of Big Data in urology has been investigated by several research groups, including addressing the diagnosis and treatment of renal cancers. The early diagnosis of renal cell cancer represents a challenge, and its incidence rate is rising in recent years, presumably due to increased incidental detection of renal masses during abdominal radiography for non-related complaints.
- Generation of big data has been utilised in the advancement of radiological imaging (radiomics), histopathological examination (pathomics), and molecular subtyping (genomics) and research is ongoing in the utility of artificial intelligence in the management of renal cell carcinoma.
- Although Big Data and AI technologies have a potential value in improving the diagnosis and treatment of patients with RCC, their incorporation in day-to-day practice is still lagging and hindered by the presence of some limitations and challenges pertaining to these techniques.
- The wide heterogeneity in the design and employed methods across these studies render the evidence derived from them inconclusive. Moreover, only few studies assessed the reproducibility of their techniques or carried out internal and/or external validation [20, 45].
- Several factors contribute to the heterogeneity of methods. For instance, in case of radiomics, the type and method of region of interest delineation/segmentation, the parameters used for CT or MR image acquisition and reconstruction, the characteristics of the lesion including its type and location as well as the software used for texture features extraction [46]. Similar challenges are met with in the field of pathomics.
- Another concern is the cost of employing AI techniques; however, the use of Big Data techniques is anticipated to reduce expenditure by identifying high risk patients, early diagnosing and characterizing malignant lesions, and designing specific therapy that suits the needs and characteristics of individual patients [47].
- In order to utilize Big Data and AI in routine clinical decision-making, these limitations and challenges should first be tackled.

References

1. Saez-Rodriguez J, Rinschen MM, Floege J, Kramann R. Big science and big data in nephrology. Kidney Int. 2019;95(6):1326–37. https://doi.org/10.1016/j.kint.2018.11.048.
2. Favaretto M, De Clercq E, Schneble CO, Elger BS. What is your definition of big data? Researchers' understanding of the phenomenon of the decade. PLoS One. 2020;15(2):e0228987. https://doi.org/10.1371/journal.pone.0228987.
3. Topol EJ. High-performance medicine: the convergence of human and artificial intelligence. Nat Med. 2019;25(1):44–56. https://doi.org/10.1038/s41591-018-0300-7.
4. Andreu-Perez J, Poon CC, Merrifield RD, Wong ST, Yang GZ. Big data for health. IEEE J Biomed Health Informatics. 2015;19(4):1193–208. https://doi.org/10.1109/jbhi.2015.2450362.
5. Shah M, Naik N, Somani BK, Hameed BMZ. Artificial intelligence (AI) in urology-Current use and future directions: an iTRUE study. Turk J Urol. 2020;46(Suppl. 1):S27–39. https://doi.org/10.5152/tud.2020.20117.
6. Mariani LH, Pendergraft WF 3rd, Kretzler M. Defining glomerular disease in mechanistic terms: implementing an integrative biology approach in nephrology. Clin J Am Soc Nephrol CJASN. 2016;11(11):2054–60. https://doi.org/10.2215/cjn.13651215.
7. Suarez-Ibarrola R, Hein S, Reis G, Gratzke C, Miernik A. Current and future applications of machine and deep learning in urology: a review of the literature on urolithiasis, renal cell carcinoma, and bladder and prostate cancer. World J Urol. 2020;38(10):2329–47. https://doi.org/10.1007/s00345-019-03000-5.
8. Siegel RL, Miller KD, Jemal A. Cancer statistics, 2018. CA Cancer J Clin. 2018;68(1):7–30. https://doi.org/10.3322/caac.21442.
9. Capitanio U, Montorsi F. Renal cancer. Lancet (London, England). 2016;387(10021):894–906. https://doi.org/10.1016/s0140-6736(15)00046-x.
10. Wuttke M, Köttgen A. Insights into kidney diseases from genome-wide association studies. Nat Rev Nephrol. 2016;12(9):549–62. https://doi.org/10.1038/nrneph.2016.107.
11. Mohan C, Putterman C. Genetics and pathogenesis of systemic lupus erythematosus and lupus nephritis. Nat Rev Nephrol. 2015;11(6):329–41. https://doi.org/10.1038/nrneph.2015.33.
12. Nakagawa H, Fujita M. Whole genome sequencing analysis for cancer genomics and precision medicine. Cancer Sci. 2018;109(3):513–22. https://doi.org/10.1111/cas.13505.
13. Varela I, Tarpey P, Raine K, Huang D, Ong CK, Stephens P, et al. Exome sequencing identifies frequent mutation of the SWI/SNF complex gene PBRM1 in renal carcinoma. Nature. 2011;469(7331):539–42. https://doi.org/10.1038/nature09639.
14. Peña-Llopis S, Vega-Rubín-de-Celis S, Liao A, Leng N, Pavía-Jiménez A, Wang S, et al. BAP1 loss defines a new class of renal cell carcinoma. Nat Genet. 2012;44(7):751–9. https://doi.org/10.1038/ng.2323.
15. Duns G, van den Berg E, van Duivenbode I, Osinga J, Hollema H, Hofstra RM, et al. Histone methyltransferase gene SETD2 is a novel tumor suppressor gene in clear cell renal cell carcinoma. Cancer Res. 2010;70(11):4287–91. https://doi.org/10.1158/0008-5472.Can-10-0120.
16. Aurilio G, Santoni M, Cimadamore A, Massari F, Scarpelli M, Lopez-Beltran A, et al. Renal cell carcinoma: genomic landscape and clinical implications. Expert Rev Precis Med Drug Dev. 2020;5(2):95–100. https://doi.org/10.1080/23808993.2020.1733407.
17. Li P, Ren H, Zhang Y, Zhou Z. Fifteen-gene expression based model predicts the survival of clear cell renal cell carcinoma. Medicine (Baltimore). 2018;97(33):e11839. https://doi.org/10.1097/md.0000000000011839.
18. Li F, Yang M, Li Y, Zhang M, Wang W, Yuan D, et al. An improved clear cell renal cell carcinoma stage prediction model based on gene sets. BMC Bioinformatics. 2020;21(1):232. https://doi.org/10.1186/s12859-020-03543-0.
19. Lubner MG. Radiomics and artificial intelligence for renal mass characterization. Radiol Clin North Am. 2020;58(5):995–1008. https://doi.org/10.1016/j.rcl.2020.06.001.
20. Ursprung S, Beer L, Bruining A, Woitek R, Stewart GD, Gallagher FA, et al. Radiomics of computed tomography and magnetic resonance imaging in renal cell carcinoma-a systematic

review and meta-analysis. Eur Radiol. 2020;30(6):3558–66. https://doi.org/10.1007/s00330-020-06666-3.
21. Bektas CT, Kocak B, Yardimci AH, Turkcanoglu MH, Yucetas U, Koca SB, et al. Clear cell renal cell carcinoma: machine learning-based quantitative computed tomography texture analysis for prediction of fuhrman nuclear grade. Eur Radiol. 2019;29(3):1153–63. https://doi.org/10.1007/s00330-018-5698-2.
22. Hindman N, Ngo L, Genega EM, Melamed J, Wei J, Braza JM, et al. Angiomyolipoma with minimal fat: can it be differentiated from clear cell renal cell carcinoma by using standard MR techniques? Radiology. 2012;265(2):468–77. https://doi.org/10.1148/radiol.12112087.
23. Abrahams NA, Tamboli P. Oncocytic renal neoplasms: diagnostic considerations. Clin Lab Med. 2005;25(2):317–39, vi. https://doi.org/10.1016/j.cll.2005.01.006.
24. Kutikov A, Fossett LK, Ramchandani P, Tomaszewski JE, Siegelman ES, Banner MP, et al. Incidence of benign pathologic findings at partial nephrectomy for solitary renal mass presumed to be renal cell carcinoma on preoperative imaging. Urology. 2006;68(4):737–40. https://doi.org/10.1016/j.urology.2006.04.011.
25. Yang CW, Shen SH, Chang YH, Chung HJ, Wang JH, Lin AT, et al. Are there useful CT features to differentiate renal cell carcinoma from lipid-poor renal angiomyolipoma? AJR Am J Roentgenol. 2013;201(5):1017–28. https://doi.org/10.2214/ajr.12.10204.
26. Sasaguri K, Takahashi N, Gomez-Cardona D, Leng S, Schmit GD, Carter RE, et al. Small (< 4 cm) renal mass: differentiation of oncocytoma from renal cell carcinoma on biphasic contrast-enhanced CT. AJR Am J Roentgenol. 2015;205(5):999–1007. https://doi.org/10.2214/ajr.14.13966.
27. Volpe A, Finelli A, Gill IS, Jewett MA, Martignoni G, Polascik TJ, et al. Rationale for percutaneous biopsy and histologic characterisation of renal tumours. Eur Urol. 2012;62(3):491–504. https://doi.org/10.1016/j.eururo.2012.05.009.
28. Kapur P, Peña-Llopis S, Christie A, Zhrebker L, Pavía-Jiménez A, Rathmell WK, et al. Effects on survival of BAP1 and PBRM1 mutations in sporadic clear-cell renal-cell carcinoma: a retrospective analysis with independent validation. Lancet Oncol. 2013;14(2):159–67. https://doi.org/10.1016/s1470-2045(12)70584-3.
29. Abel EJ, Carrasco A, Culp SH, Matin SF, Tamboli P, Tannir NM, et al. Limitations of preoperative biopsy in patients with metastatic renal cell carcinoma: comparison to surgical pathology in 405 cases. BJU Int. 2012;110(11):1742–6. https://doi.org/10.1111/j.1464-410X.2012.11124.x.
30. Holdbrook DA, Singh M, Choudhury Y, Kalaw EM, Koh V, Tan HS, et al. Automated renal cancer grading using nuclear pleomorphic patterns. JCO Clin Cancer Inform. 2018;2:1–12. https://doi.org/10.1200/cci.17.00100.
31. Ding J, Xing Z, Jiang Z, Chen J, Pan L, Qiu J, et al. CT-based radiomic model predicts high grade of clear cell renal cell carcinoma. Eur J Radiol. 2018;103:51–6. https://doi.org/10.1016/j.ejrad.2018.04.013.
32. Kocak B, Durmaz ES, Ates E, Kaya OK, Kilickesmez O. Unenhanced CT texture analysis of clear cell renal cell carcinomas: a machine learning-based study for predicting histopathologic nuclear grade. AJR Am J Roentgenol. 2019;W1–8. https://doi.org/10.2214/ajr.18.20742.
33. Lin F, Cui EM, Lei Y, Luo LP. CT-based machine learning model to predict the Fuhrman nuclear grade of clear cell renal cell carcinoma. Abdom Radiol (New York). 2019;44(7):2528–34. https://doi.org/10.1007/s00261-019-01992-7.
34. Sun X, Liu L, Xu K, Li W, Huo Z, Liu H, et al. Prediction of ISUP grading of clear cell renal cell carcinoma using support vector machine model based on CT images. Medicine (Baltimore). 2019;98(14):e15022. https://doi.org/10.1097/md.0000000000015022.
35. Schieda N, Lim RS, Krishna S, McInnes MDF, Flood TA, Thornhill RE. Diagnostic accuracy of unenhanced CT analysis to differentiate low-grade from high-grade chromophobe renal cell carcinoma. AJR Am J Roentgenol. 2018;210(5):1079–87. https://doi.org/10.2214/ajr.17.18874.

36. Vendrami CL, Velichko YS, Miller FH, Chatterjee A, Villavicencio CP, Yaghmai V, et al. Differentiation of papillary renal cell carcinoma subtypes on MRI: qualitative and texture analysis. AJR Am J Roentgenol. 2018;211(6):1234–45. https://doi.org/10.2214/ajr.17.19213.
37. Bodalal Z, Trebeschi S, Nguyen-Kim TDL, Schats W, Beets-Tan R. Radiogenomics: bridging imaging and genomics. Abdom Radiol (New York). 2019;44(6):1960–84. https://doi.org/10.1007/s00261-019-02028-w.
38. Karlo CA, Di Paolo PL, Chaim J, Hakimi AA, Ostrovnaya I, Russo P, et al. Radiogenomics of clear cell renal cell carcinoma: associations between CT imaging features and mutations. Radiology. 2014;270(2):464–71. https://doi.org/10.1148/radiol.13130663.
39. Kocak B, Durmaz ES, Ates E, Ulusan MB. Radiogenomics in clear cell renal cell carcinoma: machine learning-based high-dimensional quantitative CT texture analysis in predicting PBRM1 mutation status. AJR Am J Roentgenol. 2019;212(3):W55–w63. https://doi.org/10.2214/ajr.18.20443.
40. Alessandrino F, Shinagare AB, Bossé D, Choueiri TK, Krajewski KM. Radiogenomics in renal cell carcinoma. Abdom Radiol. 2019;44(6):1990–8. https://doi.org/10.1007/s00261-018-1624-y.
41. Goh V, Ganeshan B, Nathan P, Juttla JK, Vinayan A, Miles KA. Assessment of response to tyrosine kinase inhibitors in metastatic renal cell cancer: CT texture as a predictive biomarker. Radiology. 2011;261(1):165–71. https://doi.org/10.1148/radiol.11110264.
42. Haider MA, Vosough A, Khalvati F, Kiss A, Ganeshan B, Bjarnason GA. CT texture analysis: a potential tool for prediction of survival in patients with metastatic clear cell carcinoma treated with sunitinib. Cancer Imaging. 2017;17(1):4. https://doi.org/10.1186/s40644-017-0106-8.
43. Yeh FC, Parwani AV, Pantanowitz L, Ho C. Automated grading of renal cell carcinoma using whole slide imaging. J Pathol Inform. 2014;5(1):23. https://doi.org/10.4103/2153-3539.137726.
44. Tian K, Rubadue CA, Lin DI, Veta M, Pyle ME, Irshad H, et al. Automated clear cell renal carcinoma grade classification with prognostic significance. PLoS One. 2019;14(10):e0222641. https://doi.org/10.1371/journal.pone.0222641.
45. Santo BA, Rosenberg AZ, Sarder P. Artificial intelligence driven next-generation renal histomorphometry. Curr Opin Nephrol Hypertens. 2020;29(3):265–72. https://doi.org/10.1097/mnh.0000000000000598.
46. Kocak B, Durmaz ES, Kaya OK, Ates E, Kilickesmez O. Reliability of single-slice-based 2D CT texture analysis of renal masses: influence of intra- and interobserver manual segmentation variability on radiomic feature reproducibility. AJR Am J Roentgenol. 2019;213(2):377–83. https://doi.org/10.2214/ajr.19.21212.
47. Palanisamy V, Thirunavukarasu R. Implications of big data analytics in developing healthcare frameworks – a review. J King Saud Univ Comput Inf Sci. 2019;31(4):415–25. https://doi.org/10.1016/j.jksuci.2017.12.007.

Index

C. Anderson, M. Afshar (eds.), *Renal Cancer*,
https://doi.org/10.1007/978-3-030-84756-2

S

GPSR Compliance

The European Union's (EU) General Product Safety Regulation (GPSR) is a set of rules that requires consumer products to be safe and our obligations to ensure this.

If you have any concerns about our products, you can contact us on ProductSafety@springernature.com

In case Publisher is established outside the EU, the EU authorized representative is:

Springer Nature Customer Service Center GmbH
Europaplatz 3
69115 Heidelberg, Germany

Batch number: 10756376

Printed by Printforce, the Netherlands